Ophthalmic Photography

About the cover

The fundus image on the cover is a multi-image computer composite from multiple 60-degree fundus photographs—a FundusMap. The original 25 images were taken on slide film by Patrick J. Saine and were scanned onto a Kodak Photo-CD. The digital images were combined into a photo-illustration by Richard E. Hackel using Adobe Photoshop on a Macintosh computer. Lines were added that indicate the alignment procedure for the seven standard fields of view (circles). The term *FundusMap* describes this computer-based photo-illustrative method of combining fundus photographs to make a map.

Ophthalmic Photography: Retinal Photography, Angiography, and Electronic Imaging

Second Edition

Patrick J. Saine, M.Ed., C.R.A., F.O.P.S.
Instructor of Surgery (Ophthalmology), Dartmouth Medical School, Hanover, New Hampshire; Manager, Ophthalmic Photography, Section of Ophthalmology, Dartmouth Hitchcock Medical Center, Lebanon, New Hampshire

Marshall E. Tyler, C.R.A., F.O.P.S.
Instructor of Surgical Sciences in Ophthalmology, Bowman Gray School of Medicine of Wake Forest University, Winston-Salem, North Carolina

Butterworth–Heinemann

Boston Oxford Auckland Johannesburg Melbourne New Delhi

Every effort has been made to ensure that the drug dosage schedules within this text are accurate and conform to standards accepted at time of publication. However, as treatment recommendations vary in the light of continuing research and clinical experience, the reader is advised to verify drug dosage schedules herein with information found on product information sheets. This is especially true in cases of new or infrequently used drugs.

 Recognizing the importance of preserving what has been written, Butterworth–Heinemann prints its books on acid-free paper whenever possible.

Library of Congress Cataloging-in-Publication Data

Saine, Patrick J.
   Ophthalmic photography : retinal photography, angiography, and electronic imaging / Patrick J. Saine, Marshall E. Tyler.— 2nd ed.
     p. cm.
   Previous ed. has subtitle: a textbook of fundus photography, angiography, and electronic imaging.
   Includes bibliographical references and index.
   ISBN 0-7506-7372-9
   1. Ophthalmic photography. I. Tyler, Marshall E. II. Title.

   RE79.P54 S25 2002
   617.7'1545—dc21

                                2001046108

British Library Cataloguing-in-Publication Data
A catalogue record for this book is available from the British Library.

The publisher offers special discounts on bulk orders of this book.

For information, please contact:

Manager of Special Sales
Butterworth–Heinemann
225 Wildwood Avenue
Woburn, MA 01801-2041
Tel: 781-904-2500
Fax: 781-904-2620

For information on all Butterworth–Heinemann publications available, contact our World Wide Web home page at: http://www.bh.com

10 9 8 7 6 5 4 3 2 1

Printed in the United States of America

Contents

Contributing Authors

Thomas M. Clark, B.S., C.R.A.
Ophthalmic Photographer, University of California at San Diego, San Diego, California

Leslie D. MacKeen, B.Sc., O.A., C.R.A.
Ophthalmic Photographer, The Hospital for Sick Children, Toronto, Ontario

Timothy J. Martin, M.D.
Assistant Professor of Surgical Sciences in Ophthalmology, Bowman Gray School of Medicine of Wake Forest University, Winston-Salem, North Carolina

Lawrence M. Merin, R.B.P., F.I.M.I., F.O.P.S.
Assistant Professor of Ophthalmology, Vanderbilt University School of Medicine, Nashville, Tennessee; Director of Vanderbilt Ophthalmic Imaging Center, Nashville, Tennessee

Paula F. Morris, C.R.A., F.O.P.S.
Chief Photographer, John A. Moran Eye Center, University of Utah School of Medicine, Salt Lake City, Utah

Michael Neider, B.A.
Associate Director of Photographic Services, Fundus Photograph Reading Center, University of Wisconsin-Madison

Patrick J. Saine, M.Ed., C.R.A., F.O.P.S.
Instructor of Surgery (Ophthalmology), Dartmouth Medical School, Hanover, New Hampshire; Manager, Ophthalmic Photography, Section of Ophthalmology, Dartmouth Hitchcock Medical Center, Lebanon, New Hampshire

Stephen J. Sramek, M.D., Ph.D.
Vitreoretinal Surgeon, Davis Duehr Dean at Dean Medical Center, Madison, Wisconsin

Marshall E. Tyler, C.R.A., F.O.P.S.
Instructor of Surgical Sciences in Ophthalmology, Bowman Gray School of Medicine of Wake Forest University, Winston-Salem, North Carolina

Preface to the Second Edition

The field of ophthalmic photography has undergone a technical renaissance since the first edition of this book was published. At that time, digital imaging was moving into its own as a new tool, affordable only for large practices and institutions. Now digital angiography is an everyday matter for large and small practices alike, with high-quality digital color fundus photography becoming more practical. The then-new technology of scanning laser ophthalmoscopy is now on the forefront of exciting new research. The clinical use of indocyanine green angiography was just gaining steam—now it is an integral part of many retina practices. When we published our first edition, the World Wide Web was uncharted—a new frontier. Now, Optimal, an Internet discussion group (http://visualeyes.upmc.edu/optimal/welcome.html), helps ophthalmic photographers solve technical problems through instant Internet connections.

You might think that all this technology would reduce the ophthalmic photographer's responsibilities, making the profession less dependent on highly trained, well-compensated individuals. However, in the authors' interactions with ophthalmic photographers around the globe, we find the opposite to be true. Now more than ever, ophthalmic photography requires astute, well-trained professionals who are technically literate, not only in matters of photography, but also in computer and digital arenas. More and more, ophthalmic photographers are becoming part of the "digital elite," the portion of our society that readily uses and understands our increasingly complex digital tools. Although the instant nature of digital imaging allows the novice to learn more quickly from mistakes, it also forces him or her to upgrade his or her skills. If one can instantly determine that an image is less than perfect, who wouldn't modify techniques and try to take a better picture?

Although the professional ophthalmic photographer is reaching new heights, some things never seem to change: the precise timing required for ocular angiography, the bright words of encouragement to the light-sensitive patient, that special feeling you get when you know you have captured a great image and helped a needy patient.

We have tried in this second edition to meld the forward thrust of our profession with the essential basics that every ophthalmic photographer must understand. We have added new images and upgraded the text. Fresh discussions highlight the new technologies of scanning laser ophthalmoscopy and extreme wide-angle fundus cameras, and we have completely upgraded the digital imaging chapter to Version 2.0.

We hope you enjoy reading this book as much as we enjoyed creating it.

Patrick J. Saine, M.Ed., C.R.A., F.O.P.S.
Marshall E. Tyler, C.R.A., F.O.P.S.

Preface to the First Edition

This book is predicated on the belief that ophthalmic photography is an exciting and challenging career. Photographing the retina has become both important and routine in the practice of ophthalmology ever since the first crude photographic attempts more than 100 years ago. The introduction of fluorescein angiography in 1961 ignited new interest in fundus imaging and has since revolutionized our understanding of the retina. Electronic imaging technology and indocyanine green angiography are examples of continued evolution in our field.

Like many photographic endeavors, the profession of ophthalmic photography is a collaborative blend of art and science. Ophthalmic photography's specific mix combines the animated art of patient interaction with the inherently formidable technical challenges of recording high-quality retinal images. To be successful, you must cheerfully convince the worried, wary, or weary patient to submit to yet another set of bright lights while you simultaneously juggle complicated technical concerns.

The best preparation for this career is college-level instruction integrating the life sciences with photography and communication skills. Increasingly, facility with computers and electronic imaging is also important.

Variety is the hallmark of every fulfilling career path. Ophthalmic photography offers many options. The subject of this textbook, imaging the retina, is but one part of the complete ophthalmic photographer's repertoire. External, corneal, and operating room photography procedures combine with the skills associated with general biomedical photography for a myriad of opportunities. Settings range from basic research laboratories to large hospitals to clinical doctor's offices. Each opportunity offers a distinctly different working environment.

This book is designed to help you use photographic expertise in the pursuit of quality ophthalmic health care. As an ophthalmic photographer, you will surely experience some thrilling moments—your first view of a vein pulsating on an optic nerve head or glimpses of fluorescein dye as it ambles through ocular blood vessels. The challenges and frustrations of photographing anxious patients with compromised media will also be a part of your professional life. We sincerely hope that your career is filled with rewarding moments. You should be proud of your role in helping save a patient's vision. We encourage you to become a vital member of your eye care team.

Patrick J. Saine, M.Ed., C.R.A., F.O.P.S.
Marshall E. Tyler, C.R.A., F.O.P.S.

Acknowledgments

We appreciate the vital contributions and continuing support of our co-authors Rosario Bate, Tom Clark, Leslie MacKeen, Tim Martin, Larry Merin, Paula Morris, Michael Neider, and Steve Sramek. We graciously thank Karen Oberheim of Butterworth–Heinemann for her encouragement and support on this and other projects. We thank Erica Broennle, Shannon Riley, and Jen Rourke of Silverchair Science + Communications, Inc. for their fine editorial and composition expertise, as well as Andrea Sherman and Jodie Allen of Butterworth–Heinemann for helping guide this project to successful completion.

We are each deeply indebted to the fine physicians with whom we work—at the Section of Ophthalmology at Dartmouth Medical School and at the Department of Ophthalmology of the Wake Forest University Baptist Medical Center. Rosalind A. Stevens, MD, Chief of Ophthalmology at Dartmouth Medical School, exudes that special quality that encourages others to reach further and climb higher. The oculoplastic surgeon Richard K. Dortzbach of Madison, Wisconsin, was also a positive influence. He taught Pat, both by example and instruction, to pursue and expect the best. We thank Richard G. Weaver, MD, for his clinical mentorship and M. Madison Slusher, MD, for providing a superb clinical setting for ophthalmic photography. Marshall also thanks Hollis N. Todd, professor at the Rochester Institute of Technology, for his foundation course on materials and processes in photography.

We are grateful to the ophthalmic photographers who have shared their expertise with us. The Ophthalmic Photographers' Society has helped us grow both professionally and personally. A special thank you to the recently departed Don Wong, R.B.P., for his continuous sharing of knowledge as well as his role as an educator and friend. We acknowledge Johnny Justice, Jr., C.R.A., F.O.P.S., for his leadership in elevating ophthalmic photography from its infancy as an offshoot of biomedical photography to a profession that significantly participates on the ophthalmic clinical team.

Special thanks go to the ophthalmic photographers and physicians who have provided specific images or information for the book: Albert Aan De Kirk, Julie Balza, Timothy Bennett, Chris Berry, Mike Borgrud, Dennis Cain, Colin Clements, Brad Clifton, Mark Croswell, Denise Cunningham, Ralph Eagle, William Fisher, Richard E. Hackel, Peter Hay, Ray Hendrickson, Charles Juarez, Csaba Martonyi, George Minstsioulis, Paul Montague, William Nyberg, Michael Palczynski, Tim Steffins, Ben Szirth, and I. Wallow.

Our families deserve a special acknowledgment. A sincere thank you to Deb, Julie, and Beth, and to Alix and Christina for their understanding and support throughout this complex process. They are to be congratulated for tolerating our continuing fascination with over-commitment and constant brushes with workaholism.

Patrick J. Saine, M.Ed., C.R.A., F.O.P.S.
Marshall E. Tyler, C.R.A., F.O.P.S.

For technical data—the camera was used faithfully.

—Minor White

Chapter 1

Landmarks in the Development of Fluorescein Angiography

Patrick J. Saine

Introduction

In 1961, two medical students from Indiana, H. R. Novotny and D. L. Alvis, wrote a paper on retinal angiography techniques still in use today.[1] They described a fundus camera equipped with an exciter filter, barrier filter, and electronic flash to sequentially document the retinal blood flow after a sodium fluorescein injection. The development of this procedure began many years before this seminal report, however.

Fluorescein angiography was developed by combining the evolution of retinal imaging with the application of sodium fluorescein to ophthalmology. This chapter reviews published landmarks in the development of the fluorescein angiography by examining the historical use of dyes to view the retina, the evolution of retinal photography, and important work contemporaneous with Novotny and Alvis (Figure 1-1). It traces the history of fluorescein angiography through selected quotes from the publications of significant contributors. A list of resources is included—you are encouraged to further explore the historical record.

Beginnings

The foundation from which fluorescein angiography arose includes anatomic drawings of the retina and the use of fluorescein dye to observe ophthalmic phenomena. Fundus photography was developed in pursuit of an accurate and specific graphic representation of the retina. Medical illustration has a long history of depicting the eye (Figure 1-2).[2] A landmark in the realistic graphic representation of the retina was an 1854 publication by Van Trigt (Figure 1-3).[3] It is here that the story of modern fundus photography begins. From Duke-Elder:

	1826 Photography invented by Niepce
1850	**1851** Ophthalmoscope introduced by Helmholtz
	1854 1st color fundus illustration published by van Trigt
1860	
1870	
	1871 Fluorescein synthesized by Baeyer
1880	**1881** Ehrlich examines aqueous flow with sodium fluorescein
1890	**1886-98** In vivo human retinal photography refined
1900	**1899** High quality fundus photographs shown by Dimmer
1910	**1910** Retina and choroid examined using sodium fluorescein
1920	**1926** First commercially available fundus camera introduced by Zeiss
	1927 First fundus photography atlas published by Dimmer & Pillat
1930	**1930** Filters used to observe dye in retina
1940	**1939** Dye described as it flows through retinal blood vessels
	1946 Electronic flash tube introduced by Edgerton
1950	**1953** Electronic flash technology applied to fundus photography
1960	**1959** Sodium fluorescein photographed in cat retina with barrier filter
	1960 Injected sodium fluorescein used to determine retinal diagnosis
	1961 Modern fluorescein angiography technique described by Novotny & Alvis

FIGURE 1-1
Timeline relating events leading to the development of fluorescein angiography.

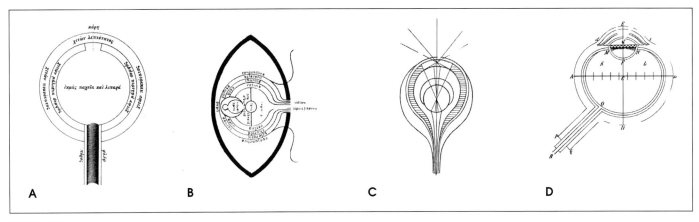

FIGURE 1-2
Medical illustration has a rich tradition of depicting the eye. Democritus (Greece, circa 400 BC) drew a simple, two-layer construction with a hollow tube connecting the eye to the brain **(A)**. Hunain Ibn Ishak (Arabia, circa 1000 AD) incorporated the layers of the retina **(B)**. Leonardo Da Vinci (Italian, circa 1500) added a three-dimensional aspect and the refraction of light to his representation of the eye **(C)**. Greater anatomic accuracy began with the work of Scheiner in 1619 **(D)**. (Reprinted with permission from S Duke-Elder. System of Ophthalmology. Vol II. St. Louis: Mosby, 1961.)

FIGURE 1-3
Reprinted with permission from S Duke-Elder. System of Ophthalmology. Vol X. London: Henry Kimpton, 1967.

A

B

FIGURE 1-4
Jackman and Webster produced the first published human fundus photograph using an albo-carbon burner, an ophthalmoscopic mirror, and a 2 ½-minute exposure **(A)**. Interpretation requires some imagination: The small upper white area is the optic disc, and the lower, larger light area is an artifact **(B)**. Blood vessels cannot be defined. (Reprinted with permission from WA Mann. History of photography of the eye. Surv Ophthal 1970;15:179.)

The frontispiece to this volume is interesting. It is a photographic represen-tation of the first coloured printed illustration of the fundus of the eye which appeared in the thesis of Adrian Christopher Van Trigt (1825–64), Dissertatio Ophthalmologica Inauguralis de Speculo Oculi *in 1853 . . .[3]*

Jackman and Webster[4] and Bedell[5] note early attempts at retinal pho-tography on anesthetized animals. The first published account of in vivo human retinal photography is by Jackman and Webster in 1886.[4] They describe the use of an ophthalmoscopic mirror (a curved mirror with a central hole) in conjunction with a 2-in. microscope objective (Figure 1-4). An albo-carbon light source provided illumination during the 2 ½-minute exposure. From their paper:

After considerable practice, and numerous experiments, we have at last succeeded in obtaining a very fair photograph of the blind spot and a few larger blood vessels of the living human retina.[4]

As important as these early attempts were, the images were blurry. Improvements in instrumentation and technique were needed before high-quality fundus photography was to become routine.

Meanwhile, Adolf Baeyer, a 1905 Nobel laureate in chemistry, described methods for producing a number of new organic dyes—including sodium fluorescein—in 1871.[6] Ten years later, fluorescein dye was used by Ehrlich to examine the flow of the aqueous humor.[7] This was the first published use of sodium fluorescein in ophthalmology. Sodium fluorescein has since become an important ophthalmic tool. Ehrlich describes his methods:

I proceeded to inject 2 cc of fluorescein, and when the yellow absorbed—this happened in a few minutes—I saw an effect nearby. After $^1/_4$ to $^1/_2$ minutes I could see a spot near the pupil border, soon the spot encircled the pupil and I saw an intense green fluorescent color which diffused through-out the anterior chamber within 2–3 minutes.[7]

Colored Dyes and the Eye

Erhlich's investigation of fluorescein in the eye was followed in 1910 by Burke's examination of the choroid and retina after the administration of fluorescein dye in coffee.[8] In 1930, Kikai viewed the retina with filtered light in an attempt to more clearly view injected dye.[9] It was not until 1939 that the path of dye in the retinal blood vessels was described.[10] While reading this next excerpt, imagine how the history of fluorescein angiography may have been changed if Sorsby had a specific interest in photographing the retina, or if his experiments had been carried out with a different patient population.

With these dyes whilst effective staining of the brain could be obtained in the intact animal, staining of the fundus was, as with the pure basic dyes, of the most transient character. The retinal vessels could be seen carrying a coloured blood stream for about two minutes, but the colouration of the fundus amounted to little more than a transient flushing. . . . The experimental observation that the damaged retina retained the colour suggested the possibility that the diseased retina in man might behave similarly.[11]

The use of fluorescein dye in circulation studies of the intestine and skin were summarized by Lange and Boyd in 1942.[11] Their technique included the rapid injection of 2–4 ml of 5% sodium fluorescein in the antecubital vein. Using a purple light for excitation, they observed the effect of fluorescein dye on multiple tissues. Except for the lack of specifics describing ophthalmic imaging, their paper describes, in very general terms, modern fluorescein angiography:

If a definite section of tissue containing a small artery and vein is observed with the aid of a low power microscope after intravenous injection, one readily can watch the stain enter the artery, pass the capillaries, stain the surrounding tissue and return through the vein.[11]

Table 1-1. Work of Retinal Photography Pioneers*

Pioneers	Publication Date
Noyes	1862
Rosebrugh	1864, 1887
Liebreich	1874
T. Stein	1877
Dor	1884
Albertotti	1884
W. T. Jackman and J. D. Webster	1886
Panel	1887
L. Howe	1887, 1893
E. Starr	1887
H. Cohn	1888, 1889
Leroy	1888
S. Segal	1888
Bagneris	1889
T. Guilloz	1891, 1893
O. Gerloff	1891
W. Thorner	1896
Guinkoff	1896
E. Borghi	1897, 1898
W. Nikolaew and J. Dogiel	1900
S. Jackson	1901

*As summarized in Dimmer's 1907 treatise on ophthalmic photography.

Fundus Photography Refined

Rapid progress in fundus photography was made in the years just after Jackman and Webster's fuzzy fundus photographs were published. Dimmer describes the work of a number of scientists who attempted retinal photography near the end of the nineteenth century (Table 1-1).[12] Howe and Barr both made progress toward better quality, as evidenced in the next three quotes[13,14]:

The photograph to which I venture to call attention is here presented. It will be seen that the disc is perfectly distinct, even the shading of the different parts is well defined. Moreover, the vessels are so clearly shown over at least a third of the fundus that the arteries can be distinguished from the veins. . . . For while it must be admitted that the results here presented are not entirely satisfactory, on the other hand this is, as far as I can learn, the first time that any photographs of the interior of the eye have been produced in which the details were even recognizable, and as such, they at least give promise of results of great practical value in the future.[13]

The next quote is taken from the uncredited discussion published directly after Howe's paper:

Letter A Carbutt's dry plate is used with ten minutes exposure to an ordinary gas light, giving an unretouched and unremagnified negative . . .

Barr wrote:

Up to the present time, so far as I am able to learn, attempts to photograph the interior of the human eye have not yielded very encouraging results. In the Philadelphia Photographer, of June 5, 1886, Drs. Jackman and Webster, of Coggestall, Essex, England, give results of their experiments. They succeeded in showing the end of the optic nerve and an indistinct

FIGURE 1-5
In 1891, Gerloff published a low-magnification retinal photograph that was much clearer than earlier efforts. (Reprinted with permission from O Gerloff. Ueber die photographie des augenhintergrundes. Klin Monatf Augenheil 1891;29:397.)

A   B   C

FIGURE 1-6
Thorner's camera **(A)** provided fundus photographs **(B, C)** with adequate detail but lacking even illumination. (Reprinted with permission from Thorner W. Ueber die Photographie des Augenhintergrundes. Berlin: C. Vogts Buchdruckerei, 1896; and F Dimmer. Ueber die Photographie des Augenhintergrundes. Wiesbaden, Germany: Bergmann, 1907.)

outline of a part of one or two large vessels. . . . I began experimenting to obtain a photograph of the interior of the human eye, and the results are better than others I have seen, showing the optic nerve and vessels quite well. . . . The lens in the camera has a focus of only three inches, and this I think is important, for it makes a very bright image, and consequently a very short exposure—six to ten seconds—is sufficient. . . .[14]

In 1891, Gerloff used flash powder to illuminate a low-magnification fundus photograph (Figure 1-5).[15] Thorner wrote a 1903 book outlining his fundus photography techniques (Figure 1-6).[16]

Accurate, high-quality fundus photography began at the turn of the twentieth century with the work of Frederick Dimmer. Bedell wrote that Dimmer "electrified the 9th International Congress (1899) with his marvelous pictures. . . ."[5] Dimmer's 1907 treatise on fundus photography described his cumbersome apparatus, which used carbon arc illumination (Figure 1-7).[12] He was the first to incorporate fundus photography into a basic ophthalmic textbook and the first to publish a photographic atlas.[17,18]

Only one of Dimmer's cameras was ever produced. Modern fundus camera design grew from the work of Helmholtz, who introduced the

A

B

FIGURE 1-7
Dimmer's fundus camera **(A)** was used to create this fine retinal photograph of a normal eye **(B)**. (Reprinted with permission from O Pes. La Photographie du fond de l'oeil. Turin, Italy: Vincenzo Bona, 1906; and F Dimmer. Demonstration von Photogrammen Des Augernhintergrundes Wiesbaden, Germany: Verlag von J.F. Bergmann, 1903.)

FIGURE 1-8
An advertisement for the Zeiss fundus camera from 1932. Fundus cameras have changed dramatically in the last 50 years. Advertising copy has not. (Reprinted with permission from American Journal of Ophthalmology, 1932;32:1214.)

direct ophthalmoscope in 1851.[19] Its design was improved by Thorner in 1899 and Gullstrand in 1910.[20,21] Nordenson introduced a camera based on Gullstrand's principles in 1925.[22] The Carl Zeiss Company marketed Nordenson's design as the first commercially available fundus camera in 1926 (Figure 1-8).[23] This camera had a 10-degree field of view and required a one-half second exposure with color film.[24]

Color fundus photography was described as early as 1929, the same year Bedell published the first stereo atlas of fundus photographs.[25,26] In June 1935, Bedell delivered the chairman's address at the Eighty-Sixth Annual Session of the American Medical Association[5] and described the then current state of fundus imaging:

Direct color photography has attracted attention and some excellent pictures have been presented, but because of the expense and the difficulty of reproduction, it is not as yet popular. Eventually, drawings will be supplanted

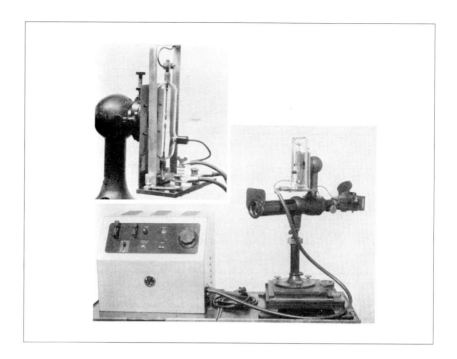

FIGURE 1-9
Hansell and Beeson adapted an electronic flash tube to a Zeiss fundus camera. (Reprinted with permission from P Hansell. A System of Ophthalmic Illustration. Springfield, IL: Charles C. Thomas, 1957.)

and even the most skillful artist will be forced to admit the superiority of photographs. For several years I have been taking colored photographs.[5]

Limitations in clinical use of fundus photography in the 1930s and 1940s can be directly attributed to the difficulty in obtaining quality images. Slow film speeds and long exposures were the rule with the then current carbon arc illumination system. Although Hartinger described a modification of the fundus camera by the addition of an electrical lamp, carbon arc fundus cameras continued to be used through the 1940s.[27,28] A bright, instantaneous light source was needed for high-quality, routine fundus photography. External eye photographs taken with a "lightning illumination process" were produced by Cohn and DuBois-Reymond in 1888.[29] In 1946, Edgerton developed the electronic flash tube, and in 1949 Rizzutti introduced its use to ophthalmology.[30,31] Electronic flash was adapted to the fundus camera in 1953 in both Britain and the United States (Figure 1-9)[28,32]:

> *The application of a new compact xenon arc lamp (FA5) to retinal photography in colour is described. The circuit required for pulse operation of the lamp is given and some modifications of the Zeiss-Nordenson retinal camera are mentioned. . . . By these means standard and comparable records of the fundus oculi may be obtained on Kodachrome colour film at exposures of $^1/_{25}$ sec.*[28]

> *By using again the ring of light just within the pupil to illuminate the retina, and photographing directly through the center of the pupil, one can obtain pictures which are reflex-free. Although some cameras use large induction coils in the flash circuits to extend the flash duration, it still remains shorter than 1/500th of a second. The use of the flash-tube technique also is less fatiguing and annoying to the patient.*[32]

By the early 1950s, fluorescein dye had been observed flowing through the retina, filters had been used to enhance the visualization of the retina filled with dye, and flash-adapted fundus cameras were a reality. A flurry of activity in the late 1950s preceded Alvis and Novotny's important paper.

Fluorescein Angiography

In early 1959, Chao and Flocks described a method for measuring the "retinal circulation time" in cats.[33] Using a stopwatch, ophthalmoscopy, and tryptan blue, they found that the circulation time of the cat retina was approximately 2 seconds. Their discussion concluded with this observation:

We do not yet know whether more innocuous indicator solutions such as fluorescein can be used so that the method could be adapted to the human retina. If it could be, it is conceivable that the study of retinal circulation time might be of value in such pathologic conditions as retinitis pigmentosa, diabetic retinopathy, and macular degeneration.[33]

Later that year, Flocks, Miller, and Chao published a refinement of their technique, including the addition of a motion picture camera, an exciter filter, and fluorescein dye[34]:

If a cobalt-blue filter is inserted in the ophthalmoscope, the retina appears dark purple in color and the vessels black. When intravenously injected fluorescein reaches the central retinal artery, it lights up the artery to a fluorescent yellow if viewed through the cobalt-blue filter. . . . The idea was conceived that the end points could be ascertained more precisely by means of motion picture photography using a motion picture film viewer and editor to examine leisurely the individual frames of the film. With this technique the unavoidable error due to the reaction time of the person pressing the stop watch would be eliminated and, in addition, a permanent objective record of the circulation time and of the retinal circulation would be obtained. . . .[34]

Their attempts at fundus cinephotography of sodium fluorescein in humans failed:

Two attempts to determine the retinal circulation times in human beings using motion pictures were unsuccessful because of insufficient light. Motion pictures of the retina of cats are much easier to make than the motion pictures of the human retina. We are currently trying to improve the optical system of our apparatus so that this method can be applied to the study of human retinal circulation time. . . .[34]

The future of fluorescein angiography was not in the determination of circulation time but rather in the evaluation and differential diagnosis of chorioretinal disease. In 1960, MacLean and Maumenee published this landmark description of fluorescein angioscopy—the first published case of sodium fluorescein being used to obtain a diagnosis[35]:

The patient, Stanford University Hospital No E-1234719 J.G., a white man, truck driver, 30 years of age, was first seen in consultation on February 16, 1955. He stated that three years prior to that time he had noted spots and flashes of light in front of his left eye. He had seen an optometrist who prescribed glasses for him. Four weeks prior to his examination visual acuity in his left eye had suddenly decreased. . . . A cobalt blue filter was placed in front of the beam of the Haag-Streit slit lamp and the patient was given 2 cc of 5.0 percent fluorescein intravenously. A dozen small spots in the central portion of the tumor fluoresced within 30 seconds. . . . A diagnosis of hemangioma of the choroid was made. . . .[35]

FIGURE 1-10
Harold Novotny produced the first fluorescein angiogram by recording fluorescein dye in the retinal blood vessels of David Alvis in 1959. Note the use of match sticks to signify print sequence. (Images courtesy of T. Steffins, University of Indiana Department of Ophthalmology.)

The final piece of the puzzle was published in the journal *Circulation* by Novotny and Alvis.[1] The description of the technique used to create the first successful fluorescein angiogram (Figure 1-10) was published in 1961:

> *The purpose of this paper is to describe a method for the study of retinal blood flow in man by the use of intravascular fluorescein and retinal photography, and to report some preliminary observations made with this method. . . . Serial fluorescence-photography of the human retinal vasculature provides a dynamic record and increased visibility of the vascular pattern and blood flow by means of a simple technique. . . . Separate arteriolar and venous filling phases, an arterio-venous shunt, sluggish choroidal circulation, stratified flow of fluorescein, and rapid central retinal circulation times were observed in normal retinas. Similar findings were seen in hypertensive and diabetic patients, and, in addition, neovascularization was clearly defined, and some cotton-wool patches, but not hemorrhages, were found to fluoresce.[1]*

Resources

We encourage you to examine the original texts of the above citations, as well as the following books and reviews:

Early Books and Photographic Atlases

Allen L, Braley AE. Stereoscopic Manual of the Ocular Fundus in Local and Systemic Disease. St. Louis: Mosby, 1964.

Bedell AJ. Photographs of the Fundus Oculi. Philadelphia: FA Davis, 1929.

Bothman L, Bennett RW. Fundus Atlas—Stereoscopic Photographs of the Fundus Oculi. Chicago: Year Book, 1939.

Cattaneo D. Oftalmoangioscopia. L. Bologna, Italy: Cappelli, 1947.

Dimmer F. Ueber die Photographie des Augenhintesgrundes. Wiesbaden, Germany: Bergmann, 1907.

Dimmer F, Pillat A. Atlas Photographischer Bilder des Menschlichen Augenhintergrundes. Leipzig, Germany: F Deuticke, 1927.

Hansell P. A System of Ophthalmic Illustration. Springfield, IL: Charles C. Thomas, 1957.

Jutte A, Lemke L. Invitalfarbung am Augenhintergrund mit Fluoreszein-Naturium. Stuttgart, Germany: Ferdinand Enke Verlag, 1968.

Matthaus W, Grotzsch K. Die Photographie in der Augenheilkunde. Leipzig, Germany: VEB Georg Thieme, 1966.

Rosen ES. Fluorescence Photography of the Eye. London: Butterworths, 1969.

Routier D. Le Fond d'Oeil des Hypertendus et des Cyanoses. Paris: Masson et Cie, 1947.

Shikano S, Shimizu K. Atlas of Fluorescence Fundus Angiography. Philadelphia: Saunders, 1968.

Shimizu K. Fluorescein Angiography. Tokyo: Igaku Shoin, 1974.

Thorner W. Die Theory des Augenspiegels und die Photographie des Augenhintergrundes. Berlin: Hirschwald, 1903.

Tillé H, Couadau A. Atlas Clinique d'Ophtalmoscopie Photographique, Syndromes Cliniques du Fond de l'Oeil. Paris: Masson et Cie, 1939.

Wessing A. Fluoreszenzangiographie der Retina: Lehrbuch und Atlas. Stuttgart, Germany: Georg Thieme Verlag, 1968.

Historical Reviews

Aandekerk AL. Ophthalmic photography in the Netherlands: past and present. J Ophthal Photog 2001;23:85.

Alvis MD, Julian KG. The story surrounding fluorescein angiography. J Ophthal Photog 1982;5:6.

Bedell AJ. Stereoscopic fundus photography. JAMA 1935;105:1502.

Dimmer F. Ueber die Photographie des Augenhintesgrundes. Wiesbaden, Germany: Bergmann, 1907.

Englebert M. Uber die photographie des augenhintesgrundes. Tecnische Roundschau 1965;39:57.

Hurtes R. Evolution of Ophthalmic Photography. In J Justice (ed), Ophthalmic Photography. Boston: Little, Brown, 1982.

Liesenfeld H. Uberblick uber die entwicklung der augenhintergrundsphotographie. Ophthalmologica 1959;137:390.

Mann WA. History of photography of the eye. Surv Ophthal 1970;15:179.

Meyer-Schwickerath GRE. Ophthalmology and photography. Am J Ophthal 1968;66:1011.

Saine PJ. Landmarks in the historical development of fluorescein angiography. J Ophthal Photog 1993;15:17.

Saine PJ. Ophthalmic photography books: an historical bibliography. J Ophthal Photog 1994;16:78.

Shatz H, Burton TC, Yannuzzi LA, Rabb MF. Interpretation of Fundus Fluorescein Angiography. St. Louis: Mosby, 1978.

Van Cader TC. History of ophthalmic photography. J Ophthal Photog 1978;1:7.

Wong D. Textbook of Ophthalmic Photography. New York: Inter-Optics Publications, 1982.

References

1. Novotny HR, Alvis DL. A method of photographing fluorescence in circulating blood in the human retina. Circulation 1961;24:82.
2. Duke-Elder S. System of Ophthalmology. Vol II. St. Louis: Mosby, 1961.
3. Duke-Elder S. System of Ophthalmology. Vol X. London: Henry Kimpton, 1967.
4. Jackman WT, Webster JD. On photographing the retina of the living human eye. Philadelphia Photographer 1886;23:275.
5. Bedell AJ. Stereoscopic fundus photography. JAMA 1935;105:1502.
6. Baeyer A. Ueber eine neue klasse von farbstoffen. Ber Dtch Chem Gzellshaft 1871;4:555.

7. Ehrlich P. Ueber provocirte fluorescenzerscheinungen am auge. Dtsch Med Wochenschr 1882;8:21.
8. Burke A. Die klinische, physiologische und pathologische bedeutung der fluoreszenz in auge nach darreichnung von uranin. Klin Monasbl Augenheilkd 1910;48:445.
9. Kikai K. Uber die vitalfarbung des hinteren bulbussabschnittes. Arch Augenheilkd 1930;103:541.
10. Sorsby A. Vital staining of the retina; preliminary clinical note. Br J Ophthal 1939;23:20.
11. Lange K, Boyd LJ. The use of fluorescein to determine the adequacy of the circulation. Med Clin North Am 1942;26:943.
12. Dimmer F. Ueber die Photographie des Augenhintergrundes. Wiesbaden, Germany: Bergmann, 1907.
13. Howe L. Photography of the interior of the eye. Trans Am Ophthal Soc 1887;23:568.
14. Barr E. On photographing the interior of the human eyeball. Am J Ophthal 1887;4:181.
15. Gerloff O. Ueber die photographie des augenhintergrundes. Klin Monat f Augenheil 1891;29:397.
16. Thorner W. Die Theory des Augenspiegels und die Photographie des Augenhintergrundes. Berlin: Hirschwald, 1903.
17. Dimmer F. Der Augenspiegel und die Ophthalmoskopische Diagnostik. Leipzig, Germany: F Deuticke, 1921.
18. Dimmer F, Pillat A. Atlas Photographischer Bilder des Menschlichen Augenhintergrundes. Leipzig, Germany: F Deuticke, 1927.
19. Helmholtz H. Bescreibung eines Augenspiegels zur untersuchung der Netzhaut in lebenden Auge. Berlin: Forstner, 1851.
20. Thorner W. A new stationary ophthalmoscope without reflexes. Am J Ophthal 1899;16:376.
21. Gullstrand A. Neue methoden der reflexlosen ophthalmoskopie. Ber Dtsch Ophth Ges 1910;36:75.
22. Nordenson JW. Augenkamera zum stationaren ophthalmoskop von Gullstrand. Ber Dtsch Ophth Ges 1925;45:278.
23. Van Cader TC. History of ophthalmic photography. J Ophthal Photog 1978;1:7.
24. Ridley H. Retinal photography. Trans Ophthamol Soc U K 1957;77:417.
25. Nida. Essai sur la photographie en couleurs du fond de l'oeil, XIII Concilium Ophthalmologicum. Hollandia 1929;1:39.
26. Bedell AJ. Photographs of the Fundus Oculi. Philadelphia: FA Davis, 1929.
27. Hartinger H. Ein neue reflexfreie ophthalmoskoplinse fur die zeiss-nordenonsche netzhautkammer. Z Ophthalmol Optik 1936;24:137.
28. Hansell P, Beeson EJG. Retinal photography in color. Br J Ophthal 1953;37:65.
29. Cohn P, DuBois-Reymond C. Photograms of the eye. JAMA 1888;10:540.
30. Edgerton HE. Photographic use of electrical discharge flashtubes. J Optical Soc Am 1946;36:390.
31. Rizzutti AB. High speed photography of the anterior ocular segment. Arch Ophthal 1950;43:365.
32. Ogle KN, Rucker CW. Fundus photographs in color using a high speed flash tube in the Zeiss retinal camera. Arch Ophthal 1953;49:435.
33. Chao P, Flocks M. The retinal circulation time. Am J Ophthal 1958;46:8.
34. Flocks M, Miller J, Chao P. Retinal circulation time with the aid of fundus cinematography. Am J Ophthal 1959;48:3.
35. MacLean AL, Maumenee AE. Hemangioma of the choroid. Am J Ophthal 1960;50:3.

Chapter 2

Fundus Photography: Instrumentation and Technique

Patrick J. Saine

A   B   C

FIGURE 2-1
A typical fundus camera **(A)** is shown with normal
fundus photographs of a right **(B)** and left eye **(C)**.

Introduction

Fundus photography documents the retina, the neurosensory tissue in the eye that translates optical images into electrical impulses the brain understands. The retina can be photographed directly, with the pupil used as both an entrance and exit for the fundus camera's illuminating and imaging light rays. Ophthalmologists use the resulting retinal photographs to follow, diagnose, and treat eye diseases.

This chapter begins by discussing the instrumentation used to perform fundus photography. A step-by-step description of clinical technique is followed by a detailed explanation of the focusing process. Practical tips for avoiding artifacts and managing challenging patients are presented. Advanced fundus photography techniques conclude the chapter.

Instrumentation

The optical instrument used to document the visual condition of the retina is called a *fundus camera*. It is a specialized low-power microscope with an attached camera (Figure 2-1).

Subsystems

All automobiles have a steering wheel, engine, and wheels. The steering wheel guides you, the engine provides the energy, and the wheels get you where you want to go. Likewise, all fundus cameras share three interrelated subsystems: mechanical, optical, and electrical. The joystick steers the camera while the optical system creates the image from light energy provided by the electrical system.

MECHANICAL
Support for the fundus camera is provided by the mechanical subsystem. The heavy optical head is mounted on a height-adjustable table, the most versatile of which is wheelchair accessible. Standardized patient interface and camera positioning are provided by the mechanical subsystem.

The chin rest and forehead rest reduce patient head movement. During the procedure, the precise positioning of the fundus camera is controlled by the joystick and optical head height control.

OPTICAL

The retinal image is accurately and efficiently transferred to both the photographer and the film using the optical subsystem. The classic fundus camera design features an aspheric objective lens precisely aligned with a 35-mm single lens reflex (SLR) camera body (Figure 2-2). Simply stated, the optical system of the fundus camera projects a ring of illumination through the dilated pupil; the light then reflects off the retina, exits the pupil through the center of the illumination ring, and continues through the fundus camera optics to form an image at the film plane. The viewfinder and the film back or digital recording device are integral parts of this subsystem.

ELECTRICAL

The fundus camera's electrical subsystem provides two sources of illumination. Distinctly different circuitry coexists for viewing the fundus and exposing the film (Figure 2-3). Viewing the retina requires a continuous light source that can be adjusted according to the patient's level of comfort and the photographer's ability to distinguish fine retinal detail. The viewing light is usually a tungsten bulb that is specific to the particular camera model and its manufacturer. Changing the viewing lamp intensity has no effect on the exposure of the final fundus photograph.

A xenon-filled flash tube provides a brief burst of intense light to expose the fundus photograph. The gas in the flash tube is ionized by the high voltage that is stored in the capacitors of the camera's power unit. Changing the intensity of the flash setting has no effect on the viewing illumination.

Types of Fundus Cameras

A number of different manufacturers make a wide variety of fundus cameras available. The particular brand of camera may be identified by its image shape and identification tab (Figure 2-4).

Fundus cameras are described by the angle of view—the optical angle of acceptance of the lens (Figure 2-5). An angle of 30 degrees, considered the normal angle of view, creates a film image 2.5 times larger than life. Wide-angle fundus cameras capture images between 45 and 140 degrees and provide proportionately less retinal magnification. A narrow-angle fundus camera has an angle of view of 20 degrees or less. Normal-angle cameras have smaller illuminating annuli, making them more suitable for patients with pupils of a smaller diameter. The inner diameter of the illuminating ring in wide-angle cameras is larger, making it more difficult to photograph patients with small pupils.

Interchangeable lenses are important tools for the general photographer. The ability to vary the angle of view allows the ophthalmic photographer the same flexibility. Fundus cameras may ("multiple-angle cameras") or may not ("single-angle cameras") have the ability to internally alter their angle of view. Accessory teleconverter-type optics can be inserted in front of the film back to increase the versatility of some single-angle cameras (Figure 2-6).

There are two strategies for obtaining multiple angles of view in an office. Either more than one single-angle fundus camera (e.g., a normal-angle and a wide-angle) or just one multiple-angle camera may be used. The optics of single-angle fundus cameras are optimized for a particu-

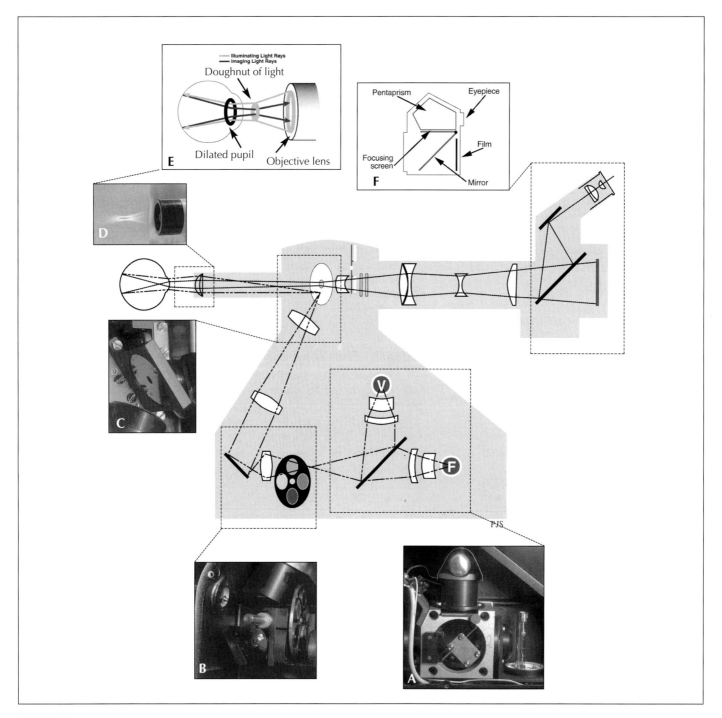

FIGURE 2-2
The optical pathway of the fundus camera. Light generated from either the viewing lamp (V) or the electronic flash (F) **(A)** is projected through a set of filters and onto a round mirror **(B)**. This mirror reflects the light up into a series of lenses that focus the light. A mask on the uppermost lens shapes the light into a doughnut. The doughnut-shaped light is reflected onto a round mirror with a central aperture **(C)**, exits the camera through the objective lens, and proceeds into the eye through the cornea. When the illuminating light is seen from the side, you can appreciate the complexity and precision of the optical scheme **(D)**. Assuming that both the illumination system and the image are correctly aligned and focused, the resulting retinal image exits the cornea through the central, unilluminated portion of the doughnut **(E)**. The light continues through the central aperture of the previously described mirror, through the astigmatic correction device and the diopter compensation lenses, and then back to the single lens reflex camera system **(F)**.

lar magnification and will provide higher-quality images than multiple-angle cameras. Multiple-angle cameras offer versatility. However, usually only one angle of view (often the widest) is sharp; alternate angles may be less critically sharp. Some cameras change optics in more than one part of the camera. These cameras may provide sharper images at

FIGURE 2-3
The flash tube (F) and the viewing lamp (V) are controlled by separate electrical subsystems. Increase the flash setting if your pictures are too dark; increase the view lamp setting if your view of the fundus is dark.

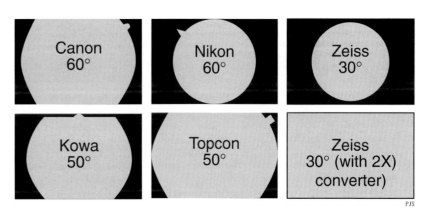

FIGURE 2-4
The shape and location of identification tabs help identify the brand of fundus camera. The actual size and shape of the image mask and the location of the identification tab may vary with the year of manufacture.

multiple angles. The choice here is the familiar dilemma, pitting high quality against convenience and cost.

There are a number of specialized fundus camera designs. Extreme wide-angle cameras have an angle of acceptance of more than 150 degrees and are used when large retinal areas need to be documented (Figure 2-7). Their small magnification minimizes fine retinal detail.

Simultaneous stereo fundus cameras use one exposure to place two images side by side on a single 35-mm frame (Figure 2-8). Their standardized stereo base allows longitudinal studies of retinal topography as well as detailed electronic analysis of retinal topography.

Hand-held fundus cameras provide maximum portability (Figure 2-9). They are useful for photographing bedridden, infant, and animal patients (see the section on Hand-Held Fundus Cameras, page 78).

Both mydriatic and nonmydriatic fundus cameras are available. Mydriatic fundus cameras require patient dilation. Their versatility allows both sequential stereo fundus photography and fluorescein angiography. Nonmydriatic fundus cameras exploit the patient's natural dilation in a dark room. The photographer views the fundus using an infrared light source and an infrared video camera. Only a single image is captured, either digitally or on instant film. Because the patient's pupil will take some time to naturally dilate again, multiple-image procedures are difficult. Nonmydriatic cameras are useful as screening devices.

Like much of the rest of the imaging world, ophthalmic photography is currently in a state of flux. Traditional silver-based imaging (film) is

A

B

C

D

FIGURE 2-5
Angles of view. The greater the angle of view, the larger the retinal area contained in the photograph **(A)**. The smaller the angle of view, the greater the magnification. The same eye is photographed at 20 degrees **(B)**, 35 degrees **(C)**, and 50 degrees **(D)**.

A

B

FIGURE 2-6
In multiple-angle cameras, select the angle of view by flipping a switch that inserts a different lens internally **(A)**. In single-angle fundus cameras, place auxiliary teleconverter-type optics between the camera body and lens to modify the angle of view **(B)**.

FIGURE 2-7
This 150-degree fundus photograph **(A)** of a tumor illustrates relative size and location. Multiple 30-degree photographs **(B)** would be needed to convey the same information.

A   B

FIGURE 2-8
Simultaneous stereo cameras record two slightly different views of the retina side by side on a standard 35-mm film.

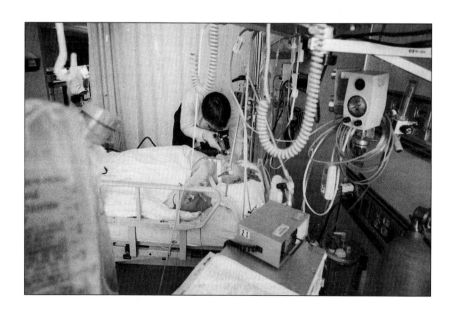

FIGURE 2-9
Hand-held fundus cameras are useful when patient positioning makes it difficult to use a standard fundus camera.

Choosing a Fundus Camera

1. How much versatility or specialization is required for your ophthalmic practice? Will the practice be growing or changing soon? Is this the practice's first or only fundus camera? If this is a second or third camera, should it be identical (for compatibility) or different (to expand the photographic capabilities or take advantage of technological advances)?

2. Will the optics of this camera provide adequate or superior sharpness and contrast? What angles of view are available and of what quality?

3. What are the clinical needs of the physician who will be evaluating the photographs? Will extremely fine macular detail be required in all images?

4. What type of patients will be photographed? Will their pupils be widely or poorly dilated? What is the minimum pupil size required for a good fundus photograph on a particular camera model?

5. Will patients be reasonably comfortable during the procedure? Can physically challenged patients be accommodated? Is portability an issue?

6. Are the camera's controls well balanced, adequately marked, and ergonomically placed? How easy or difficult is the viewing or focusing system to use?

7. Is this a reliable model? How sturdy does the camera feel? If this camera breaks down, how will it be repaired? How much time is involved? What is the cost, expected life, and availability of viewing lamps and flash tubes?

8. What is the initial cost of the unit? Is a used camera of the same model available?

9. What experience have other photographers had with this camera model? Is the photographer's preference to view with or without the barrier filter during fluorescein angiography?

10. Will the photographer using the camera be pleased with it?

Cleaning Your Lens

The best fundus photographs are taken using a fundus camera with a clean front element (Figure 2-11). Recommendations for cleaning your objective lens are available from your fundus camera manufacturer. Most lenses will not be harmed by over-the-counter "photographic" or "coated lens" cleaners and good-quality photographic lens cleaning tissue. Avoid products that leave a residue.

Begin cleaning your lens by inserting the negative diopter lens and focusing on the dust on the front element. Use a bulb syringe to blow off any loose dust. Place a few drops of lens-cleaning solution on a piece of lens tissue or natural cotton (never on the lens itself, and never on a commercial cotton swab manufactured with glue). Using gentle pressure, wipe in circular motions beginning in the center of the lens and spiraling to the outside.

(continued)

being challenged by the silicon-based technology of electronic imaging using computers. See Chapter 7 for a discussion of this technology.

Selecting a Fundus Camera

Choosing a fundus camera is similar to buying an automobile. A family minivan is selected because of its versatility: It can transport people and haul larger loads. It's not flashy, nor particularly fast, and it won't get the best gas mileage. A minivan is most like a medium-priced multiple-angle fundus camera. It offers respectable sharpness in a variety of optical angles and is suitable for the general ophthalmic practice.

A minivan will never outrace a sports car. Built for performance first and price second, the sports car is analogous to the normal-angle fundus camera favored by the retinal specialist. It is designed to produce sharp photographs of the macula and does so extremely well. Its small illumination doughnut facilitates photographing through narrow pupils, and the astigmatic compensation device is useful for peripheral views.

Special-use fundus cameras can be compared to pickup trucks or all-terrain vehicles. These include extreme wide-angle, simultaneous stereo, and hand-held fundus cameras. Minimal-feature, entry-level cameras and used models are inexpensive purchase options.

Pay careful attention to your specific needs when surveying the market. Compare and test drive competing camera models during fundus photography workshops such as those sponsored by the Ophthalmic Photographers' Society. The questions in the sidebar on choosing a fundus camera may help you prioritize fundus camera features and your practice's needs.

Fundus Camera Controls

Each time you perform fundus photography, you will be adjusting a complex optical instrument in a darkened room filled with patients. Your mission: to completely familiarize yourself with each of your camera's controls. The alternative? Turning the light repeatedly on and off while searching for the appropriate setting, all the while cursing under your breath. Not a pretty picture.

Read your manual cover to cover. Memorize it. Contact the manufacturer to obtain a copy of a missing manual.

Figure 2-10 provides an overview of the controls found on most fundus cameras. Rely on your manual for the location and function of specific or specialized controls.

Fundus Camera Maintenance

The proper maintenance of a fundus camera involves skills as simple as changing a light bulb and procedures as complex as aligning optics.

A properly maintained fundus camera will provide years of reliable service. You should be able to handle simple maintenance such as cleaning the front surface of the objective lens or cleaning the film transport chamber (Figure 2-11) (see the sidebar on cleaning your lens). Surfaces that come into direct contact with the patient should be disinfected after each procedure and at the end of every day. Consult a member of your infection control team or your physician for current recommendations of appropriate antimicrobial agents.

Always have two spare viewing lights, flash tubes, and fuses readily available. Know when and how to change them. Your fundus camera's instruction manual should contain detailed installation procedures. Alternately, contact the manufacturer's technical representative.

The 35-mm camera body is the fundus camera's most frequently repaired component. Its shutter fires and its film transport gears rotate each time a photograph is exposed. Keep a spare camera body available.

Fundus cameras that are used daily should have yearly inspections by factory-trained technicians. Consider returning your camera to the factory for complete optical realignment and refurbishment every 5–10 years. Mobile cameras may need service more often.

Fundus Photography Technique: Step by Step

The time involved in obtaining a good fundus photograph is significantly longer than the tiny fraction of a second it takes to expose the film. Like the athlete who is judged on split-second decisions, you should recognize that proper preparation, standardized technique, and careful follow-through are vital to successful fundus photography.

Fundus photography is actually a multistep procedure (Table 2-1). We explore each of the following four major steps in detail:
- Prepare
- Align
- Expose
- Follow-up

Prepare

1. *Prepare the room.* The room should be clean and tidy. All billing, departmental, and other paperwork should be completed before escorting the patient to the camera. Adjust the stool height and the fundus camera's mechanical controls to their approximate midpoints. Select the appropriate camera back and load it with color slide film (Figures 2-12 through 2-14) (see the sidebar on choosing

FIGURE 2-10
Controls on three different fundus cameras are labeled to correspond with the numbered descriptions below **(A–D)**. Your controls may vary according to the specific make and year of your fundus camera. You should be completely familiar with the function of all of your fundus camera's dials, knobs, and switches; consult the manual or the manufacturer if you are not. (Images courtesy of Canon, USA, Topcon USA, and Humphrey Instruments/Carl Zeiss).

1. **Angle selection lever.** Inserts lenses into the optical pathway, which either increases or decreases the angle of view (or magnification). You should be familiar with the retinal area circumscribed by each setting, as well as the relative sharpness of each.
2. **Anterior segment lens.** Inserts a positive lens into the optical pathway, allowing for a more accurate imaging of the external eye or name tag. The diopter compensation lens performs this function on some cameras.
3. **Astigmatism compensation control.** Inserts an adjustable cylindrical lens into the optical pathway. It is especially useful when patients have a large amount of astigmatism or when photographing the periphery of the retina.

A

FIGURE 2.10 *(continued)*

4. **Barrier filter slide.** Positions a yellow barrier filter (for fluorescein angiography) in front of the film, but after the image has left the patient's eye. Some camera models position the barrier filter directly in the throat of the 35-mm camera back; some place it further forward in the optical system.

5. **Camera back.** Conventionally, this is a light-tight container that holds the film and contains the shutter. Modern fundus cameras offer a choice of film (silver-based imaging), video, or a digital chip (electronic imaging). Use separate camera backs for color film (for fundus photography) and black and white film (for fluorescein angiography). An instant film back may also be available.

6. **Camera back selection switch.** Selects between multiple camera backs. This is one of those simple switches that, if left in the incorrect position, can sabotage your session by sending images to the wrong camera body. Not shown.

7. **Chin rest.** Stabilizes the patient. This should be cleaned between each patient.

8. **Data card port.** Positions a patient data card for recording information on the film next to the fundus images. Most photographers prefer to expose a separate name tag between patients.

9. **Diopter compensation lens.** Places positive and negative lenses into the optical pathway, extending the focusing range to permit the photography of patients with unusually long or short eyes. The plus setting can also be used for external or anterior segment photographs.

10. **Eyepiece diopter adjustment.** Sets the eyepiece, allowing the photographer to view the reticle in sharp focus. The eyepiece must be correctly set and the reticle must be in sharp focus to obtain sharp fundus photographs. Proper adjustment of the eyepiece is a critical element in successful fundus photography.

11. **External fixation light.** Used to direct patient fixation, this small light is universally positionable. Fixation lights can be green, red, or white; can have a focusable target; and sometimes blink.

12. **Filter slide.** Allows the addition of optional filters into the optical pathway (see number 13, filter wheel, for insertion of standard filters). These filters affect the light that enters the eye.

13. **Filter wheel.** Inserts the clear (color fundus photographs), green ("red-free" photographs), blue (exciter filter for fluorescein angiography), or red (choroidal photography) filter into the optical pathway in front of the light source (i.e., before the light enters the patient's eye).

14. **Flash intensity control.** Adjusts the amount of illumination emitted from the electronic flash. This control has no effect on the viewing illumination.

15. **Focusing knob.** Adjusts the distance between the front element and the focusing screen/film plane to maximize sharpness.

16. **Forehead rest.** Stabilizes the patient. It should be cleaned immediately after patient contact.

17. **Forehead rest adjustment.** Moves the patient toward and away from the front element. Used to position the fundus camera's illumination system with the patient's eye. Not shown.

18. **Fuse.** Know the location of all of your camera's fuses and keep spares readily available. If the fuses on your power supply are unmarked, label them for future reference.

19. **Instruction booklet.** Full of important information, this should be read studiously from cover to cover. Not shown.

20. **Internal fixation device.** Small pointer that can be introduced into the optical pathway. It is useful for obtaining fixation in the eye you are photographing, for recording the retinal location of patient fixation, or as a pointer in a teaching slide. When not serving a specific purpose, it should be removed from the optical pathway before the picture is taken.

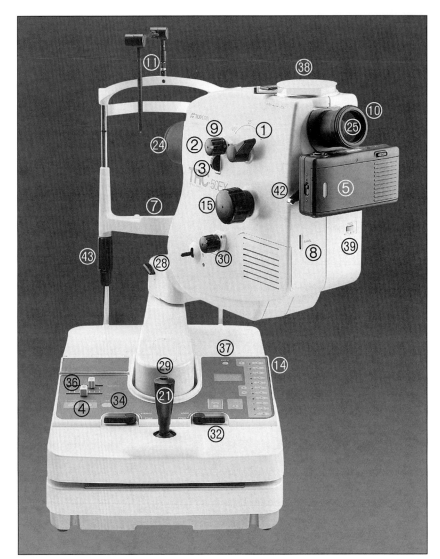

B

film). Check that the illumination and flash settings, the filter wheel, and the diopter compensation control are in their standard positions.

2. *Adjust the eyepiece.* Follow the step-by-step procedure described in the sidebar on setting your reticle. Each time you look through the fundus camera, you should see the reticle in sharp focus. A full explanation of how the reticle system works is found below in the section on focusing the fundus camera, page 42. Photograph a name tag before the patient enters the room. A name tag is simply a photograph of the patient's name and chart number; you may use the patient's chart or routing slip or, alternately, handwrite or type the information. The name tag assures you that the camera is functioning properly and serves as a guidepost during editing. You won't be looking into the eyepiece again until Step 9.

3. *Plan the photographs.* Take a moment to prepare yourself for the procedure. You should be familiar with the basic anatomy of the eye (Figure 2-15). Review the photo request form (Figure 2-16), consulting with the referring physician as needed. Remember that you will be creating a permanent record of the patient's fundus at a particular moment in time. Your photographs should be complete enough

FIGURE 2.10 *(continued)*

21. **Joystick.** Controls the side-to-side and forward-to-backward motion of the optical head during photography. Using this control becomes second nature with experience.
22. **Joystick tension control.** Adjusts the ease of moving the joystick. Not shown.
23. **Lens cap.** Protects the front element. It should be placed over the lens whenever photographs are not being taken and immediately after each patient session. Not shown.
24. **Objective lens.** The expensive, aspheric lens that is primarily responsible for imaging the retina. Both the front and the rear surface should be kept scrupulously clean and dust-free.
25. **Ocular (eyepiece).** Allows you to view and judge the image before it is exposed. During fundus photography, keep both of your eyes open, relaxed, and focused on infinity. (See also number 10, eyepiece diopter adjustment.)
26. **On/off power switch.** Obvious, but essential—master switch that controls all electrical functions.
27. **Optical head height adjustment.** Raises or lowers the optical head in relation to the patient's eye.
28. **Pivot point.** The fundus camera rotates about this point, facilitating the visualization of nasal or temporal retina.
29. **Shutter release.** When pressed, exposes the photograph by initiating a series of events that includes raising the eyepiece mirror and opening the shutter, which triggers the flash.
30. **Small pupil device.** Slightly decreases the diameter of the illumination ring on a wide-angle camera, improving photographs imaged through a smaller pupil. This device is usually ambitiously named; a single, normal-angle camera is the best choice in small pupil situations.
31. **Table adjustment.** Raises or lowers the table height manually or with an electric motor.
32. **Table lock.** Holds the table steady during photography or while transporting the fundus camera.
33. **Tilt mechanism.** Rotates the camera up and down, facilitating inferior or superior retinal views.
34. **Timer reset.** Resets the angiogram timer to zero.
35. **Timer start.** Begins the angiogram timer.
36. **Viewing illumination control.** Adjusts the intensity of the viewing light. It has no effect on the brightness or darkness of the final fundus photograph.
37. **Flicker.** Turns on flicker function for external fixation light. Not shown.
38. **Camera port.** Second active port for digital, second 35-mm, or Polaroid camera.
39. **W.D.** Turns on and off the working distance dots.
40. **Front toggle.** Turns on flicker function for external fixation light. Not shown.
41. **Stereo lock.** Turns on flicker function for external fixation light. Not shown.
42. **Camera release lever.** Locks camera in mount. Pull down to release. Not shown.
43. **Chin rest height.** Rotate to raise and lower the chin rest.
45. **B&W digital capture.** Records electronic images.

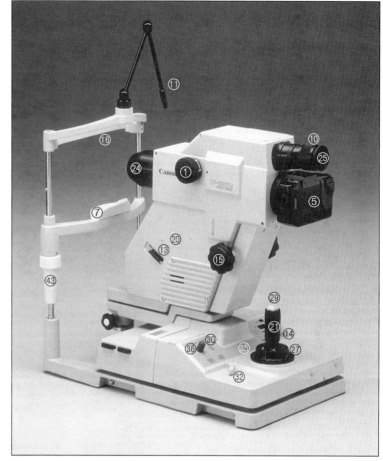

C

to convey the condition of the retina to the physician. Examine prior photographs and notes made by the previous photographer or the physician. Note the patient's visual acuity and working diagnosis. Will the patient have trouble fixating because of a macular problem? Which fields should be photographed? On which retinal level should the camera be focused? Should the periphery be scanned for retinal changes? Will another photographic procedure better document this particular disease entity? Should today's images match the magnification and fields of previous photographs? You should have a photographic plan in mind before you escort the patient into the room. This plan should include your camera and angle of view selections, the areas of the patient's retina you intend to document, and any specialized techniques that may be useful.

4. *Escort the patient.* Your patient's pupils must first be dilated in accordance with the attending physician's orders (Figure 2-17; Table 2-2) (see the sidebar on dilating your patient's pupils). Mentally evaluate your patients while escorting them to the fundus camera. Do they seem to be in good or poor general health? Are there any obvious physical disabilities? Retinal photography patients are often mature: Familiarize yourself with typical age-related hearing and visual changes. Become aware of your patient's disposition. Some patients will be uncomfortable merely because they are in a doc-

Which Film Should I Use?

Choosing a film involves making two decisions. First, the general type must be determined, and then a specific brand must be chosen.

One way to describe film is by listing opposing characteristics (Figure 2-12). You know that film is available in black and white and color. It is also available as positive (or slide film: black records as black) and negative film (black records as white). Of course, both black and white film and color film are available in positive and negative emulsions. Slow film (ISO 25: less sensitive to light but finer grain and better image quality) and fast film (ISO 400: more sensitive to light but coarser grain and lesser image quality) are options in each of the above categories. Finally, film can vary in its spectral sensitivity or light balance—daylight, tungsten, and infrared emulsions being available. Most ophthalmic photographers choose a 35-mm slow (ISO 25) or medium (ISO 100) speed transparency film balanced for daylight for routine fundus photography.

If you are unsure about the film characteristics described above, a basic photography course will help.

Which specific brand or speed of film should you use? That question is best answered through empirical testing. Although each film records physical reality, no pair of films ever records it in quite the same way. Each brand and speed of film has its own specific color cast, resolution, acutance (the transition between black and white when a straight edge is imaged), and "look" (Figure 2-13). The same brand of film (e.g., Kodachrome) is sold in different film speeds (e.g., 25, 64, and 200), each of which has different image characteristics.

Before settling on a film, perform a film test. Photograph the same volunteer or patient using a number of different films (keeping other factors constant, of course). Both you and the physician should evaluate the choices without knowing the names of the films used, using a daylight balanced light box. After selecting the best choice, determine its practicality: Is the film and processing readily available at a reasonable price? Are the archival properties of the chosen film adequate (Figure 2-14)?[1]

Film manufacturers are continually improving their film stocks. We suggest keeping current with emulsion changes and testing new films regularly.

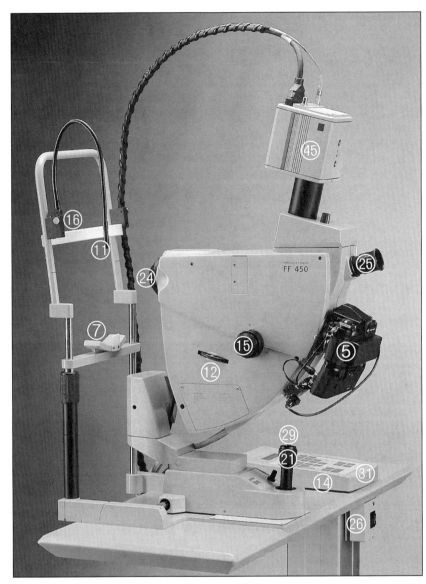

D

FIGURE 2.10 (continued)

FIGURE 2-11

This fundus photograph was not taken during a blizzard. Keep your front element scrupulously clean. Blurry white circles appearing in the image are images of dust, dirt, or tears on the front of your objective lens. Dirty lenses are more noticeable in photographs of patients with smaller pupils and with off-center camera alignment.

Setting Your Reticle

To obtain a sharp view of the reticle, your eyepiece must be correctly set. Here is a step-by-step procedure for eyepiece adjustment:

1. Have your eyes corrected for their best visual acuity. You may choose to photograph with or without glasses or contact lenses if your correction is spherical. Remember, however, that the correct eyepiece setting will be different depending on whether you wear your corrective lenses. If you have astigmatism, you should wear your corrective lenses while adjusting the eyepiece. Alternatively, correct the eyepiece itself by securing the appropriate trial lens directly over the eyepiece.[2] Do not wear reading glasses.

2. Eliminate any subject matter from the camera's field of view. Set your camera to the farthest focusing extreme and hold or tape a piece of white cardboard in front of the objective lens. When you look through the viewfinder, you should see a blurry reticle on a white field. The illumination level should be adjusted to a medium or low setting (approximately the same intensity as when viewing the retina). If the picture is too bright, it may cause your pupil to constrict, bringing depth of field into play and making an accurate setting difficult.

3. Set the eyepiece adjustment to the maximum plus diopter setting. This will blur any image of the focusing reticle. When looking through the viewfinder, you should see an evenly illuminated white field.

4. Relax your eyes. Blink and look at something far away—perhaps down a long hall or at a reflection. It is extremely important that your eyes be focused on infinity to obtain the correct setting. Keeping both eyes open may help keep you from accommodating.

5. Peer through the viewfinder and begin turning the eyepiece ring toward the zero setting. Smoothly rotate the ring. Rotate at a slow enough rate that you perceive the reticle becoming sharper, but not so slowly that your eyes accommodate for the change. Remember to keep both eyes open and focused at infinity.

6. **Stop** rotating when the reticle is **just** in sharp focus. If you continue to rotate the reticle after you achieve sharp focus, or if you begin to search for sharpness by rotating the reticle back and forth, then accommodation may be influencing your decision. If your eyes are at their best correction, your setting will probably be within a diopter or so of the zero mark. If your diopter setting is a high minus, chances are that you have accommodated. If you are wearing no correction, the setting should be within a diopter of your best correction.

7. *Repeat, repeat, repeat.* Continue setting the eyepiece until three successive, near-normal settings agree. Note the most consistent position of the eyepiece ring. Remember to correctly set the eyepiece before each patient session. New photographers should repeat this exercise daily until they are confident that their eyepiece setting is accurate.

(continued)

Table 2-1. Fundus Photography: Step by Step

Prepare	Prepare the room
	Adjust the eyepiece
	Plan the photographs
	Seat the patient
	Inform the patient
	Position the patient
	Position the photographer
Align	Establish fixation
	Focus the illumination system
	Adjust the joystick
	Select the area of interest
	Select the angle of view
	Check the focus
Expose	Double-check everything
	Expose the film
	Close the session
Follow-up	Process the film/edit the images
	Edit the film/archive the data
	Deliver the finished product
	Review your work

Note: Review these steps before or during the procedure to help establish your routine. Post a copy of these steps near your fundus camera for reference.

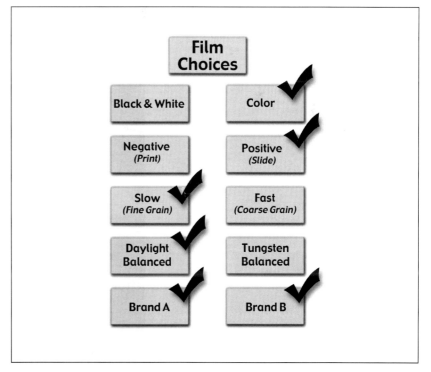

FIGURE 2-12
Choosing a film. Listing opposing characteristics will help you identify the film of choice for a particular application. With your final application in mind, follow the check marks: fundus photography requires a color film that is positive (slides), has a slow or medium speed (for fine grain), and is daylight-balanced (flash illumination). Once these broad characteristics are defined, the choice of brand is a practical matter. Select the film with the best image quality, truest color balance, greatest convenience, and best value.

Setting Your Reticle   *(continued)*

Each fundus camera should be set individually by each photographer. The correct setting for each camera (especially if brands vary) may be slightly different for the same photographer, and the correct setting for a single camera will vary between photographers in the same office. If an instrument has more than one user, a signal can be developed to alert alternate users of possible eyepiece setting changes (perhaps an empty film box placed over the eyepiece).

Check the eyepiece setting and reticle before each patient. It cannot be overemphasized that once your personal setting has been ascertained, it is imperative to check it before each patient. Be aware of the focusing screen's reticle throughout each photographic procedure. *Only conscientious use of the eyepiece/reticle focusing system will assure consistently sharp fundus photographs.*

A

B

FIGURE 2-13
Comparing different films. Film and processing have a major impact on the color of your final fundus photographs. These three photographs **(A–C)** of the same patient were exposed with the same camera on the same day but using different brands of film. Because commercially available film emulsions may change frequently, regularly test new film products.

C

FIGURE 2-14
Archival properties of film. Are your images exposed on color film that will not fade or discolor with time? Both of these fundus photographs were exposed in the 1960s. By the mid-1990s, **B** has faded considerably while **A** has not. Investigate the archival properties of your film of choice.

A

B

tor's office. Others may be in low spirits because they just received some unpleasant news from the doctor. Your demeanor should be bright but professional. Offer to take a coat or other personal items, setting them on the available shelf or hook. Invite your patients to be seated and introduce yourself with a smile. ("My name is ____, and I'd like to take some pictures of your eyes for Dr. ____.") Speak in a clear, calm voice to put your patients at ease. Remember that this may be their first experience with fundus photography—they will be looking to you to guide them through the procedure. Talk to your patients throughout the procedure; reassure them and let them know what to expect.

5. *Inform your patient.* Informed patients are cooperative patients. Ask your patient if they have had their eyes photographed before. Explain the procedure, acquainting them with the impending bright flashes and with your expectations. Let them know that it is

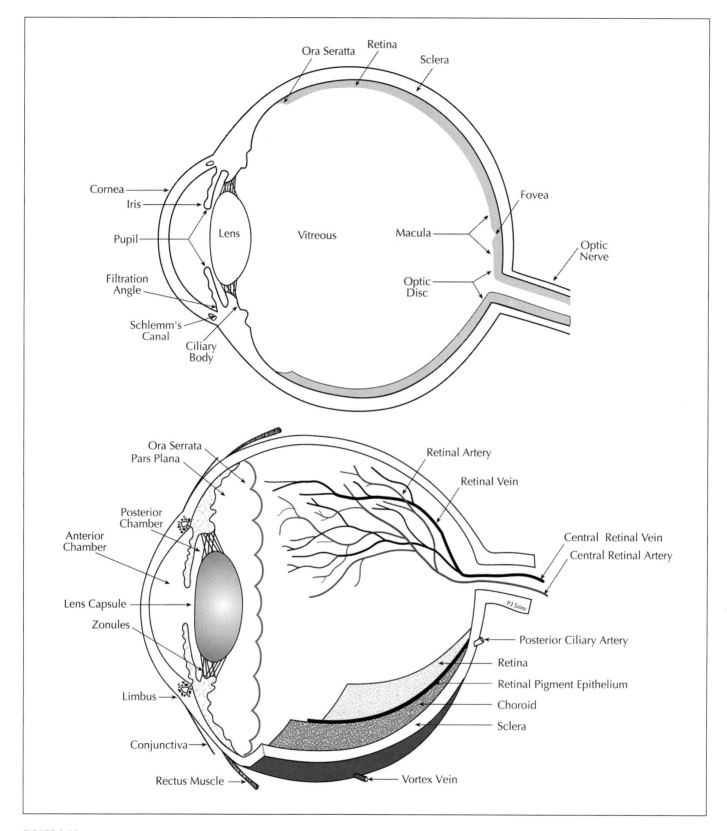

FIGURE 2-15
Basic eye anatomy. A thorough knowledge of the anatomy of the eye is a prerequisite for successful fundus photography.

RETINAL PHOTOGRAPHY

Name _____ Chart # _____ MD _____

Date _____ Dilated (Time) _____ **MD Signature** _____ ☐ **No Charge**

Brief History and Clinical Findings: _____ Dx code number _____

This patient has had previous photographs: ☐ Yes ☐ No   Allergies? _____

Fundus Photography
(Sketch as Necessary)

Field
Disc   1 OD OS
Macula 2 OD OS
       3 OD OS
       4 OD OS
       5 OD OS
       6 OD OS
☐ **2 Sets** 7 OD OS

Wide Angle
☐ Also
☐ Only

Filters
☐ Red
☐ Green
☐ Blue

Processing
☐ Digital ☐ ASAP   ☐ Pt. Wait
☐ Film   Time Back: ☐ Pt. Go
☐ Either ☐ Next Day ☐ Will Call

☐ Save Extras

Fluorescein Angiography

Earlies (Choose **One** Only) | **Lates** (Circle as needed)

Field   Field
1 OD OS   **Disc**   1 OD OS
2 OD OS   **Macula** 2 OD OS

(Please choose earlies and lates.)

_____
Other (Please Sketch or Describe)

LATES (min.) 1 3 5 10 15 (Circle as needed)
☐ Wide Angle Fluorescein   ☐ ICG (_____ min. lates)

PJS

Photographer's note   Reaction:
Initials _____

Ocular Media: **Cooperation:** **Fixation:** ☐ IOL
☐ Clear   ☐ Good   ☐ Good   ☐ Small Pupil
☐ Hazy   ☐ Fair   ☐ Fair   ☐ Cataract
☐ Very Hazy ☐ Poor ☐ Poor   ☐ Light Sensitive

FIGURE 2-16
Photography request form. Using a photography request form facilitates communication between the physician and the photographer. One form should be completed for each patient photography session. (ICG = indocyanine green; IOL = intraocular lens; OD = right eye; OS = left eye.)

fine for them to blink and breathe normally. Reassure them that the multicolored spots they will see afterward are nothing to worry about. Remind them that it is just like looking into a flash when they are having their picture taken and that no x-rays are involved. A mounted photograph should be available for simple explanations. Invite questions and answer them appropriately. Remember, however, that your role as a photographer precludes you from dispensing specific medical information. Diplomatically refer appropriate questions back to the referring physician.

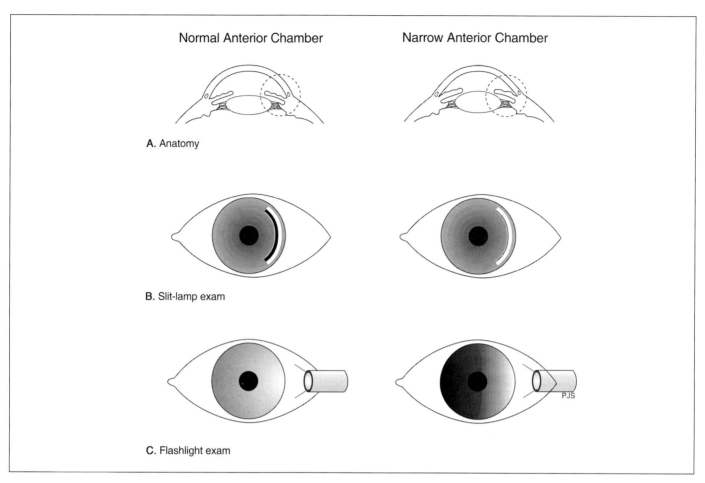

FIGURE 2-17
Estimating anterior chamber depth. The anterior chamber depth of each patient should be estimated before introducing dilation medication. Normal anterior chambers will not close during routine dilation. Narrow anterior chamber angles, however, may close on routine dilation, causing increased intraocular pressure and the possibility of an episode of medication-induced closed-angle glaucoma. Anatomically, the normal iris is well separated from the trabecular network **(A)**. The iris and trabecular meshwork are more closely positioned in patients with narrow angles. Angle depths are estimated using a 0 (closed angle) through 4 (large, fully open angle) scale. Slit-lamp examination is the best method for estimating anterior chamber depth. If a slit beam is projected at a 45-degree angle, then the aqueous space is indicated by unilluminated space (the black line between the two white lines) between the corneal reflection and the beam's projection on the iris **(B)**. The normal anterior chamber will reveal a wide space, the narrow anterior chamber, a narrow distance. A flashlight projected at the limbus in the same plane as the iris can also be used to estimate the depth of the anterior chamber (note: the flashlight technique has fallen out of favor with many ophthalmologists). Normal chambers cast little or no shadows. A bowed iris in a shallow anterior chamber projects a wide shadow across the pupil to the limbus **(C)**. Careful slit-lamp or flashlight examination is necessary on all patients before dilation. Always check with the ophthalmologist before dilating a patient with a narrow anterior chamber angle.

Table 2-2. Medications Used for Routine Dilation

Generic Name	Trade Name	Action	Maximal Effect	Duration
Tropicamide	Mydriacyl Opticyl Tropicacyl	Mydriasis and cycloplegia	20–30 mins	4–6 hrs
Cyclopentolate hydrochloride	AK-Pentolate Cyclogyl	Mydriasis and cycloplegia	15–30 mins	24 hrs
Phenylephrine	AK-Dilate	Mydriasis	20–40 mins	3 hrs
Hydrochloride	Efricel Mydfrin Neo-Synephrine	—	—	—

FIGURE 2-18
Seating the patient. Patient comfort is affected by the height of the patient's chair and the height of the fundus camera. Both the chair and the camera are adjusted to their midpoint for the average-sized patient **(A)**. Lower the stool and raise the camera for tall or long-bodied patients **(B)**. Raise the stool and lower the camera for heavy or short patients **(C)**. A child's height will dictate the best seating strategy. The child may be comfortable while standing flat on the floor or on a short step stool **(D)**. Younger children may sit or kneel either on their parent's lap or directly on a raised patient chair. Remove the head rest and lay papoosed babies on their side, or use a hand-held fundus camera for infant fundus photography.

Dilating Your Patient's Pupils

DILATION MEDICATION

An obvious prerequisite to creating any photograph is the ability to record the light that reflects off of the subject matter. This is taken for granted under ordinary circumstances. We are confronted with a biological system that is designed to counteract our best efforts when we attempt to photograph the retina, however. Because the eye has no internal light source, to photograph the retina we must shine a light into the patient's eye. This causes the iris to constrict—in effect, closing the window through which we are attempting to view. Extinguishing the light allows the pupil to become larger; however, then we are unable to record or even see in the resulting darkness. Clearly, we must counteract the iris' natural reaction to light if we are to obtain retinal photographs.

The solution to this fundamental problem is to artificially dilate the patient's eyes using topical medication. When we "dilate a patient," we instill drops that counteract the patient's normal reaction to light. This increases the size of the patient's pupil, allowing the illuminating light rays to be projected in and the imaging light to independently exit the eye.

The size of the pupil is controlled by the ciliary muscle, the iris sphincter muscle, and the dilating muscle. We can manipulate the normal reactions of these muscles by using two different types of medications: mydriatics and cycloplegics (Table 2-2). Mydriatics are sympathomimetics that dilate the pupil (or affect mydriasis) by causing the dilator muscle to contract. They also cause vasoconstriction and should be used with caution in individuals with a history of hypertension or heart problems. A commonly used mydriatic is phenylephrine. Available in both 2.5% and 10% solutions, maximal pupil dilation begins in 20 minutes and lasts for approximately 3 hours.

Cycloplegics are parasympatholytics that cause mydriasis by relaxing the iris sphincter muscles. They also arrest accommodation (or cause cycloplegia) by paralyzing the ciliary muscle. A commonly used cycloplegic is tropicamide. Available in 0.5% and 1% solutions,

(continued)

6. *Position your patient.* Comfortable patients are cooperative patients. Adjust the patient's chair height, then the height of the camera, and finally the height of your chair (Figure 2-18) (see sidebar on patient seating). Instruct the patient to place his or her chin in the chinrest and forehead against the bar. Raise or lower the table height or adjust the chinrest as needed. When correctly positioned at the fundus camera, your patient should have a straight back and be leaning slightly forward. The height of his or her eyes should approximately correspond to the height of the objective lens. A mark on the side of your headrest may indicate this height. (Some photographers place a mark at the lowest and highest lens objective height setting to help gauge appropriate patient alignment at a glance.) Be sure to ask the patient whether he or she is comfortable. ("Can I raise or lower the camera to make you more comfortable?") This question helps put your patient at ease by extending the same courtesy we would expect if we were in the patient's position.

7. *Position yourself.* After the patient has been made comfortable, you should do likewise. Your eye should be at the same height as the viewfinder; raise or lower your seat as appropriate. A typist uses the "home row" to standardize interaction with the keyboard. In the same way, you are encouraged to find your own "home keys." Grip the joystick with your dominant hand. If the optical head height adjustment is a separate control, place your other hand on it. The second hand also easily extends upward to the focusing knob or the external fixation device. The index finger of the joystick hand or the right foot triggers the shutter release. The hand closest to the power supply is used for any adjustments there.

Align

8. *Establish fixation.* Slide the fundus camera in front of the eye to be photographed (see the sidebar on which eye should be photographed first). Ask the patient to look straight ahead. Present the external fixation device to the eye that is not being photographed. Ask the patient if he or she can see the little light straight ahead. You may need to move the external fixation device quickly back and forth to gain the patient's attention (see the sidebar on establishing patient fixation). Ask the patient to keep looking at the little light while you shine another light into the other eye. Let the patient

Dilating Your Patient's Pupils *(continued)*

maximal pupil dilation occurs at approximately 30 minutes and lasts for 4–6 hours. Some offices prefer cyclopentolate. Available in 0.5%, 1%, and 2% solutions, it causes pupil dilation in 15–20 minutes and lasts for 24 hours. Other cycloplegics include atropine, homatropine, and scopolamine; each is available under various trade names.

A word of caution and an editorial: It is important to recognize the photographer's role in the health care setting. Ophthalmic photographers are surrounded by licensed individuals who specialize in understanding drugs and their effect on the body. These individuals should guide us in the use of all of the medications we administer to our patients. No drug should be administered to any patient without a physician's order. If a reaction occurs, refer the patient to a licensed health care worker. This does not mean that as ophthalmic photographers we are "just photographers." Ophthalmic photographers are highly trained professionals who specialize in acquiring images of the eye. We should use the strengths of other health care workers just as we expect them to recognize our areas of expertise.

INSTILLING EYE MEDICATION

Some important cautions: Read the medication insert completely for a description of contraindications and side effects. The administration of dilating drops is contraindicated in patients who are at risk for narrow-angle glaucoma. Estimate the anterior chamber depth before instilling dilation medication (Figure 2-17). Check with your physician before dilating patients with iris-fixated intraocular lenses. Children and infants should be dilated using ophthalmic medications that contain lower concentrations of active ingredients; consult the physician for specific instructions.

Educate your patients about the normal side effects of dilation. Remind them that the drops may sting (we jokingly remind patients that "these drops just sting on (insert day of the week)" and tell older pediatric patients ("close your eyes and count backwards from 20: the stinging will be over by then")). Warn the patients of increased light sensitivity due to their enlarged pupils. Offer them inexpensive, disposable sunglasses. Patients should be counseled that reading may be difficult because their near vision will be blurry. Reassure them that their distance vision should not be affected. We suggest patients bring a driver if they will be dilated.

Begin by washing your hands with soap and water and instructing the patient to tilt his or her head back. Gently pull the lower eyelid down slightly to create a small space between the lid and the globe. Place a single drop in this

(continued)

FIGURE 2-19
This diagram illustrates the normal patient's view when the retina is photographed. The patient will fuse the bright fundus camera light with the less bright fixation light. When fused, the small light will be perceived to be inside of the large light. The small light will be centered for macula photographs.

know that the small light will be in the middle of the bigger light once you have everything centered (Figure 2-19).

9. *Position the illumination system.* Turn the room lights down. Grossly align the fundus camera from side to side until the viewing light is centered on the cornea. Keep the joystick upright and use the optical head height adjustment as needed. Position the illumination system by moving the forehead rest adjustment (and patient) toward or away from the objective lens until the doughnut of light is centered on the pupil and focused on the cornea (or eyelid). On looking through the viewfinder with your dominant eye, you should see a blurry fundus image with an overlapping reticle (Figure 2-20). The image you see will probably be out of focus and may have a crescent-shaped artifact. Focus quickly (keeping the image of the reticle sharp and turning the focusing knob until the retina looks sharp), knowing that you will make fine focusing adjustments later. The crescent-shaped artifact indicates that the distance between the objective lens and the cornea is nearly correct.

FIGURE 2-20
Just after aligning the optical system, your look through the viewfinder will probably look blurry and contain artifacts **(A)**. After a quick focus **(B)**, move up and down or side-to-side to eliminate all crescent artifacts **(C)**, then move forward and backward to find the maximum color saturation **(D)**. Finally, focus carefully on the retina.

A

Dilating Your Patient's Pupils   *(continued)*

pouch, being careful not to contaminate the bottle by allowing it to touch the patient. (The drop may be applied inside the lower eyelid, on the sclera, or on the cornea. The patient's blink will distribute the medication.) Instill a second drop if you are not sure that the first was successful. One properly placed drop is sufficient: Avoid flooding the patient's eyes. After the drop has been instilled, ask the patient to close his or her eyes for a moment (without squeezing the eyelids). Blinking in moderation is acceptable. Patients may gently dab their closed eyes with a clean tissue but should avoid applying pressure. Replace the cap or dropper immediately after use. Wait 1 or 2 minutes between different eye medications.

Pay careful attention to the expiration date of your dilating medications. Never instill outdated or discolored medication. Consider dating the bottles when opened and then disposing of opened bottles after 30 days of use.

DIFFICULT CLINICAL SITUATIONS

Large pupils permit easier fundus photography. However, dilating medication is not equally effective in all individuals. Be prepared to photograph through smaller pupils in patients who

- Have darkly pigmented irises
- Are older
- Are taking glaucoma medication
- Have iritis with posterior synechia
- Have diabetes

You may encounter patients whose pupils constrict when you begin fundus photography. This could be the result of a number of different clinical situations. For example, the patient may have been dilated only with tropicamide. This dilation regimen is appropriate for routine direct ophthalmoscopy but inadequate for fundus photography. Patients being examined for closed-angle glaucoma are often dilated with only tropicamide. Another example is the patient who has been dilated much earlier that day. Routine dilation medication can last as little as 4–6 hours; if a patient has been dilated more than 3 hours earlier, his or her pupils may constrict during fundus photography. The patient may have a darkly pigmented iris and require a second set of drops for adequate dilation. Our routine for all of these situations is identical: We consult with the referring ophthalmologist to determine whether additional dilating drops may be safely administered. If so, fundus photography is resumed approximately 15 minutes after their administration. If additional dilating drops are not recommended, then fundus photography is resumed, the most important fields being imaged first. A note concerning the poor dilation is made on the order sheet, as it may affect the quality of the photographs.

B

C

D

FIGURE 2-20 *(continued)*

Establishing Fixation

There are a number of reasons why your patient may not be able to fixate on the external fixation light, the most obvious of which is that your patient probably has vision problems! If you are having trouble establishing fixation using the external fixation device, try one of the following practical suggestions:

1. *Clarify your instructions.* Patients may look to the side and see the fixation light with the eye you are photographing (as opposed to the fixating eye). They will ask you which of the two lights you want them to look at—the one to the side or the one straight ahead. Instruct them to look at the little light in the middle of the big light, or at the small light straight ahead, not at the light to the side.

2. *Alter the visual stimulus.* A moving or blinking stimulus commands attention better than a stationary stimulus. Try moving the fixation light from side to side using short, quick movements. If your camera doesn't have a blinking fixation light, then simulate blinking by rapidly moving your finger back and forth in front of the fixation light.

3. *Change the fixation light location.* Younger patients may attempt to fixate with both of their eyes. These patients will cross their eyes, making it difficult for you to obtain the proper field of view. If your instructions to look straight ahead fail, try adjusting the distance between the fixation light and the patient's eye. Some patients will straighten their eyes if you move the fixation light further away, effectively hiding it from the eye being photographed. Alternately, rotate the fixation light in slightly and move it closer toward the inner canthus. The fixating eye will remain crossed, but the eye being photographed will be looking straight ahead.

4. *Use the internal fixation device.* Insert your internal fixation device into the optical pathway where it will cast a shadow onto the patient's fundus. This stick-like shadow will look in focus to the patient when it looks in focus to you. In most cases you will want to remove the internal fixation device before the fundus photograph is exposed. This fixation strategy is especially useful if the eye being photographed has better vision than the fixating eye, or when the patient is monocular.

5. *Instruct the patient verbally.* If you have difficulty obtaining fixation with either fixation target, try asking the patient to look straight ahead in the middle of the light (for macula views). Alternately, have the patient look straight ahead at you (or your nose, voice, or the back wall). Simple directions (left, right, up, and down) or clock hours may help when peripheral photographs are requested. The patient's hand or thumb can be used to direct the patient's gaze.

6. *Move the camera.* If no reliable fixation can be obtained, simply instruct the patient to hold his or her eyes still. Use your fundus camera's adjustments to swing, tilt, or otherwise move until you locate the area of interest.

(continued)

An unsharp or fuzzy artifact implies that the illumination system is improperly aligned.

10. *Adjust the joystick.* The location of the crescent indicates your centration within the pupil (Figure 2-21). If the crescent is found on the right side of the fundus image, the camera is off-center to the right side of the pupil. In this case, use the joystick to shift the camera slightly to the left, centering the doughnut in the pupil. These crescent artifacts can occur above, below, and to each side. Using the joystick, move in the opposite direction of the crescent to recenter the camera in the pupil (and eliminate the artifact). (See Chapter 3 to learn the importance of finding and using these artifacts for stereo fundus photography.) Once your view is free from crescent-shaped artifacts, seek proper color saturation. Moving the joystick toward and away from the patient, check for the most even, most fully saturated view. Remember that the reticle and fundus should both still be sharp.

Two simple guidelines affect positioning artifacts during fundus photography: (1) moving the joystick from side to side and moving the optical head up and down controls the centration of the illuminating ring in the pupil and therefore controls the presence or absence of crescent-shaped artifacts, and (2) moving the joystick in and out focuses the illumination and controls the color saturation of the image.

11. *Select the area of interest.* Your photographic plan (step 3) should specify the areas you intend to photograph (Figure 2-22). If no posterior pole photographs have been requested, we routinely photograph the macula of the right eye first to ensure a familiar landmark during the editing process. Adjust the external fixation device until the area of interest is centered in the field of view. Some patients may require just disc photographs, whereas others need complete documentation of the posterior pole and periphery. Glaucoma and age-related macular degeneration are examples of conditions that may only require posterior pole photographs. Diabetic retinopathy, artery and vein occlusions, and retinitis pigmentosa are examples of conditions that may need peripheral documentation. When recording a peripheral nevus, be sure to include a photograph of the posterior pole and a photograph that contains both the nevus and a major blood vessel for orientation. All borders of a nevus should be visible in the final set of photographs. It is usually better to err on the side of too many photographs than too few.

12. *Select the angle of view.* Your choice of magnification depends on both the patient and the characteristics of the pathology. A normal angle of view is used to document fine retinal details (Figure 2-23). Recording the extent of a retinal condition requires a wide angle of view (Figure 2-24). Consider using multiple angles of view (Figure 2-25): Fundus photographs depicting the extent of a vein occlusion may benefit from a wide angle of view, whereas photographs of macular edema in the same eye may be more appropriate using a narrower angle of view.

Alternate factors may affect angle selection. A small pupil may preclude the use of a wide-angle camera, as the larger doughnut may not evenly illuminate the retina. You may choose to photograph an uncooperative child with a wide field of view to improve the chance that the final photograph will include a specific area of interest.

13. *Check the focus.* Look critically at the reticle and the fundus image. Adequate tear film is important to maximize clarity: Ask the patient to blink if he or she is not doing so naturally. Begin turning the

Establishing Fixation *(continued)*

7. *Nystagmus.* Attempt to define a null point (the position of gaze at which the patient's eye movement decreases or stops) in patients with nystagmus. Alternately, adjust the camera to image the fundus at an extreme of travel (the furthest point at which the eye moves and must reverse direction), and time your photographs to coincide with the patient's eye movements.

8. *Do your best.* Some of your most challenging patients will be those that your ophthalmologist could not examine. The hope is that you will be able to provide at least one good photograph to help your physician examine the patient's retina. Young patients may not have reliable fixation. Using a wide angle of view maximizes the possibility that your final photograph will include the area of interest (assuming appropriate dilation). Use your ingenuity in other difficult cases. Adopt the attitude of the Canadian Mounties: *always get your fundus photograph.*

Selecting a Patient Chair

Patient comfort and patient stability are two important considerations when selecting a patient chair. Height should be adjustable for multiple patient sizes (Figure 2-18), seats should be wide and padded for large patients. Wheeled stools with backs allow mobility between multiple cameras in a single room; locking casters promote patient stability. Motorized reclining patient examination chairs (with footrests removed) have been adopted in many clinics. [3]

FIGURE 2-21
Centering the camera. When the camera is centered on the pupil (A), you will see no position-related artifacts. Moving the camera slightly to the left (B) causes a reflection from the edge of the dilated pupil. Moving slightly further to the left (C) eliminates this reflection but results in a slightly darker, unevenly illuminated image (the result of a smaller portion of the doughnut being used to illuminate the retina). Further movement to the left (D) places the illuminating doughnut outside the pupil, effectively eliminating the retinal image. This same phenomenon happens along each axis. If we were to imagine a plane containing all centered and decentered fundus photographs of a specific retinal field, their composite would form a bull's eye (E). This bull's eye is narrower in poorly dilated patients. Reproducing this series (with both a well-dilated and a poorly dilated patient) is a useful exercise for the intermediate photographer. Each fundus camera's angle of view and illuminating circle make the specific bull's eye different for each camera model (F). Normal-angle cameras have wider concentric rings of acceptable imaging, allowing a wider stereo base. Wide-angle cameras generally have narrower "bull's eye" rings. This results in less potential for side-to-side movement and therefore a smaller stereo base.

A B C D E

F

A Anterior/Posterior

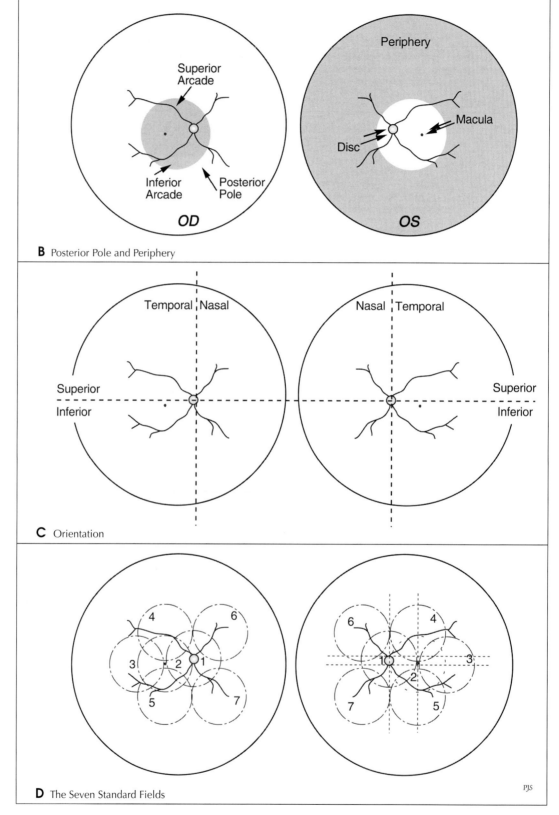

B Posterior Pole and Periphery

C Orientation

D The Seven Standard Fields

PJS

FIGURE 2-22
Finding your way. Items located in the front half of the eye are labeled *anterior*; those in the rear half of the globe are labeled *posterior* **(A)**. A retinal lesion may be located in the posterior pole (the disc, macula, and the area enclosed within the inferior and superior arcades) or within the periphery (the area outside of the arcades) **(B)**. Directions, such as temporal (toward the temple), nasal (toward the nose), inferior, and superior, allow greater specificity **(C)**. Clock hours can also be used to specify location. Disc diameter (the width of the disc) is a convenient measuring stick. In a normal patient, the macula lies approximately 2.5 disc diameters temporal to the disc and just below the a line that bisects the disc. The seven standard fields describe specific retinal locations as imaged by a 30-degree fundus camera **(D)**. (OD = right eye; OS = left eye.)

Which Eye Should Be Photographed First?

When both eyes are to be photographed, one convention dictates that the macula of the right eye (OD) be photographed first. This establishes a routine introduction to the patient both at the camera and at the editing table. This approach is often favored for novice fundus photographers because of its simplicity.

Another approach is to photograph the affected eye first. This is the eye the physician is most interested in; it may have been chosen for the transit phase of a fluorescein angiogram. In this system, if the session ends early (e.g., if the camera breaks or if a very young patient declines further photography), the most important images have been captured. Additionally, the second eye photographed often exhibits increased light sensitivity.

It matters little which specific system you choose as long as you establish a logical and systematic approach to your patients.

FIGURE 2-23
Normal- or narrow-angle fundus photographs excel in showing the fine details of a retinal problem. This 30-degree photograph **(A)** reveals more macular detail than this 60-degree photograph **(B)**.

FIGURE 2-24
Wide-angle cameras are useful for showing the extent of a retinal problem. Here, a single 60-degree fundus photograph **(A)** tells the same story as three 30-degree fundus photographs **(B, C, D)**.

focusing knob and the retinal image will sharpen. While remaining aware of the focusing reticle, keep turning the knob, and the major blood vessels will become sharp. Concentrate on the next smaller blood vessel branches, and then the next smaller branches. In very clear eyes, you may be able to distinguish extremely fine blood vessels. Eyes with cataracts or other media opacities may reveal only the major blood vessels. Focus as best as you can, remembering that not every patient has clear media.

A brighter viewing light may make retinal details easier to distinguish; however, you should balance this need with patient comfort and cooperation. If you need a brighter light to focus with, try

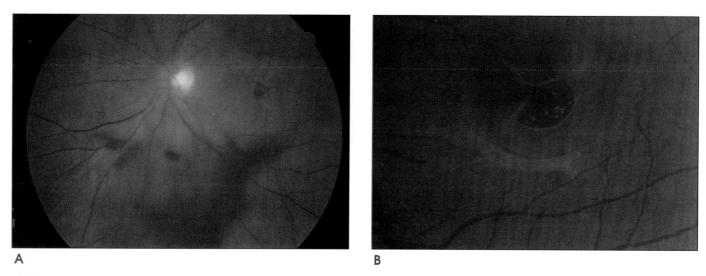

A

B

FIGURE 2-25
Consider using multiple angles of view in the same patient. Combining a wide-angle view **(A)** with a narrow-angle view **(B)** is effective in showing the retinal damage from this industrial laser accident.

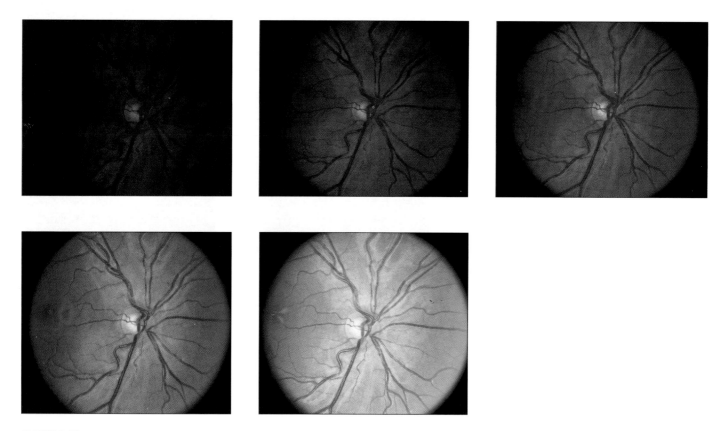

FIGURE 2-26
Exposure test. Create a series of photographs using each of the flash settings on your power pack. Carefully evaluate the pictures with the physician to determine a standard exposure.

Determining the Correct Exposure

The correct exposure for a fundus photograph is the exposure that most clearly communicates the visual condition of the retina to the referring physician. Many factors influence the exposure. The photographer chooses the film stock and selects the flash intensity. Pupil size and fundus coloration are patient-related exposure factors. The judgment of the interpreting physician is important—does the physician prefer fully saturated or lighter fundus images?

Determining the correct exposure for fundus photography is an empirical process. First determine your standard exposure (Figure 2-26). Choose a slow or medium-speed color slide film and a standardized processing method. Using a well-dilated volunteer, expose two fundus photographs at each of your fundus camera's flash settings. Some fundus camera power supplies are calibrated in full stop increments, whereas some change by one-third or one-half stop between settings. A neutral-density filter (available from a photographic retailer) may assist you in achieving a precise exposure. Review this series of photographs with the physician to determine the best standard exposure.

Note the date and the exposure in the front of your camera manual. File the photographs for future reference.

Use the standard exposure on all patients who have the same pupil and fundus coloration characteristics as your model. You may need to increase this exposure by one or two steps if a particular patient

- Has a small pupil
- Has a retina with significantly darker pigmentation
- Has a large retinal hemorrhage
- Needs higher magnification (e.g., 2×) photographs

Decrease your exposure for:

- Young children
- Patients with significantly lighter pigmentation than your standard subject
- Patients with highly reflective fundi (e.g., Coats' disease, choroideremia, albinism).

Repeat this test each time you make a significant change in your procedure (e.g., a change in film types or processors). Individually test each of your fundus cameras; each fundus camera–power supply combination can exhibit unique exposure characteristics. If you notice an exposure drift toward darkened images over time, consider scheduling a thorough cleaning of your fundus camera's internal optics.

FIGURE 2-27
This unusable fundus photograph was damaged (*arrow*) by the film processor.

turning the viewing light up to focus and then turning it down again for final alignment.

A full discussion of focusing technique (including the rationale, a description of the mechanism, and a guide for focusing on different layers of the retina) is found later in this chapter.

Expose

14. *Double-check everything.* Develop the habit of quickly reviewing major variables just before the exposure. Make sure that both the reticle and the retina are in focus. Double-check the flash setting (Figure 2-26) (see the sidebar on determining the correct exposure). Fine-tune your focusing and field of view. Monitor the image for maximum color saturation and the absence of artifacts.

15. *Expose the film.* Press down on the shutter release button to take a picture (it's as easy as that!). Take multiple photographs of all necessary fields in each eye (see the sidebar on how many pictures to take), then proceed with the patient's other eye.

16. *Close the session.* Let your patients know that they did well (even if they did not) and that you obtained the needed photographs (which you should have). Remind them that the colors they are seeing are normal. Reassure them that the spots will go away soon. Suggest that fundus photography is just like looking into a flash when they get their picture taken. Release the patient with a smile, making sure that he or she feels fine and knows where their next clinic stop is. Complete all paperwork, including signing the chart. An uncharted procedure is an incomplete procedure. To avoid confusion, finish completely with one patient before beginning another.

Follow-Up

1. *Process your film.* Have your color film promptly developed by a professional processing laboratory. Quality processing and timely delivery are two important factors to consider when selecting a film processing vendor. Remember that the quality of your work will be judged by the quality of their processing (Figure 2-27).

2. *Edit and label your photographs.* Edit the film promptly after it is returned from the processor; keep the best images and discard the rest. If only a single mediocre photograph of a needed retinal field

How Many Photographs Should I Take?

The answer to this question depends on the patient, your skill level, and your practice. The desired outcome of the procedure is a good fundus photograph. Patients routinely blink, shift fixation, move their head, and in general make it difficult to guarantee that any single exposure will succeed. Most experienced photographers expose at least two photographs (or two stereo pairs) of each requested retinal field. It is less expensive to use an extra frame of film for insurance than to repeat the session. Film is actually a small part of the total procedure cost, especially when you consider the capital expense for the fundus camera and the wages and benefits of a skilled ophthalmic photographer.

A young child or an extremely light-sensitive patient may make it difficult to expose multiple photographs. In these cases, you should attempt to capture the best single image you can, concentrating all of your patient management and camera-positioning skills on the few photographs you will be able to expose.

Novice fundus photographers may need to expose more images to obtain a single good fundus photograph. This is encouraged: Experience is your best teacher. Film use will decrease as skill level increases.

Interesting or rare pathology deserves a few additional photographs. If your practice includes physicians or photographers who routinely lecture or publish, increase your number of exposures. Originals are always better than duplicate slides for teaching, reproduction, or sending to a referring physician.

You will need additional original exposures to build a portfolio of interesting patient photographs displaying fine technique. A portfolio is required for certification and for most job interviews.

is available, then by all means include it. Otherwise, do not dilute your good photographs with poor images. Remember that good photographers don't just take good pictures; good photographers show good pictures. Label each slide with the patient's number, the date taken, and the referring physician. Some offices label each slide with the patient's diagnosis, others place unmounted strips of slide film in negative sleeves—labeling only the sleeves. Always take some time during the editing process to examine your work with an eye toward quality control. How could this photograph have been more effective? What could have been done to eliminate that artifact?

3. *Deliver the finished product.* Deliver the patient's photographs and chart for physician review in a timely manner.
4. *Review your work.* You should endeavor to understand not only pertinent photographic principles but also the various disease processes and their effect on the eye. Learn to look at photographs from your physician's point of view. Schedule regular conferences or ask impromptu questions, but regularly review your work with your employer. Your professional competence will benefit from this dialogue, as well as your value to your practice or institution.

Record Keeping Essentials

Visualize the sheer quantity of images a moderately busy ophthalmic photography practice can generate: If two or three patients fit on each roll of color film, and 12 patients are photographed each day, then four to six rolls of film are generated daily. In a week, that is 20–30 rolls of 36 images. Expressed differently, the clinical setting we have just described generates more than 1,000 different images each week. We are required to precisely match the appropriate patient's image to their medical record for each of these 1,000 images. This process demands the integration of a number of record keeping tools: patient logs, patient identification on the actual film, consecutive numbering of film rolls, and accurate slide labeling. Appropriate billing sheet and chart notations must be made if your photography procedures are to be billed (Table 2-3).

A patient logbook is essential, whether it is of the old-fashioned bound sort or a customized computerized database. Your procedure log will act as a guide during the editing and labeling process, allow you to check whether images from a particular patient are ready, and help you retrieve patient photographs with a particular diagnosis.

Patient information should be entered before clinical photographs are exposed. After completing the procedure, document in the chart and on the billing slip that the procedure was performed. Pertinent logbook information to consider gathering includes procedure date (e.g., 2-27-2003), patient name and medical record number (e.g., Smith, Joe, 541212312-5), the procedure performed and its location (e.g., fundus photography OU), diagnosis (e.g., glaucoma suspect), and referring practitioner or clinic (e.g., Dr. Jones, Northern Eye Clinic). Consider adding columns in the database for "Photographs Processed" or "Photographs Edited" and "Photographs Delivered" or "Photographs Filed." A column for "Photographer Notes" (e.g., good patient, save extras for teaching, send a set to Dr. Smith) is a good idea. Relational databases used with networked office computers allow you to customize multiple variations on this basic scheme.

Photograph each new patient's name or medical record number before you photograph each new patient's fundus. This provides identification on the film, which will act as a guidepost as you edit. It also allows you

Table 2-3. Ophthalmic-Related *Current Procedural Terminology* Codes (CPT Code) and Modifiers (2001)

92135	Scanning computerized ophthalmic diagnostic imaging (e.g., scanning laser) with interpretation and report, unilateral
92235	Fluorescein angiography (includes multiframe imaging) with interpretation and report
92240	Indocyanine green angiography (includes multiframe imaging) with interpretation and report
92250	Fundus photography with interpretation and report
92285	External photography with interpretation and report for documentation of medical progress (e.g., close-up photography, slit-lamp photography, gonio photography, stereo photography)
92286	Special anterior segment photography with interpretation and report; with specular endothelial microscopy and cell count
92287	With fluorescein angiography
922499	Unlisted ophthalmologic service or procedure
Modifiers	-22 Unusual procedural services
	-26 Professional component
	-50 Bilateral procedure
	-51 Multiple procedures
	-52 Reduced services
	-90 Reference (outside) laboratory
	-99 Multiple modifiers

to confirm that the fundus camera is indeed working, that the correct camera back has been attached, and that film is loaded. Most practices photograph the name again if a patient photograph session continues to the next roll of film. The small price you pay for the extra frame of exposed film is more than made up in the efficient manner in which you can identify patient photographs.

Each roll of film should be labeled or numbered sequentially. Color-coded twin check labels, available commercially from film processing supply houses, are ideal for this. Alternately, a pen and simple stickers will suffice. Use these numbers to track the film as it is processed and returned for editing.

With your logbook handy and your processed film laid sequentially next to the light table, it is a simple matter to follow the name tags, edit, and label each patient's slides. Inspect each image using a loupe or stereo viewer for magnification. Discard subpar photographs, keeping the better extras for the office teaching file or your portfolio. Slides may be labeled by hand, with specialized slide imprinters, or by using computer-generated sticky labels. Each slide is labeled with the clinic name, patient name, medical record number, date the photograph was taken, and diagnosis; the specific eye, photographer, and satellite location are other information options. Remember that each specific multicenter clinical trial has its own guidelines for slide labeling. Once each slide is labeled (and each slide should be labeled), place the images in a storage page for filing. Check off in the log that the images are ready.

Labeling slides can be a time-intensive task. Consider involving secretaries, students, or hospital volunteers to ease the workload. If labeling each slide is impractical, consider placing unmounted color slide film in negative protector sleeves and labeling the sleeves. This arrangement works best if the reviewing physicians do not routinely use mounted slides for projection.

Once labeling and editing of the images is completed, retrieve the patient chart and deliver it with the slides to the referring physician for review. Some offices file patient photographs directly with the chart, whereas others have a separate "Photography File" which is organized and maintained by the photography staff.

Of course, using color digital imaging simplifies many of the preceding tasks: but it is not without its record-keeping responsibilities. Archival media, whether it be magnetic media CD-ROM or DVD, must be written, labeled, and stored. Check Chapter 7 for more specifics on archiving electronic images.

A last paperwork essential that is often overlooked can be described as a meeting report or an annual report. Take some time after returning from a continuing education meeting and create a report for your employer. Include specific items you learned that may help you or the practice offer better or more efficient care. You should consider generating a similar yearly report that details the improvements you have made, special projects you have worked on, and talks or publications you have participated in. Identify specific increases in the number of photography procedures you have performed this year. Keep your employer informed of your professional efforts.

Focusing the Fundus Camera: A Clinical Approach

Ophthalmic photography is a system of information transfer. Fundus photography transfers a visual description of the retina onto film. This two-dimensional representation is used by the physician to make judgments about the health and treatment of the patient's retina. Your goal is an accurate representation of the three-dimensional retinal and choroidal tissues. A sharp, well-focused retinal image is essential to successful fundus photography.

This section describes the fundus camera's aerial image-focusing system and its correct use. The well-focused fundus photograph is described, and proper focusing technique is related to retinal anatomy and pathology.

The Fundus Camera's Focusing System

In their most basic form, optical systems require light, a subject, a lens, a receiving plane, and an observer. Light reflects off the subject, is refracted (bent) by the lens, and is projected onto a receiving plane, where it is viewed. In fundus photography, the patient's retina becomes the subject, the optics of the patient's eye and the fundus camera replace the simple lens, the focusing screen or the film becomes the receiving plane, and you, the photographer, become the observer (Figure 2-28). Focusing the fundus camera consists of adjusting the relationship between the subject and lens so that the subject lies within the lens' depth of field and the receiving plane lies within the depth of focus of the image.

Most fundus cameras use a SLR viewing system. You should become familiar with the SLR design and the fundus camera's aerial image-viewing system (Figure 2-29).

SINGLE LENS REFLEX VIEWING SYSTEM
The objective lens of the fundus camera transmits light for both viewing the subject and exposing the film (Figure 2-30). The hinged mirror is positioned differently for viewing and taking the picture. First the image is evaluated through the viewfinder with the mirror in the down position. Then the mirror flips up and out of the way, the shutter opens, the flash is tripped, and the film is exposed to light.

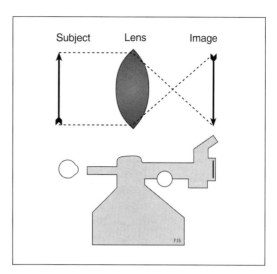

FIGURE 2-28
A sharp fundus photograph is created when a specific retina layer is the object, the fundus camera optics serve as a lens, and the film plane coincides with the plane of sharp focus.

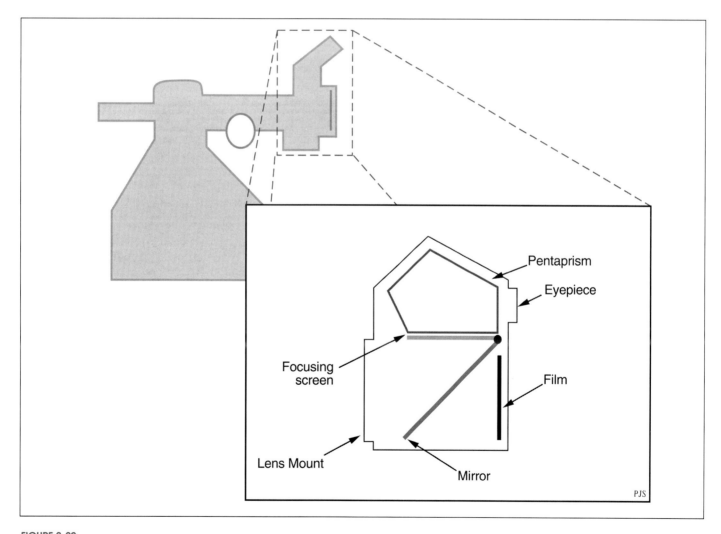

FIGURE 2-29
Most modern fundus cameras use a single lens reflex (SLR) system for viewing the fundus image. Standard components of an SLR are identified in this simplified version of the fundus camera's SLR viewing system.

FIGURE 2-30
Using a single lens reflex (SLR) camera. **A.** To preview a scene before you take a photograph, the light from the lens enters the camera body and reflects off the hinged, 45-degree mirror through a prism and to the focusing screen. You view the image on the focusing screen while looking through the viewfinder. **B.** When you choose to expose an image, depress the shutter release. This initiates a series of steps (specifics may vary according to the particular camera and flash) that includes the mirror flipping up and out of the way, momentarily darkening the viewfinder. This allows the same light that you saw to expose the film. **C.** An SLR system is basically a "what-you-see-is-what-you-get" system. The distance between the focusing screen and the lens system is equal to the distance between the film plane and the lens system. When the image appears sharp on an SLR camera's focusing screen, it will also appear sharp on the film.

The focusing screen helps the photographer judge image sharpness before exposing the film. It is always located the same distance from the objective lens as the film plane. When an object appears sharp on the focusing screen, its image will also be sharp at the film plane. In standard 35-mm cameras, the focusing screen glass is ground glass either with or without a Fresnel surface.

Light intensity decreases as it is scattered by a standard patterned glass focusing screen, an effect that is of little importance to most photographers. In fundus photography, however, a number of factors make it difficult to use these focusing screens.

1. *Relatively small amounts of light must be used when viewing the eye*. The possibility of retinal damage increases as the quantity and duration of illumination increases.[4] Many patients are sensitive to bright lights, making examination with bright light difficult.
2. *High magnifications* (e.g., 2.5× in a 30-degree fundus image) are used to photograph the retina. Light energy from a small portion of the subject is distributed over a physically greater image area when the image is magnified. This results in a relatively lower level of light available for imaging any particular portion of the subject.
3. *The grainy structure of a ground-glass focusing screen breaks up the fine detail of the fundus image*. The relatively large size of the grains in a ground-glass focusing screen make it difficult to focus on the fine

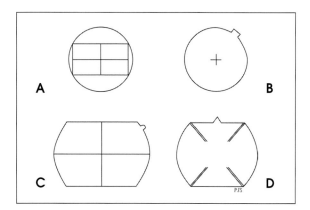

FIGURE 2-31
Various designs of focusing reticles. The reticle for your specific camera may vary according to manufacturer, camera model, and date. **A.** Zeiss 30°. **B.** Topcon. **C.** Canon. **D.** Kowa.

retinal blood vessels. The main reason not to use a ground glass is that it absorbs too much light.

Fundus cameras replace the patterned glass of a standard 35-mm SLR camera system with a clear glass-focusing screen containing etched lines (Figure 2-31). The clear glass maximizes the light entering the photographer's eye. The etched black lines (called the *focusing reticle*) assist the photographer in focusing on the correct plane.

Because the image in the viewfinder is not "captured" by the focusing screen, but rather floats in the air space both in front of and behind the clear glass, it is termed an *aerial image*. Learning to focus this aerial image using the reticle is essential to obtaining sharp images with a fundus camera.

VIEWING THE AERIAL IMAGE

When you look through the fundus camera's viewfinder with your best corrected vision, you will see one of four possible views. The image inside the viewfinder may be totally out of focus, without distinct reticle lines or sharp areas of retina. The image alone may be in focus, only the black reticle lines may be in focus, or both the image and the black reticle lines may be in focus. Only in the last case will a sharp retinal image be recorded on film (Figure 2-32).

If both the focusing reticle and the fundus image are completely out of focus, then one of two conditions may exist. First, your eyes may not be corrected for their best visual acuity. A routine eye examination is recommended when you begin your career and at regular intervals thereafter. Second, the fundus camera's reticle and focus adjustment may be improperly set (see the section on obtaining a sharp fundus photograph below). Of course, a combination of the preceding circumstances may occur.

ACCOMMODATION

Accommodation is the normal mechanism your eye uses for focusing on near objects. In simple terms, the ciliary muscle tugs or releases tension on the lens zonules, modifying the refractive power of the lens. At the same time, the near reflex causes miosis and convergence. The ability to accommodate lessens with age.

A significant cause of unsharp fundus photographs is accommodation by the photographer during the focusing procedure. When you look through the camera eyepiece and accommodate, you may see a sharp image of the retina but not see a sharp image of the focusing reticle. If you accommodate to perceive a sharp image of the retina, then the optical system of your eye is used to obtain sharpness, rather than the optical system of the fundus camera. You may attempt to sharpen the image using the focusing knob, but a blurry photograph results.

PHOTOGRAPHER'S VIEW IN EYEPIECE	DIAGRAMMATIC EXPLANATION	FINAL FILM IMAGE

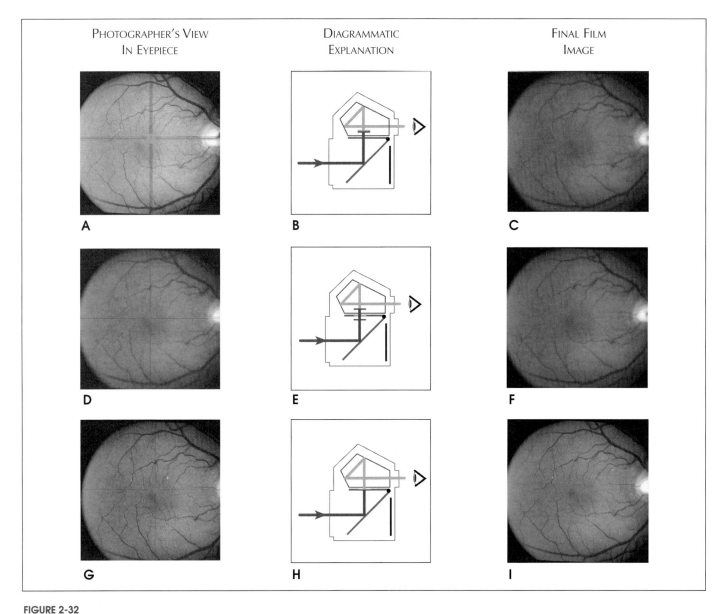

FIGURE 2-32
Using the reticle to focus. This figure illustrates the relationship between sharpness in the reticle, your fundus view, and the sharpness in the final fundus photograph. When you focus the image without regard to the sharpness of the focusing reticle, you will perceive the fundus image as sharp while the reticle image appears blurry **(A)**. The image you see is focused by your eyes above the focusing screen, closer than infinity **(B)**. Even though you see a sharp image in the viewfinder, the exposed photograph will be blurry **(C)**. When you view through a correctly adjusted eyepiece before the fundus has been focused on, the fundus appears blurry while the reticle is distinctly sharp **(D)**. You have correctly focused on the reticle, but the camera's image has not yet been adjusted to coincide with the receiving plane **(E)**. If a picture is taken, the resulting image will be as unsharp as you see it in the viewfinder **(F)**. After correctly adjusting the eyepiece and the fundus camera's focusing mechanism, both the fundus image and the reticle appear sharp and clear **(G)**. Your eyes are focused on the reticle, and the image from the fundus camera corresponds with the film plane **(H)**. Only this final combination yields a sharply focused fundus photograph **(I)**.

The tendency to accommodate when focusing is especially prevalent in fatigued or novice fundus photographers, and in experienced photographers who are younger than approximately 40 years of age. Strategies for safeguarding against accommodation problems during fundus photography procedures include the following:

1. Highly trained photographers can "feel" themselves accommodate. You may want to test this yourself. Find a quiet room with no distractions. Fully relax your mind and body while focusing your eyes on an object at least 20 feet away. Bring your index finger approximately 18 in. from your nose. When you focus on your index finger, notice that the background becomes unsharp. Keeping your finger in

focus, move it toward your nose slowly. The background will become increasingly less sharp and the edges of your visual field will constrict. You will feel your eyes converge, and you may feel a sensation in the anterior section of your eyes. Focus on the distant object again and repeat. With practice, you will become more aware of your personal sensation during accommodation. Awareness of this sensation during fundus photography will alert you to the possibility of accommodation and the unsharp photographs that may result.

2. If you think you are accommodating during a procedure, look away from the eyepiece. Merely blinking or closing your eyes may help reset their focus. On looking again into the viewfinder, concentrate on the thin black lines of the focusing reticle. Intentionally blurring the fundus image (move the plane of focus into the vitreous by rotating the focusing knob) may help you concentrate on the reticle image.

3. Try to keep both eyes open throughout the procedure, preferably with the non-eyepiece eye focused across the room. A well-placed visual (of a landscape or distant scene) on the opposite wall of the fundus photography room will promote distance focusing. If the room is especially small, a mirror (or the glass from the above print) may be used to reflect the image from a visual hanging directly behind the photographer. Glancing at this reflection will better approximate distance focusing in a small room. Viewing exciting scenery through a window in a fundus photography room may seem tempting. However, the darkness necessary during procedures precludes this option.

4. A full day of fundus photography may distort the normal accommodative process, causing your eye to be "stuck" in near-focus. Accommodative excess is the result of "prolonged and intense periods of near work," which may result in eyestrain and headaches.[5,6] Persistent focusing on infinity may help retard this near-focus spasm. Consciously focus across the distance of the waiting room (or down a long hall) when you call patients. Practice distance focusing out a window during breaks or at lunch. Make a point of looking at distant scenery or buildings while commuting to and from work.

Of course, your eyes should always be corrected to their best visual acuity. You may find that one eye is sharper than the other. Keep your eyeglasses or contacts scrupulously clean.

Certain physiologic conditions may also distort the focusing process. Extreme changes in blood sugar may alter the thickness of the diabetic photographer's lens, making distance vision unsharp. Certain drugs may produce pseudopresbyopia.[7] Dry eyes can be a problem if you find yourself blinking less frequently when looking through the fundus camera viewfinder. Use artificial tears or contact lens wetting solution as needed. Maintaining a healthy diet and good physical condition will also help your focusing abilities.

Sharp Fundus Photographs

DEFINITION

Sharpness in a photograph is a visual phenomenon that is difficult to quantify. Both contrast and resolution play a role in our subjective evaluations of sharpness. An image is described as sharp when the borders defining the subject are distinct and clear. An unsharp image contains borders between adjacent areas that are double, overlap, or are difficult to distinguish. A sharp fundus photograph results when the fundus camera's plane of sharp focus coincides with the specific pathology in question.

LAYERS

Vitreous

Internal Limiting Membrane
Nerve Fiber Layer
Ganglion Cell Layer

Inner Plexiform Layer

Inner Nuclear Layer

Outer Plexiform Layer

Outer Nuclear Layer

External Limiting Membrane
Rods and Cones
Pigment Epithelium
Bruch's Membrane

Choriocapillaris

Choroidal Vessels

LEVELS

VITREOUS

INNER RETINA

CENTRAL RETINA

OUTER RETINA

CHOROID

PJS

FIGURE 2-33
Layers and levels. A 10-layer histologic representation of the retina and choroid is related to the five levels that may be distinguished when viewing either through a narrow-angle fundus camera viewfinder or the final stereo fundus photograph. Each of these five levels may or may not be able to be distinguished depending on the thickness and pathology of a particular patient's retina.

When photographing the retina, remember that, like most photographic subjects in our three-dimensional world, the posterior segment of the eye has depth. The vitreous, retina, and choroid may be described histologically as overlapping layers of gel, tissue, and blood vessels that are located at specific levels* within the eye (Figure 2-33).

Five distinct levels (the vitreous, inner retina, central retina, outer retina, and choroid) may be distinguished using white-light, 30-degree stereo fundus photography in many patients with diseased or swollen retinas.

Short wavelength color filters (e.g., exciter and barrier filters for fluorescein angiography, blue filters for retinal nerve fiber layer photography, and green filters for "red-free" photography) enhance the photographic separation of retinal levels.[8] Thickened diseased retina, normal-angle fundus camera optics, and stereo imaging also facilitate the recognition of retinal levels and expedite their differential focusing (Figure 2-34).

Monocular (single-image) photography, wide-angle fundus cameras, and inaccurate focusing inhibit the ability to distinguish five separate

*The term *layer* is used when referring to histologic sections, whereas the term *level* is reserved for discussion of the fundus camera image.

FIGURE 2-34
Multiple retinal levels may be appreciated when this photograph is viewed in stereo.

FIGURE 2-35
This eye was photographed at three different planes of focus. All three images contain areas that may be considered sharp. If the macula is the intended subject of the photograph, however, only the center image can be judged a sharp fundus photograph.

retinal levels. The levels' thinness combined with the depth of field of the fundus camera may make it difficult to distinguish each of the five levels in patients with normal or thin retinas.

A sharp fundus photograph is precisely focused on a specific subject within a specific level of the retina. The objective appearance of clear, distinct borders in a fundus photograph does not in itself certify the sharpness of that photograph. A fundus photograph may be sharp, but not at the appropriate retinal level (Figure 2-35). Focusing too far forward (into the vitreous) or too far backward (into the outer retina or choroid) results in a fundus photograph that does not accurately document the pathology of concern.

How can optimal focus at the appropriate layer within the eye be achieved? An understanding of retinal anatomy is essential to achieving sharp fundus photographs.

RETINAL ANATOMY: LAYERS AND LEVELS

Accurately adjusting the fundus camera's focus requires an awareness of the layered aspect of the eye's anatomy. The vitreous gel fills the posterior segment of the eye. The retina is a three-dimensional tissue described histologically as 11 separate layers. The choroid contains two layers of blood vessels.

The vitreous is positioned anterior to the retina. In the normal eye, the vitreous cannot be imaged with a standard fundus camera. However, when documentation of a diabetic neovascular frond, a retinal detachment, or asteroid hyalosis is necessary, the fundus camera should be focused "up" into the vitreous, rather than "down" on the retina (Figure 2-36).

The internal limiting membrane, the nerve fiber layer, and the ganglion cell layer combine to form the inner retina. It is visualized as the nerve fiber layer and the reflections from the large retinal blood vessels. Cotton-wool spots, nerve fiber defects, myelinated nerve fibers, and flame-shaped hemorrhages occur at this level.

The inner and outer plexiform layer and the inner and outer nuclear layer form the central portion of the retina. The central retina contains the smaller blood vessel branches, hard exudates, and diabetic microaneurysms. The capillary net surrounding the foveal avascular zone is imaged during fluorescein angiography when the fundus camera is properly focused on this middle level of the retina.

The outer retinal level includes the rods and cones, the retinal pigment epithelium, and Bruch's membrane. Subretinal neovascular membranes, drusen, presumed ocular histoplasmosis scars, and angioid streaks occur at this level.

The choriocapillaris and major choroidal blood vessels lie below the retina. The surface of nevi and choroidal tumors can be imaged by focusing "down" into the choroid.

TARGETING FOCUS

It is difficult to distinguish 10 different retinal layers when looking through the eyepiece of the fundus camera. However, you can target the focus of the final fundus photograph to a specific level by recognizing its visual contents. Table 2-4 relates common retinal disorders, the affected retinal level, and examples of possible corresponding retinal abnormalities. Targeting focus to a specific level is a matter of recognizing retinal pathology and optimizing the focus to the appropriate retinal depth.

Focusing on the highlights reflected from the large blood vessels results in a sharp photograph of the inner retina. The central retina appears clear in the fundus photograph if the photographer first seeks sharpness in the larger blood vessels, then their branches, and their branches, and so forth. If the granular appearance of the pigment epithelium is focused on, then the outer retina becomes the subject of the photograph. When photographing a subretinal neovascular membrane (located in the outer level of the retina), an unsharp photograph of the offending blood vessels results if you focus on the larger, main retinal blood vessels (found in the inner level of the retina). A sharp image can be obtained by focusing on the drusen that lay directly on the pigment epithelium.

Multiple levels of focus may be chosen in a retina with diabetic macular edema (Figure 2-37). If you focus on the inner surface of the retina, the photograph will document the elevation of the retina but may render much of the posterior pole blurred. A deeper focus may depict the surface of the swollen macula unsharply but will clearly reveal any hard exudates or blot hemorrhages, or both. Focusing in the central retina will accurately document the leaking retinal blood vessels in a fluorescein angiogram.

The fundus camera's depth of field is a focusing consideration. When focusing a fundus camera, only the single level that has been targeted will be in critically sharp focus. When the final photograph is viewed,

FIGURE 2-36
Clinical examples of focusing on different levels of the retina are demonstrated in the following images. **A.** Focusing the fundus camera "up" in the vitreous documents neovascularization at disc and neovascularization elsewhere. **B.** The nerve fiber layer, accentuated with a blue 490-nm filter, is the object of focus. **C.** The avascular zone surrounding the fovea may be best appreciated when the central portion of the retina is the object of focus. **D.** Focusing on the retinal pigment epithelium or outer retina results in a sharp image of these drusen. **E.** Maximum information at the level of the choroid is achieved through the use of a red (650-nm) filter and careful focusing on the choroidal nevus.

Table 2-4. Patient Diagnosis and Retinal Levels

Patient's Diagnosis	Examples of Possible Abnormalities	Retinal Level
Asteroid hyalosis	Lipid deposits	Vitreous
Diabetic retinopathy	Neovascular fronds	
Retinoschisis	Elevated retinal sensory layers	
Retinal detachment	Elevated retina	
Diabetic retinopathy	Cotton-wool spots	Inner retina
Glaucoma	Nerve fiber layer defects, optic disc borders	
Hypertensive retinopathy	Cotton-wool spots	
Macular hole	Edges of macular hole	
Pre-retinal membrane	Cellophane maculopathy	
Retinal hemorrhage	Pre-retinal hemorrhage, sub-hyaloid hemorrhage	
Retinal vein occlusion	Flame-shaped hemorrhages	
Cystoid macular edema	Swelling	Central retina
Diabetic retinopathy	Microaneurysms, hard exudates, dot and blot hemorrhages, macular edema	
Retinal artery occlusion	Blocked artery	
Retinal vein occlusion	Neovascularization	
Retinitis pigmentosa	Bone-spicule–like pigment	
Age-related macular degeneration	Subretinal neovascular membranes, drusen	Outer retina
Central serous retinopathy	Pigment epithelium defect	
Hereditary abnormalities	Angioid streaks	
Presumed ocular histoplasmosis syndrome	Subretinal neovascular membranes, punched out hypopigmented areas	
AMPPE	Choroidal disturbance	Choroid
Nevus	Surface texture	
Optic nerve head drusen	Drusen under disc	
Choroidal tumor	Surface texture	

AMPPE = acute multifocal placoid pigment epitheliopathy.

Note: Sample patient diagnoses are listed and related to the retinal layers visible through the fundus camera. Examples of possible retinal abnormalities (which may or may not be evident in each specific patient) are correlated. To target the focus to a specific layer, note the patient's diagnosis, and focus on the specific abnormalities. If the retina is abnormally thick, you may be able to focus on the same retinal field at different levels. Double-check the focus with each field change.

A   B

FIGURE 2-37
With significant retinal elevation, should you focus on the highest elevation **(A)** or the general level of the retina **(B)**? Use professional judgment or expose multiple photographs.

however, more than one level may appear acceptably sharp. This range of acceptably sharp focus extends both in front of and behind the actual plane of sharp focus.

Wide-angle fundus cameras produce a greater depth of field than do normal-angle cameras if the same eye is photographed, and the exposed film area is identical (Figure 2-38). It is not the angle of the optics but

FIGURE 2-38
When narrow **(A)** and wide-angle **(B)** photographs of this eye with asteroid hyalosis are compared, the wide-angle image appears to have greater depth of field because of its smaller magnification.

FIGURE 2-39
Images from a well-corrected fundus camera closely match the curvature of the retina. Learn the limitations of your particular camera by carefully focusing on the fovea of a clear eye and then evaluating the actual sharpness at the edges of the processed photograph.

rather the decrease in magnification that contributes to the increased impression of sharpness.[9]

A working knowledge of depth of field helps when documenting the retina. Focusing on the central retina (in a normal, clear eye) yields a final photograph in which the outer and possibly the inner retina are acceptably sharp. However, if you focus on the granular appearance of the retinal pigment epithelium, then the inner retina will most likely not be in sharp focus.

Depth of focus is found at the film plane and usually mirrors the depth of field located at the subject plane. The depth of focus in most traditional imaging systems is relatively flat. This corresponds with the flatness of the film that is used as a receiving plane (Figure 2-39). The depth of field in most fundus camera lens systems is curved to mimic the shape of the normal retina. In well-corrected fundus camera optical systems, the curved plane of the subject's detail is translated into a flat plane for maximum interface with the film plane. In less well-corrected fundus camera lens systems, the plane of the depth of focus is just as curved as the depth of field. Fundus cameras that exhibit this curved depth of focus yield film images that are unsharp at the edges when the camera is focused centrally (and are unsharp centrally when focused on the edges). The intended subject will appear sharp on the film only with careful composition and focus.

SHARPNESS LIMITATIONS OF THE CAMERA

The sharpness of a final fundus photograph is, of course, limited by the sharpness of the specific camera's optical system. Objective tests comparing the relative sharpness of various fundus cameras are unavailable. However, experience with multiple cameras in a clinical setting has yielded some general guidelines.

Resolution of fine detail decreases as the magnification decreases because less film area is used for creating an image of a particular detail.

FIGURE 2-40
Carefully focus and photograph a sampling of clear-eyed patients with each angle of view. Examine the images together to discern the sharpness and contrast characteristics of each angle choice.

FIGURE 2-41
Although the sharpness and contrast of magnified images are compromised, they may still provide useful information.

When two fundus cameras have imaging circles of equal size, the wide-angle fundus camera (greater than 45 degrees) will be less able to resolve fine detail than the normal-angle camera (30 degrees). When two fundus cameras have optics of equal quality, the fundus camera with higher magnification will achieve better definition of fine retinal details.

Resolution and contrast decrease with the introduction of angle-changing lens systems (Figure 2-40). Multiple-angle cameras typically have one best setting—often the widest angle. An optical departure from this angle of view degrades image quality. However, greater magnification may yield details not perceived under low magnification (Figure 2-41). Use your professional judgment to determine the most appropriate angle of view for a specific fundus photograph, or expose multiple images for later editing.

Wide-angle cameras suffer greater losses in resolution from local areas of potential blurriness (e.g., a cataract or a corneal scar) than do normal-angle cameras. This phenomenon is due to the larger bundle of returning image-forming rays that constitute the wide-angle image. The thinner bundles of normal-angle camera optics are more likely to permit you to select small pockets of clear media.

Remember that newer fundus cameras of the same design may be sharper than older cameras (Figure 2-42) and that "identical" cameras of the same design and vintage may produce images with slightly different results.

A fundus camera's cost is not directly proportional to the sharpness of its optics. Lens performance, cost, and ease of use must each be considered separately. Although a low price and ergonomic design should be considered when purchasing a fundus camera, actual lens performance is critical.

Only the publication of unbiased data detailing the actual performance of many different fundus cameras allows fair comparisons to be made. Until such tests are designed and implemented, the opinions of other ophthalmic photographers and personal experience must guide us.[10]

A   B

FIGURE 2-42
Although of identical optical design, it is probably not surprising that the brand new fundus camera image **(A)** is sharper than the image from the older fundus camera **(B)** which has been moved, disassembled, and cleaned multiple times in 15 years.

Focusing Technique

If you conscientiously use the reticle and practice a deliberate focusing procedure, you will produce consistently sharp fundus photographs. The eyepiece must be correctly set to obtain a sharp view of the reticle. Instructions for adjusting the eyepiece are found in the sidebar on setting your reticle. A suggested focusing procedure is as follows:

1. Review the patient's photograph request form and prior photographs. Note the working diagnosis.
2. Seat the patient at the instrument and explain the procedure.
3. Adjust the headrest, chinrest, joystick, and camera head height while looking around the side of the camera. Align the patient and camera so that the retina and the film plane are parallel. Project the doughnut of light into the center of the dilated pupil. Position the illumination system by obtaining a sharp image of the viewing light's filament on the cornea or closed outer eyelid.
4. Turn out the room lights. Your view through the viewfinder will brighten, and your eye's depth of field will decrease as a result of your slightly dilated pupils. It will be easier for you to discriminate between retinal layers with this shallower depth of field. In addition, the darkened room enhances the figure-ground relationship between the external fixation light and its background. This allows the patient to follow the external fixation device more easily.
5. Establish patient fixation (focusing on a moving target is difficult).
6. Look through the ocular and visualize the focusing reticle. Constant awareness of this reticle throughout the focusing procedure is necessary for obtaining sharp fundus photographs. Dust specks may be visible in the viewfinder. If these dust specks are on the same plane as the etched lines, use them like the reticle. If you are unsure of their precise location, consult a knowledgeable service technician to either clean the dust specks or to determine the specific plane on which they rest.
7. Adjust the image for maximum color saturation and minimum artifacts. Move the fixation light to visualize the requested retinal field.
8. Begin turning the focusing knob. You will see the retinal image begin to sharpen. Check the sharpness of the focusing reticle and decide on which retinal level to focus. Myopic, hyperopic, and aphakic patients may require you to adjust the compensation lens system (diopter control). Myopic patients (long axial length) may need a minus diopter compensation. Hyperopic patients (short axial length) and patients without their natural lenses may require a plus diopter cor-

A   B

FIGURE 2-43
If the fundus looks stretched or just slightly out of focus, consider using the astigmatic compensation knob. This control is useful for patients who have large amounts of astigmatism (e.g., after surgery) or when photographing the periphery. Seek your best focus **(A)** and then visually determine whether rotating the knob will be beneficial **(B)**.

rection. A small black antireflection dot in the front element may be imaged by some cameras when patients with high myopia are photographed. Both this artifact and the use of the diopter compensation lens system can be eliminated by requesting highly myopic patients to wear their contact lenses while being photographed.[11]

9. As the plane of sharpness travels inward with the rotation of the focusing knob, the vitreous, inner retina, central retina, outer retina, and finally choroidal levels will become sharp in turn. The focusing reticle must always remain sharp.

10. Stop focusing inward as the targeted level is passed and becomes unsharp again.

11. "Rock" the focus (with tiny forward and backward movements of the focusing knob) until the sharpest focus has been obtained. Re-check the sharpness of the focusing reticle.

12. Patient fixation or camera position is adjusted until the precise field of view is obtained. Re-check crosshair sharpness and retinal focus. The area of primary importance should be photographed first, as the best images are often obtained at the beginning of the photo session when both you and the patient are fresh. Many patients require photographs of both the macula and disc. Focusing on the macula first will approximate more closely the general depth of the retina.

13. Evaluate the need for the astigmatism control (if available). If the image of the fundus seems not quite sharp, or if the blood vessels appear elongated in a single direction, then adjusting the astigmatism control may be useful (Figure 2-43). Sharp posterior pole photographs of patients with keratoconus, patients with large amounts of corneal astigmatism, and peripheral photography may require astigmatic correction. Imaging rays traverse an oblique cross section of the lens and cornea in peripheral fundus photography, creating an image that may appear smeared or stretched in a single direction.

14. Constantly monitor the focus throughout the procedure. Re-check the focus each time you change fields; a diseased retina may or may not be elevated in different areas (Figure 2-44). Monitor the focus during side-to-side changes in camera position during stereo photography. Peripheral fundus photography necessitates a change in the camera-cornea distance and will require focus adjustment. The axial length of most patients' eyes varies slightly from right to left. If alternating photographs of the right and left eye are required and a large focusing discrepancy exists between the two eyes (e.g., OD aphakic, OS intraocular lens), then a small piece of tape on the right and left focusing knobs may be used to mark each side's correct adjustment.[12] Although these landmarks will help you adjust the

FIGURE 2-44
Be prepared to alter your focus or alignment to capture items of interest extending into the vitreous. As the camera is pulled back, the yellow artifact in this posterior pole photograph **(A)** of a patient with cytomegalovirus retinitis **(B)** is revealed to be a ganciclovir implant **(C, D)**.

camera more quickly as the alternate eyes are photographed, always check your viewfinder for a final focus.

Assuming a par-focal digital/film system, red-free photographs may be used to obtain instant feedback as to focusing accuracy.

Focusing is an acquired skill requiring both practice and a keen understanding of the retinal landscape. Constant awareness of the focusing reticle and precisely targeting the focus to a specific retinal level are keys to success.

Errors in Fundus Photography: Artifacts

Successful fundus photographs are obtained through the mutual interaction and proper alignment of the patient, the camera, and the photographer. The patient contributes a cooperative attitude and clear media. The camera must faithfully translate the fundus image using integrated optical, mechanical, and electrical subsystems. The photographer must elicit a cooperative response from the patient, correctly align and set the camera controls, and make decisions concerning film choice and processing procedures. Each of these factors must be taken into consideration when evaluating a fundus photograph.

Causes of Artifacts

The ideal fundus photograph is an accurate visual representation of the retina. Of course, as with any complex process, many things may go wrong. If the error alters the ideal image (i.e., if the error can be seen in the final fundus photograph), it is called an *artifact*. Artifacts are portions of the image that arise from the process—not from the patient's retina. Typical artifacts include yellow or orange crescents, white or blue haze at the edge of the photograph, blinks, dust on the front element, and poor focus (Figure 2-45).

The fundus camera generates a flash that is projected into the patient's eye, reflects off the fundus, and then travels through the camera's opti-

FIGURE 2-45
Typical artifacts. The most common artifacts are related to position errors or interruptions in the imaging path. Crescents can appear on any side of the image and indicate off-center camera alignment **(A)**. A light, slightly unsharp area surrounding a fully saturated center indicates incorrect camera-to-cornea distance **(B)**. Short, light-colored streaks arising from the top or bottom of the frame are stray patient lashes or hair **(C)**. Bright spots indicate dust on the front objective **(D)**.

cal system to the film. Each step in this process has the potential to compromise image quality. If we follow the pathway of image-forming energy from its point of origin (the electrical wall socket) to its final destination (the finished fundus photograph), we can identify specific problem areas where technical difficulties could occur.

Electrical energy flows from the electrical outlet to the camera's power pack, where it is stored until a signal is given for its release (an interruption in any of these circuits is possible). The photographer properly adjusts the camera to the patient's eye (incorrect positioning and focusing are possible). A switch is closed and then stored electrical energy travels to the flash tube where it is transduced into light energy (a misaligned or nonworking flash tube is possible). This light energy passes through a series of optical condensers and imaging lenses (all potentially dirty or out of alignment, or both), out of the camera through the front element (a literal dust magnet), and across the air space between the camera lens and cornea (which can be obstructed by hair, eyelashes, or eyelids). The projected light passes through the cornea, anterior chamber, lens, and vitreous (all in various possible states of opacification) and reflects off the retina (which may be swollen or hidden from view by hemorrhage). The reflected light projects back through the vitreous, lens, anterior chamber, and cornea into the front element of the camera lens (multiplying any previous negative effects). The light is refracted through another series of lenses toward the camera. Just as the light reaches the camera body, the shutter opens and closes (the shutter may malfunction or timing may be off), allowing the light to modify the chemical nature of the film (assuming the film is cor-

Table 2-5. Descriptors for Fundus Photography Artifacts

Extent	Full frame	There is no useful information in any part of the frame. The picture may be completely black or white.
	Full image area	The standard fundus image area contains no useful information, but black surround (unexposed because of the fundus camera's mask) and the film frame numbers are left unaffected.
	Partial image area	The artifact obscures a portion of the retinal image area; the remaining retinal image is of adequate quality.
Character	Location	The artifact can be described as central or peripheral; superior, inferior, to the right or left.
	Shape	Circular, crescent, or rectangular artifacts with sharp or blurry borders are possible.
	Exposure	The overall photograph may be too light or dark, or it may be a double exposure.
	Color	The artifact may be any color: white, yellow, orange, and blue are common. Multicolored artifacts are also seen.
	Sharpness	The full image area may be sharp or unsharp, as may portions thereof.
Distribution		The artifact can be found at the beginning, the middle, or the end of the roll.
Frequency		The artifact may be observed randomly or regularly, throughout a single roll or a single patient, or crossing several rolls or patients. Artifacts can be seen frequently, occasionally, or just once.

Note: Providing a complete description of fundus photography artifacts helps us reason or intuit their cause. Use the vocabulary from the table above when describing artifacts.

rectly manufactured, chosen, and loaded). Once sensitized, the emulsion is processed (another complex procedure with its own long list of possible errors). This image pathway is, of course, dependent on a camera that is aligned correctly with the patient and a patient-photographer relationship that will enable this alignment.

Describing Artifacts

If artifacts are described systematically, we learn about the subtleties of the image and will more likely reason or intuit the artifact's cause. Just as a correct diagnosis from a fluorescein angiogram requires first a proper description of hypo- or hyperfluorescence, describing artifacts is the first step in determining the cause of fundus photograph errors.

Four essential details should be included in each description of the imperfect fundus photograph: the extent and character of the artifact and the distribution and frequency of the affected slide in relation to other fundus photos in the same or adjacent rolls (Table 2-5). Some common artifacts are illustrated in Figure 2-46. The legends indicate the correct use of descriptors and note the cause of the illustrated artifact.

Managing the Challenging Patient

Successful fundus photography with a cooperative patient who has clear media and widely dilated pupils becomes routine with practice. Not all patients are ideal, however. Patients with glaucoma and diabetes generally have smaller pupils. Elderly patients often have cataracts. And light-sensitive patients may have difficulty cooperating. In many clinics, fundus photography is performed at the end of the patient's appoint-

FIGURE 2-46
Describing artifact examples. Extent describes the area the artifact occupies in the photograph. **A.** This processing error involves the full frame. **B.** A vitreous hemorrhage would obscure only the full image area, and notably not the black surround. **C.** "Intraocular lens shimmer" fills the frame when off-center camera alignment is pursued in a patient whose pupil is larger than the outer diameter of the intraocular lens. **D.** The same retina is better photographed using central alignment. **E.** Search for a clear area, shooting around, as opposed to through cataracts **(F). G.** This multicolored crescent variation is an example of a partial image area artifact. The rest of the fundus photograph is usable. The character of the artifact is a set of distinguishing features that describe location, shape, color, exposure, and sharpness. **H, I.** The location of the white artifact (caused by a smudge on the lens) in both these photographs was identical—even with a significant field change. **J.** Excessive camera-to-cornea distance results in a centrally located spectral reflectance and haze along the periphery of the image area. The crescent shape **(K)** and linear shape **(L)** are position-related artifacts. Move the camera in the opposite direction of the artifact to eliminate.

FIGURE 2-46   *(continued)*
M. This irregularly shaped blob was from a blast of freon from "canned air." Artifacts come in all colors. **N.** This blue haze can be eliminated by changing the objective lens-to-cornea distance. **O.** Always look for an even, deep color through the viewfinder. An often overlooked artifact is the greenish cast that occurs when color fundus photographs follow an intravenous injection of sodium fluorescein. **P.** Proper technique requires exposing color photographs before the dye injection. **Q.** This local overexposure is the result of taking fundus photographs while a patient's glasses are on (it is fine to photograph through contact lenses, however). **R.** The light area represents a patient's eyelash or hair. Unsharpness can be caused by a number of situations, including incorrect eyepiece settings and hazy media. Another setting that has an effect on sharpness is the astigmatism compensation control: correctly **(S)** and incorrectly **(T)** set. Distribution. **U.** Loading film incorrectly can cause artifacts in the beginning of the roll. **V.** Opening the camera back will cause a light leak in the middle of the roll. **W.** A poorly adjusted motor drive can cause double exposures at the end of the roll.

X   **Y**   **Z**

FIGURE 2-46   *(continued)*
Some artifacts occur with constant frequency. **X.** When an incorrect shutter speed is set, the shadow of the shutter curtain will obscure a portion of the fundus in each and every succeeding frame until proper sync speed is restored (a faulty camera flash sync may cause intermittent problems and indicate the need for service to the camera body). Artifacts may be confined to just one roll or to one patient. **Y.** A photo-sensitive patient can cause blink artifacts more often than other patients. **Z.** Light leaks from an unsealed camera will continue throughout fundus photographs regardless of a change in patient or film magazine.

FIGURE 2-47
Dark clouds. If a patient's pupil is significantly smaller than the outer diameter of the illuminating doughnut, a portion of the retina will receive inadequate illumination. The resultant "dark cloud" shifts as the camera's position changes. If you cannot eliminate the underexposed area, minimize its interaction with pathology.

ment. By the time patients are ready to be photographed, they may be tired and irritable. How can we take successful photographs in difficult clinical situations? Some common problems and their solutions are suggested below.

Illumination Problems

Maximum pupil dilation allows the entrance and exit of the fundus camera's illuminating and imaging light rays without interference. Work together with your referring physician to establish a dilating regimen that is safe and provides adequate dilation. Expect widely dilated pupils in young patients who are not taking medications, especially if they have light irises. Expect smaller pupils in older patients, in patients who have diabetes or who are being medicated for glaucoma, and in patients with dark irises. Less than maximum dilation will make accurate focusing and alignment difficult.

Your images may be locally underexposed, especially with wide-angle fundus cameras (Figure 2-47). Increase your flash setting, decrease your angle of view, or insert the "small pupil" diaphragm for a more evenly illuminated final photograph. Decentering the fundus camera may result in better illumination (Figure 2-48). If the "black cloud" continues to persist, avoid placing it over important pathology.

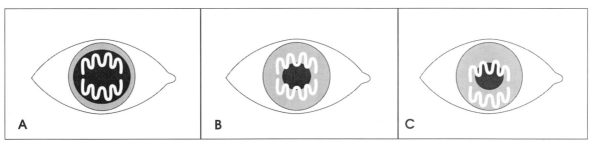

FIGURE 2-48
Decentering the fundus camera may help illuminate the fundus through a small pupil. Normally, the doughnut of the viewing light readily fits within the dilated pupil when centered **(A)**. If the dilated pupil is very small, centering the doughnut may exclude illumination **(B)**. Lowering or raising the camera axis **(C)** again divides the pupil evenly between viewing illumination and imaging rays. Be sure to increase the exposure to compensate for the smaller amount of illumination.

A   B

FIGURE 2-49
Look for local areas of sharpness in patients with cataracts. Initial alignment indicated a blurry fundus photograph **(A)**, but careful searching revealed a clear view **(B)**.

Unsharp Subjects

The bundle of illuminating and imaging rays must twice pass through the patient's tear film, cornea, anterior chamber, lens, and vitreous. The clarity of the final fundus photograph is directly related to the clarity of each of these layers.

Specific areas of the cornea and lens may affect the passage of light. Maneuver around local areas of unsharpness such as central cataracts, corneal scars, and pterygia. The key to success is positioning the central imaging light rays through a clear portion of the media (Figure 2-49). Spend time exploring all possible camera positions.

A dry, swollen, or hazy cornea, asteroid hyalosis, and vitreous hemorrhage represent conditions that can blur the entire fundus photograph. Adequate tear film is essential for corneal clarity and a sharp fundus image. Encourage your patients to blink frequently. Instill artificial tears in patients with dry corneas. Topically applying glycerin (under the physician's supervision and with a topical anesthetic) to an edematous cornea may help sharpen the image.[13]

Corneal manipulation diminishes corneal clarity. Applanation tonometry disturbs the corneal epithelium and discolors the cornea with topi-

A

B

FIGURE 2-50
Document compromised media or a small pupil using an external photograph **(A)**. Although the resulting fundus photograph may not be a prize-winner, it may contain adequate diagnostic information **(B)**.

cal fluorescein. Examination by diagnostic contact lenses may cause slight corneal edema and introduce topical methylcellulose. Fundus photography should be performed before any contact lens examination is undertaken. For optimal quality, reschedule patients who have undergone a procedure that involves corneal applanation. If postlaser photographs are requested, multiple rinses with commercially available eyewash preparations may clarify the image.

There is little you can do to sharpen the final photograph if dense asteroid hyalosis, vitreous hemorrhage, or a mature cataract exists. Indeed, obtaining a view of the retina can be a feat in itself. When general haziness is a problem, focusing with a green filter (540–570 nm) may help increase the contrast between the blood vessels and the retina. If blood vessels are indistinguishable, begin by locating the disc: It will look like a bright, blurry circle. Focus as best you can and then, using the disc as your landmark, locate the requested field. Your final photograph will almost always contain retinal details not perceived through the viewfinder (Figure 2-50).

Documenting hazy media or a small pupil will assist in evaluating photographer performance, especially if the question of poor dilation or hazy media versus poor photographic technique arises. Adjust the fundus camera for external photographs by moving the patient's headrest away from the camera's objective lens, inserting the plus diopter setting, and increasing the exposure. Focus should correspond with the level of the opacity. Use the optic disc as a reflector by centering it directly behind the pupil (Figure 2-51).

The Light-Sensitive Patient

Most people have a natural aversion to bright lights. Light-sensitive patients blink and tear excessively when looking in the fundus camera. Avoidance behavior by these patients may make aligning the fundus camera difficult. Younger patients are often more light-sensitive than older patients. Aphakic and pseudophakic patients are in general more light-sensitive, having lost the filtering qualities of their natural lens. Patients with cataracts may be quite light-sensitive. Patients with cone dystrophy, albinism, or blepharospasm may be extremely light-sensitive.

FIGURE 2-51
Using the optic disc as a reflector may help to better identify compromised media.

A

B

C

D

FIGURE 2-52
Dimming the viewing light. If the viewing light has been turned down to its minimum setting and your light-sensitive patient is still uncomfortable, decentering the illumination bulb may provide relief. When the illuminating bulb is correctly mounted **(A)**, the illuminating circle is centered within the dilated pupil **(B)**. Pulling the illuminating housing slightly out **(C)** decenters the illumination doughnut **(D)**, decreasing the amount of light used to focus. As the position of the electronic flash tube has not changed, the film image will be correctly exposed.

Prepare your patient for multiple bright flashes by accurately explaining the procedure. Inform the light-sensitive patient of your progress throughout the photographic session; provide gentle verbal encouragement or praise regularly. Patients may complain of dry corneas: instill artificial tears in both eyes to reduce discomfort of dry corneas. An alternate option for the frequent blinker and light-sensitive patient is a drop of topical anesthetic.

Many fundus cameras have an illumination intensity knob that adjusts the focusing illumination from virtually nil to very bright. Use the lowest illuminating intensity at which you can clearly distinguish retinal detail. You may find it useful to turn the viewing light up while focusing, then down to a minimal level while photographing. If, at its lowest setting, the illumination still bothers your patient, decentering the illuminating bulb may help (Figure 2-52).

The light-sensitive patient may more easily tolerate focusing when a green filter (540–570 nm) is placed in the illumination path. Remove the filter just before the exposure.

A

B

C

FIGURE 2-53
To retract the upper lids with a cotton-tipped applicator, have the patient look down and place the cotton tip at the lid margin **(A)**. Rotate the applicator (clockwise right eye, counterclockwise left eye) **(B)**. Instruct the patient to look straight ahead **(C)** and continue fundus photography.

Be constantly aware of your patient's disposition throughout the procedure. Frequent rest breaks (between, not within stereo pairs) help keep the patient fresh. Tension-relieving techniques, including deep breathing, shoulder relaxation, and humor are useful. Remember that patients are usually trying to do their best—even when it seems that they are not. Use positive reinforcement and praise to help your patients work with you, rather than against you.

You must remain in control of your demeanor throughout the procedure. Patients will often adjust their disposition according to your behavioral cues. If you exhibit calmness and patience, your patient will make an effort in that direction. If you become exasperated and exhibit threatening or obnoxious behavior, your patient will often react in a like manner. Don't be afraid to call a time-out if either you or the patient needs some time to regain composure.

Eyelids

A cooperative light-sensitive patient will allow you to lift his or her upper eyelid with a cotton-tipped applicator. An uncooperative light-sensitive patient will require you to depend on an assistant to hold both the upper and lower lids. Use cotton-tipped applicators or a gloved finger for lid manipulation. Place the tip of an applicator at the bottom of the upper lid and rotate up and in to raise the lid (Figure 2-53). Rotate the swab clockwise (as seen temporally) for the right eye and counterclockwise for the left eye. The globe should not be depressed during lid manipulation, as this may induce astigmatism.

Lid speculum use is not usually recommended: An uncooperative patient may sustain a corneal abrasion. Some photographers suggest the patient hold his or her own eyelids.[14] Be aware that the patient may be more interested in avoiding bright lights than in ensuring that the procedure is successfully completed.

Eyelids may present a mechanical (rather than behavioral) barrier to fundus photography. Lid elevation is necessary for the patient with blepharoptosis. Manage excess eyelid skin with the creative use of tape (Figure 2-54).

Children

Retinal photography challenges quickly mount when the patient is a child. One difficulty is that the equipment is designed for the "average-sized" adult. Specific suggestions for accommodating the smaller bodies of your younger patients are found below.

FIGURE 2-54
"Instant lid lifts" with adhesive tape are useful with some ptotic eyelids.

Good pediatric fundus photography depends on conveying the proper attitude. Successful patient management techniques in the young patient vary with the age of the patient. Infants, toddlers, grade-schoolers, and teenagers all require specific strategies.

Babies are both the easiest and most difficult patients to photograph. Those who have just nursed are cooperative and sleepy, while those who have missed their naps are invariably cranky and extremely challenging. Patience and good humor are your only means of taming the uncooperative child. Your most emotionally challenging photographic subjects will be the retinas of children who have been abused.

For babies, use a hand-held fundus camera. Alternately, the forehead rest may be removed from the standard-angle fundus camera and your young patients laid on their side.[15] A pediatric speculum provides access to the pupil. Speculum use requires topical anesthesia and a balanced salt solution to keep the cornea moist. A standard mummy wrap with two or three volunteers (for head, torso, and legs) stabilizes the child. Remember to take into account both the decreased pupil size and the shorter axial length in children younger than 3 years old when setting your flash exposure. Expose several photographs if you can, bracketing toward the lower flash settings. Use your general or external camera and flash to document abnormalities in abused children.

Verbal communication may be used to your advantage with toddlers and grade-schoolers. Speak directly to the patient, as opposed to communicating through the parent. Introduce yourself directly to the child with a smile to help establish trust. Remind young children of the special events (such as birthdays or holidays) that are usually associated with picture taking. Explain the intended procedure as just as necessary (using a nod and eye contact to make sure the parents understand). Speak slowly and distinctly. Although all patients like to know what to expect, younger children especially fear the unknown. Sharing a frank overview of the process informs children and allays their fears. Let your patient have some fun: Our young patients like to experience photography from the "taking" end. We waste a frame of film but gain their friendship by letting them press the shutter release. An instant film image or digital print may be used to elicit a cooperative spirit and creates a great giveaway for show-and-tell. Spend as much time as needed to obtain the best photographs.

Difficulties may be encountered during your straightforward attempts at photography. Remember to respect each family's specific disciplinary system. Don't bribe or threaten to punish—other alternatives are available. Games help focus the child's attention on something other than the procedure. The child may "pretend to be a statue" or "find the bunny in the middle of the lens."

Try setting a mutual goal with the patient. Ask the child to count aloud with you to three. Tell them you will be taking three pictures and have them count each one along with you. You may want to cushion this figure; most children will only allow the negotiated number.

Actively solicit suggestions from the patient. Ask the child "what can I do to make this easier for you?" Appeal to his or her friendship with the doctor or parent ("Dr. ____ thinks these pictures are important. Will you help me get them?"). If lids need to be held, employ a technician who has previously worked well with the particular child. Above all, remain calm and patient throughout the procedure.

Older children who are difficult may require you to announce, in a firm voice, that "we are going to take these pictures before you leave. Let's work together to get this completed." If you feel yourself losing control of the situation, sometimes it is better to leave the room and have the parent and child negotiate the terms of pictures. Be sure to leave with these verbal messages: "Dr. ___ thinks these picture are important. When I come back, we'll be ready to finish the pictures." On returning to one 6-year-old girl, I discovered that the parent had agreed to pay the child $1.00 for each of three photographs.

It is especially important not to distress the child if you see the patient before the physician has completed the examination. As important as good photographs are, the doctor's examination takes precedence. The photographer may be the last health professional to see the child on a particular day. You have the opportunity to make future visits easier by parting with the patient on good terms.

Patient Communication

During fundus photography, the patient and photographer are thrust together for a brief time during which the photographer explores a very private part of the patient: the eyes. In this setting, the photographer must act in a variety of technical and communicative roles. Besides obtaining technically correct photographs, the photographer acts as the initiator, information giver, and coordinator. Ophthalmic photographers must be good communicators.

Show your patients respect by calling them from the waiting room using their first and last name and addressing them with their title (Mr./Mrs.) as appropriate. Be aware of the patient's body language throughout the procedure. Make conscious use of your body language, voice, word choice, and touch to keep your patient and their companions at ease. Be generous with positive feedback, especially if the patient is having trouble with the procedure. Keep a smile in your voice.

Communicate with patients using plain, straightforward English. Avoid street lingo and medical jargon. If the patient does not speak English, arrange for a translation. A relative or friend may be available, or your medical center or clinic may keep a list of employees with second-language talents. Keep in mind that a certified medical translator may be required for some procedures. Alternately, refer to Table 2-6 for a succinct listing of familiar ophthalmic photography phrases in alternate languages.

Table 2-6. Alternate Languages

English	Spanish	French	Greek
Hello	Hola	Bonjour	Yia sas
Good morning	Buenos días	Bonjour / Au revoir	Kalh mepa
Good afternoon	Buenas tardes	Bonjour / Au revoir	Kalo apogevma
Good evening	Buenas noches	Bonjour / Au revoir	Kalh spera
Mr.	Señor	Monsieur	Kyrios
Mrs.	Señora	Madame	Kyria
Miss	Señorita	Mademoiselle	Despinis
Please come with me	Por favor venga conmigo	Veuillez me suivre s'il vous plaît	Parakalo elate mazi mou
How are you today?	¿Como está Ud. Hoy día?	Comment allez-vous aujourd'hui?	Pos eisthe shmera?
Is this your first visit here?	¿Es ésta su primera visita aquí?	Est-ce que c'est votre première visite ici?	Eine afth h proth sas episkepsh?
Have you had this test before?	¿Le han hecho éste test antes?	Avez-vous subi cet examen auparavant?	Exate afth thn exetash prohgoumenos?
Please sit down	Tome asiento por favor	Veuillez vous asseoir s'il vous plaît	Kathiste parakalo
How can I help you?	¿Cómo le puedo ayudar?	Comment puis-je vous aider?	Pos mporo na sas bohthiso?
What is the reason for your visit?	¿Cuál es la razón de su visita?	Quelle est la raison pour votre visite?	Pios einai o logos ths episkepsis sas?
When did this problem start?	¿Cuando empezó éste problema?	Depuis quand avez-vous constaté ce problème?	Pote arxise afto to problhma?
Look up to the ceiling	Mire al techo	Regardez au plafond s'il vous plaît	Koitaxte thn orofh
Cover your right eye	Cubrase el ojo derecho	Couvrez votre oeil droit	Skepaste to dexi sas mati
Cover your left eye	Cubrase el ojo izquierdo	Couvrez votre oeil gauche	Skepaste to aristero sas mati
What letters do you see in this line?	¿Qué letras ve en ésta linea?	Quelles lettres parvenez-vous à déchiffrer sur cette ligne?	Poia gramata vlepete safth thn grami?
Look down	Mire hacia arriba	Regardez vers le bas	Koitaxte kato
Look up	Mire hacia abajo	Regardez vers le haut	Koitaxte epano
Look to the right	Mire a la derecha	Regardez à droite	Koitaxte sta dexia
Look to the left	Mire a la izchierda	Regardez à gauche	Koitaxte sta aristera
I will put drops in your eyes	Voy a poner gotas en sus ojos	Je vais appliquer des gouttes dans vos yeux	Tha balo stagones sta matia sas
These drops will sting a bit	Estas gotas arden un poco	Ces gouttes vont causer une légère sensation de brulure	Aftes h stagones tha anixoun thn koph tou matiou
These drops will dilate your pupils	Estas gotas dilatarán sus pupilas	Ces gouttes vont dilater vos pupilles	Aftes h stagones tha anixoun thn koph tou matiou
Your vision will be blurry for a couple of hours	Su visión será borrosa por un par de horas	Vous aurez la vue trouble pendant deux heures	H orasi sas tha tholosi gia liges ores
These drops will freeze your cornea	Estas gotas son para anestesiar su cornea	Ces gouttes servent à anesthésier la cornée	Aftes h stagones tha anesthetopihsoun ta matia sas
Do not rub your eyes for 20 minutes	No se restriegue los ojos para veinte minutos	Eviter de frottez vos yeux pendant vingt minutes	Mhn trypsete ta matia sas gia 20 lepta
This is normal	Esto es normal	C'est tout à fait normal	Afto einai physiologico
Rest your chin on the chin rest	Ponga el mentón sobre éste pedestal	Poser votre menton sur la mentonnière	Valte to sagoni sas sto mixanima
Lean your forehead against this bar	Apoye la frente sobre ésta barra.	Poser votre front contre cette barre de soutien	Akoumpiste to metopo sas safto to meros
Open your eyes as wide as you can	Abra los ojos lo más que pueda	Ouvrez vos yeux aussi grand que possible	Anoixte ta nmatia sas oso poli mporite
Raise your eyebrow	Eleve las cejas	Soulevez vos sourcis	Sikosete psyla to fridi sas
Do not move your head	No mueva la cabeza	Veuillez ne pas bouger la tête	Mhn kounate to kefalh
Keep your upper and lower teeth together	Mantenga los dientes de arriba y abajo juntos	Errez vos dents	Krathste ta epano kai kato donntia mazi
Follow the red light	Siga la luz roja	Suivez la lumière rouge	Parakolouthiste to kokino fos
Follow the green light	Siga la luz verde	Suivez la lumière verte	Parakolouthiste to prasino fos
There is a black pointer at the center of the light in front of you	Hay un puntero negro al centro de la luz en frente suyo	Vous verrez un index noir au centre de la lumière devant vous	Hparxy mia mavrh koukida sto kendro tou fotos
Your skin will turn a bit yellow for about six hours	Su piel se tenirá un poco amarilla por cerca de seis horas	Pendant six heures environ, votre peau sera jaunâtre	To derma sas tha kitrinish gia merikes ores
Your urine will turn orange for a day or two	Su orina se tenirá naranja por un día o dos	Pendant un ou deux jours, votre urine sera orangée	Ta oura sas that ginoun portakali xroma gia merikes meres
This is because of the dye	Esto ocurre por el colorante	C'est à cause du colorant	Afto eine apotelesma ths xrostikhs
Place your arm here	Ponga el brazo aquí	Posez votre bras ici	Topothetiste to xeri sas edo
Make a fist	Empune la mano	Faites un poing avec votre main	Sfyxte thn grothia sas

Table 2-6. (continued)

English	Spanish	French	Greek
We will inject fluorescein dye in your hand or arm	Ahora vamos a injectar el colorante en una vena en el brazo o en la mano	Nous allons injecter un colorant dans la main ou le bra	Tha baloume fluorecein xrostikh sto xeri h sto braxiona
It takes a few seconds for the fluorescein to reach your eyes	La fluorosceina se demora unos pocos segundos en llegar a el ojo	En quelques secondes, le colorant apparaitra dans les vaisseaux sanguins de l'oeil	Tha pari liga deftero deftero lepta gia na ftash sto mati sas
It is essential that you remain still while we take the pictures	Es esencial que permanezca sin moverse durante la toma de fotos	C'est essentiel que vous ne bougiez pas pendant la séance photographique	Eina hpoxreotiko na min kiniste
Do not move	No se mueva	Veuillez ne pas bouger	Mhn khneste
You can blink, but do not move your head	Puede pestanear, pero sin mover la cabeza	Vous pouvez cligner des yeux, mais ne bougez pas la tête	Mporite na anigoklisete ta matia xoris na kinesete to kefali
Now I will start taking the pictures	Ahora voy a empezar a tomar las fotos	Maintenant je vais commencer à prendre les photos	Mporite na anigoklisete ta matia xoris na kinesete to kefali
Breath slow and deep	Respire profundo y lento	Respirer lentement et à fond	Anapnefste siga and bathia
Relax	Relajese	Détendez-vous	Ksekourasteite
The nausea will pass soon	La nausea pasará pronto	La sensation de nausée est transitoire	Tha perassi grigora
How do you feel?	¿Cómo se siente?	Comment vous sentez-vous?	Pos esthaneste?
Keep your eyes wide open	Mantenga los ojos bién abiertos	Garder vos yeux grand ouvert	Krathste ta matia sas telios anixta
You can sit back and relax	Ahora puede descansar	Vous pouvez vous reposer	Kathiste piso kai hremiste
We will take a few minutes' break	Ahora tomaremos unos minutos de descanso	Nous allons prendre quelques minutes de pause	Tha kanoume dialima gia liga lepta
We will continue with the pictures now	Ahora continuaremos con las fotos	Maintenant nous allons continuer à prendre des photos	Tha exacolouthisoume me ths fotographies tora
We are done with the pictures	Hemos terminado con las fotos	Nous avons terminé la séance photographique	Teliosame me tis fotographies
The test is finished	El test ha terminado	L'examen est conclu	H exetasi teliose
It is necessary for you to come back to this clinic	Es necesario que usted regresa a la clinica	Il fra revenir à la clinique	Eina aparetito gia sas na elthete sthn kliniki
Tomorrow	Mañana	Demain	Avrio
On Monday	El Lunes	Lundi	Thn deftera
On Tuesday	El Martes	Mardi	Thn triti
On Wednesday	El Miércoles	Mercredi	Thn tetarth
On Thursday	El Jueves	Jeudi	Thn pempth
On Friday	El Viernes	Vendredi	Thn paraskevy
On Saturday	El Sabado	Samedi	To savato
On Sunday	El Domingo	Dimanche	Thn khriaki
The doctor will explain the result of your test in a few minutes	El doctor le va a explicar el resultado de el test en unos minutos	Le médecin vous expliquera le résultat de votre examen d'ici quelques minutes	O giatros tha sas exigisi ta apotelesmata ths exetasi sas se liga lepta

Note: This table, prepared by Rosario Bate, RN, CRA, presents common patient phraseology in multiple languages. If you are not familiar with the pronunciation, point to the phrase and have the patient or companion read the appropriate words in the same row.
Translations—Spanish: Rosario Bate, RN, CRA; French: Bernard C. Szirth, PhD; Greek: George Minstsioulis, MD.

Advanced Techniques

The Periphery

Many retinal diseases may manifest changes outside of the posterior pole. Peripheral fundus photography is used to image these areas. The retina described by the standard fields 3–7 is referred to as the *mid-periphery*; retina nearer the ora serrata is termed the *far periphery*. This section begins by explaining the basics of peripheral photography and concludes by suggesting tips for the experienced photographer.

Two basic techniques allow you to move beyond posterior pole fundus photography: off-center fixation and fundus camera movements. You know that obtaining straight-ahead fixation and centering the illumination doughnut in the patient's pupil will result in a macular photograph. You can visualize the peripheral retina by moving the fixation light off center and then recentering the doughnut of light (usually by

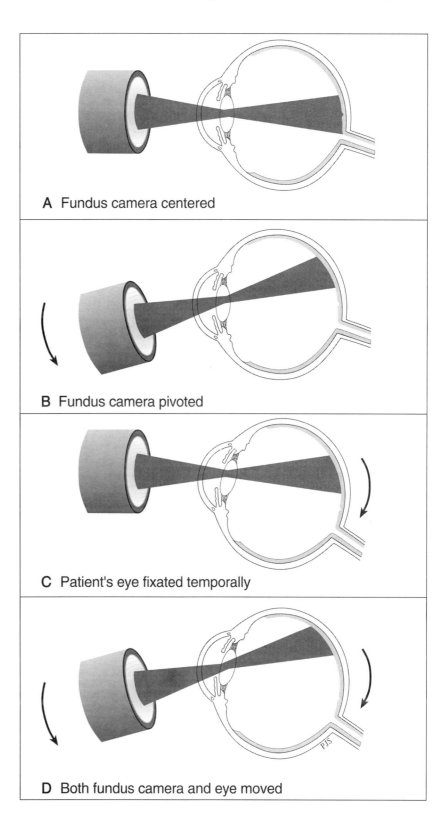

A Fundus camera centered

B Fundus camera pivoted

C Patient's eye fixated temporally

D Both fundus camera and eye moved

FIGURE 2-55
Imaging the periphery. When the fundus camera and the patient's eye are aligned squarely, the macula is centered **(A)**. Swing the camera to one side to photograph the periphery **(B)**, adjusting the distance between the objective lens and the cornea and recentering the doughnut of light on the pupil. Alternately, change patient fixation, rotating the patient's eye up and to the side until the proper field is obtained **(C)**. Use both techniques for far peripheral views **(D)**. A combination of swinging the camera to the side, tilting the camera up or down, and oblique patient fixation may be needed for some peripheral views. Evaluate the need for using the astigmatism compensation control when working in the far periphery.

looking to the outside of the camera) on the pupil. You can also photograph the peripheral retina by obtaining straight-ahead fixation (using the external fixation device) and then swinging or tilting the fundus camera. Using either one of these techniques results in midperiphery photographs; using both helps you image the far periphery (Figure 2-55).

The "seven standard fields" describe a uniform method of photographing the midperipheral fundus. Standardized field definition was

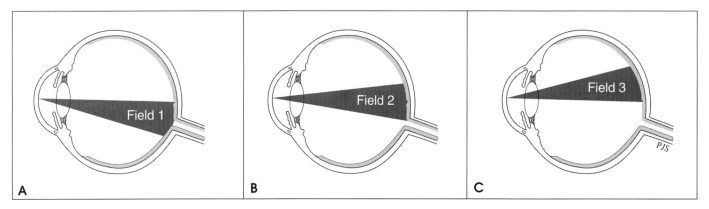

FIGURE 2-56
Seven standard fields. Visualized on a cross section of the eye from above, field 1 is centered on the optic nerve **(A)**. For field 2, the camera is centered on the fovea **(B)**. The nasal edge of field 3 intersects the fovea **(C)**. Field 4 is directly superior to field 2; field 5 is directly inferior. Field 6 is superior-nasal to field 1. Field 7 is inferior-nasal to field 1. Field 8 is a "wild card" field that is assigned to any needed retinal position.

A   B

FIGURE 2-57
The seven standard fields. These are photographic examples of the seven standard fields in the right **(A)** and left **(B)** eyes. FundusMap illustrations courtesy of Richard Hackel of the University of Michigan.

developed to assess the peripheral retina for multicenter studies. It allows the comparison of similar retinal fields, whether they be exposed at your office on different visits, or by ophthalmic photographers in different parts of the world. You should standardize your midperiphery photographs by learning the anatomic landmarks that define each field (Figure 2-56).

Field 1 is centered on the disc (Figure 2-57). Field 2 is centered on the macula with the disc in the 3:00 (OD) or 9:00 (OS) position. Field 3 is temporal to the macula, including the fovea at the 3:00 (OD) or 9:00 (OS) position. In the right eye, field 4 is superior to the macula and includes the 12:00 position of field 2 at its 6:00 position. Field 5 is inferior to the

---

FIGURE 2-58
When photographing the periphery, begin with a macula photograph **(A)** or include a landmark in your photograph **(B)**.

A B

macula and includes the 6:00 position of field 2 at the 12:00 position. Field 6 is superonasal to the disc, including the 1:30 position of field 1 at 7:30. Field 7 is inferonasal to the disc and includes the 4:30 position of field 1 at 10:30. Most photographers image these fields "out of order," proceeding thusly: 2-1-6-4-3-5-7 or 2-1-3-5-7-6-4.

The seven standard fields are considered the gold standard for documenting the midperiphery and hence are utilized widely in a number of multicenter clinical trials. Alternative schemes for documenting the midperiphery include a standardized nine fields for wide-field cameras and a short three-field screening protocol.[16,17] A typical clinical shortcut when using wide-angle cameras is to expose for central fixation, then superior, inferior, nasal, and temporal fields.

Because practical experience is your best teacher, begin by photographing the retinal periphery of an office volunteer. Alternatively, expose some peripheral photographs of your patients who need only macula or disc photographs, polishing your skills before you need them.

Obtaining high-quality peripheral fundus photographs can be a challenge. Factors that are optimized for posterior pole photography become mediocre when photographing the far periphery. A circular, widely dilated pupil becomes an ellipse. The retina is imaged through an oblique cross section of the lens. Your camera position, once simple, is now complex. Peripheral fundus photographs may not seem as sharp as your posterior pole photographs. The following practical techniques may help improve their quality:

1. Begin with an establishing shot. Document the eye (OD or OS) by photographing the posterior pole before you image the periphery or include a landmark (such as the disc) in the photograph (Figure 2-58).
2. Don't limit yourself when positioning the patient's eye or the camera for peripheral fundus photography. Both the internal or external fixation device can be used to obtain fixation. If peripheral photographs are requested of monocular patients, you can use the external fixation device on the eye being photographed. Try verbal instructions if targets do not work; clock hours or simple directions (up, down, right, left) may be helpful. Ask the patient to imagine looking in the center of a square; asking the patient to look to "the upper left hand corner" will result in a superior temporal view (OD). If reliable fixation cannot be obtained, request the patient to look straight ahead (at the wall or at you) and swing or tilt the camera until the proper field is visualized. You may need to stand or crouch when the camera is tilted or swung to its extreme position. If the patient's fixation has reached its limits and you still need to see "just a little bit more," ask the patient to look "beyond the light"

FIGURE 2-59
Photographing the periphery: wide angle or normal? The peripheral fundus can be imaged with both wide-angle and normal-angle fundus cameras. Choose the angle that best documents the patient's condition.

to reveal more peripheral retina. In the extreme cases, the patient may need to rotate his or her head to the right or left or move his or her head away from the forehead or chinrest. A combination of off-center fixation, camera head movement, and patient head tilt extends your range further into the periphery (note: using all three of these options at the same time is possible only with the most widely dilated pupils).

3. Scleral depression (by the photographer or the physician) and extremely wide-angle contact cameras (e.g., the Pomerantzeff or RetCam) can yield photographs that include the ora serrata.

4. Should a normal-angle or a wide-angle camera be used in peripheral photography? Normal-angle cameras always image better in tight spaces. Because the round pupil becomes a narrow ellipse as the eye is rotated, the smaller imaging circle of the normal-angle camera makes it the camera of choice for peripheral photographs in patients with a small or medium-sized pupil. In patients with large pupils, however, an elliptical pupil may still be large enough for a wide-angle camera. These cameras may reveal more of the peripheral retina with their larger angle of view and closer working distance. One wide-angle picture may take the place of several 30-degree pictures. Attempt peripheral photographs using both fields of view if possible (Figure 2-59).

The astigmatic correction device helps correct the paraxial astigmatism that results from the oblique angles at which the cornea and lens are approached.[18] Rotate the angle of the astigmatic correction device to the same axis as the patient's gaze, and then twist or rotate, or both, the astigmatic correction slowly until a sharper image is seen. Check the unmodified view before the exposure to be certain that the change is beneficial. If only a portion of the picture becomes sharper, make the adjustment with the lesion in mind.

Photographs after Laser Treatment

Fundus photography is often used to document recent laser treatments (Figure 2-60).[19] The overlay function of newer digital imaging systems readily compares the area of treatment with angiographic information, making electronic postlaser photographs clinically advantageous. However, the quality of postlaser fundus photographs may be compromised because of the contact lens and lubricant used during the laser procedure. Increase the clarity of your postlaser photos by rinsing the eye thoroughly with commercially available eyewash. We rinse the eye three separate times, asking the patient to blink in between each. Allowing

FIGURE 2-60
Rinse the cornea with commercially available eyewash before attempting postlaser fundus photography.

some time (at least 10 minutes) to pass after the treatment helps to resolve corneal edema from the contact lens use.

Fundus Photography with Filters

Two principles enable specific retinal details to be enhanced by using monochromatic filters during fundus photography. First, when used with black and white film, monochromatic filters lighten objects of their own color and darken objects of the complementary color (Figure 2-61). Second, longer and shorter wavelengths of light penetrate the retina to different levels (Figure 2-62). The effects of monochromatic light when photographing the normal and abnormal retina have been described by Ducrey and Delori.[20, 21] In clinical practice, blue, green, and red filters have gained wide usage.

Use your blue fluorescein exciter filter (490 nm) to enhance information from the nerve fiber layer of the retina or vitreoretinal interface (Figure 2-63). Select a slow, fine-grain black and white film such as Kodak Technical Pan or Ilford Pan F film.[22] Focus carefully on the uppermost layer of the retina by first focusing on the retinal blood vessels and then moving the focus slightly "up" toward the vitreous. High-contrast development and printing techniques accentuates the nerve fiber layer.

The monochromatic green filter (often archaically termed a "red-free filter") transmits either 540- or 575-nm wavelengths of light. These wavelengths enhance the visualization of the retinal vasculature and hemorrhages by increasing the contrast between the retinal blood vessels and the retinal pigment epithelium (Figure 2-64). Using these filters with black and white film results in the best monochromatic representation of the physician's view with an ophthalmoscope. Traditionally, the photographs before a fluorescein angiogram are taken with this filter. Focus on the central retina for vascular studies. Parenthetically, using a green filter when black and white internegatives of color slides are made results in a more pleasing separation between the retinal blood vessels and the choroid.

A red monochromatic filter (640 nm), when coupled with precise focusing, highlights choroidal details (Figure 2-65). This technique can define the borders of pigmented lesions or document choroidal vasculature or vascular details before indocyanine green angiography. Focus first on the major retinal blood vessels and then continue focusing slightly "down" toward the choroid.

Although colored filters may not be useful with every patient, they can selectively highlight specific fundus details in particular cases.

Fundus Photographs for Torsion

Fundus photography can be used to document the objective presence or absence of ocular torsion in patients with vertical strabismus (Figure

FIGURE 2-61

Monochromatic filters. A 12-hue color wheel **(A)** was photographed on panchromatic black and white film with blue **(B)**, green **(C)**, and red **(D)** filters placed in front of the lens. Note that colored filters lighten the reproduction of similar colors and darken complementary hues. Normal and abnormal fundus characteristics can be selectively emphasized using monochromatic filters. A blue, 490-nm filter highlights the nerve fiber layer; highlighting epiretinal membranes (*arrow*) **(F, J)** which may be difficult to evaluate in the color fundus photographs **(E, I)**. The green, 540-nm filter darkens the veins and increases contrast: emphasizing a macroaneurysm **(G)** and macular hole **(K)**. The red, 640-nm filter reveals the choroidal vasculature, lightens the arteries, and defines the borders of a pigmented nevi (*arrow*) **(H, L)**. Targeting focus to the appropriate level is essential when using monochromatic filters.

FIGURE 2-62
The wavelength of monochromatic light determines its capacity for retinal penetration. Shorter wavelengths (e.g., blue) scatter more easily and reveal the surface of the retina. Longer wavelengths (e.g., red) scatter less easily, allowing deeper imaging. (Courtesy of B. Clifton, University of Washington.)

FIGURE 2-63
Your blue exciter filter can highlight changes in the top layer of the retina, as is seen in this example of a nerve fiber layer sector defect. This patient with primary open-angle glaucoma was photographed with Kodak Tech Pan film and a 490-nm filter. (Courtesy of B. Clifton, University of Washington.)

FIGURE 2-64
Your green filter highlights changes in the retinal vasculature by increasing contrast. This arteriovenous malformation was documented using a 540-nm filter. (Courtesy of B. Clifton, University of Washington.)

FIGURE 2-65
A red filter (this photograph used a 640-nm filter) penetrates through the retina to the choroid, in this case documenting a choroidal nevus. (Courtesy of B. Clifton, University of Washington.)

FIGURE 2-66
Document torsion with fundus photography by inserting the internal fixation device and centering the disc within the height of the frame. Compose to include both the macula and disc. The macula in a normal eye falls slightly below the line that bisects the disc; the macula of the abnormal eye is positioned above (incyclotropia) or below (excyclotropia) this line.

2-66).[23] Take extra care to position the patient's head squarely in the head rest for torsion photography. Frame the posterior pole, aligning the center of the disc on the midline of the frame at the 3:00 (OD) or 9:00 (OS) position. Insert and focus the internal fixation device. Double-check that the patient's head has not tilted before exposing the film.

Hand-Held Fundus Cameras

Portable, hand-held fundus cameras are useful in a variety of situations—for babies and small children who are too small for the standard headrest and for supine patients—whether bedridden, undergoing surgery, or being examined under anesthesia. Animal fundus photography is often performed using hand-held fundus cameras (Figure 2-67).

Positioning the hand-held fundus camera requires skill and practice. The patient should be stationary (papoose small babies and have one person to stabilize the head and one for the feet) and with lids retracted (either by a helper or with a speculum). Hold the camera in your left hand, using your thumb for the shutter release and your right hand for the film advance. Position the front element of the camera approximately 2 in. away from the cornea. Center on the exterior of the eye and focus on a retinal blood vessel or the optic disc. Move the camera closer to the cornea, allowing the fundus to fill the frame. Refocus, optimize color saturation, and minimize the artifacts. Tilt the camera or have your assistant manipulate the eye with a cotton swab for disc or peripheral photographs.

Condensing lenses used for indirect ophthalmoscopy may be used with the hand-held fundus camera to alter the field of view or to view through a particularly small pupil. Position these lenses close to the cornea while you view through the fundus camera at arm's length. Increase the expo-

A

B   C

D   E

FIGURE 2-67
Fish fundus photography using a hand-held camera
and a condensing lens **(A)**. First obtain a red reflex
(B), then optimize the distance for fundus imaging
(C). An owl retina **(D)** and rat retina **(E)** complete this
fundus menagerie. (Courtesy of M. Croswell, Henry
Ford Health System.)

sure to compensate for the greater flash-to-subject distance. Tilt either the
lens or the camera until reflection artifacts are minimized.

If you are using a hand-held fundus camera to perform fluorescein
angiography on small animals, refer to Table 5-4 for weight-specific 10%
fluorescein dosage.

Not Necessarily the Fundus

If a slit-lamp camera is unavailable, a fundus camera may be used to record
pathology in the anterior segment. Increase the patient-objective lens dis-

FIGURE 2-68
External photography with the axial illumination of a fundus camera is helpful when documenting leukokoria or a "white pupil."

A

B

C

D

E

F

FIGURE 2-69
A photo slit-lamp can extend your photographic range. A macular hole **(A)** is better appreciated with slit illumination **(B)**. This wide-angle fundus photograph **(C)** does not quite match the reach of a 90-D condensing lens **(D)** in these photographs of a dislocated intraocular lens. A relatively small portion of the choroidal detachment is documented with a 60-degree view **(E)**. A more comprehensive view is obtained at the photo slit-lamp using a wide-angle contact lens **(F)**.

tance and dial a plus lens into the diopter compensation setting. Increase the exposure to compensate for the increased distance the light must travel. Focus on the cornea, iris, or lens as appropriate. If the area of interest is translucent, arrange patient fixation to permit the optic disc to act as a reflector. External photographs are useful in documenting patients with compromised media or patients with leukokoria (Figure 2-68).

Auxiliary Lenses at the Photo Slit-Lamp

Diagnostic lenses permit fundus photographs to be taken with a photo slit-lamp (Figure 2-69). Condensing lenses (e.g., a 60- or 90-D lens) help capture a wide-angle peripheral fundus view or slit images of the retina. A Goldmann three-mirror lens is useful for narrow-angle views in the

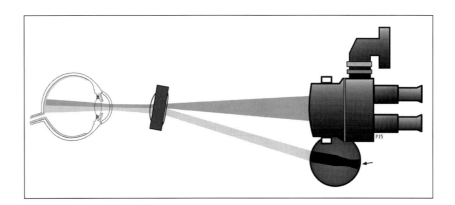

FIGURE 2-70
When imaging the fundus using a condensing lens at the photo slit-lamp, direct the illumination slightly off axis. Place the lens approximately 6-mm from the cornea and tilt as needed to reduce reflections. A lens holder (available from the manufacturer) simplifies the procedure.

retinal periphery. Slit views of the posterior pole are obtained with the Goldmann fundus lens. The Rodenstock Panfundoscope lens is useful for extremely wide-angle views. We encourage you to experiment with the specific lenses available in your office.

The basic technique for using condensing lenses is illustrated in Figure 2-70. Select and clean a lens, recalling that the higher the diopter, the larger the field and smaller the magnification. After seating the patient comfortably at the slit-lamp, begin with a wide slit beam at a low or medium magnification. Swing the slit illumination housing slightly off center temporally and de-center the beam in the same direction. Hold the lens approximately 6 mm from the cornea and adjust the slit-lamp to obtain a red reflex. Focus by moving the condensing lens or the joystick, or both, forward and backward. Select a wide or narrow slit beam as dictated by the subject matter. Adjust the angle of the auxiliary lens and the angle of illumination to minimize reflections. Change to a medium or high magnification to fill the frame before your exposure. Bracket exposures around your standard slit-lamp exposure.

Step-by-step instructions for using diagnostic contact lenses at the slit-lamp can be found in slit-lamp photography texts.[24] Remember that careless use of diagnostic contact lenses can result in corneal damage. We routinely obtain approval from the attending ophthalmologist before our photographers perform contact lens procedures. Have your physician train you in the proper use of diagnostic contact lenses before attempting to photograph a patient.

Prepare the patient by briefly explaining the procedure. Confirm that the patient is not wearing contact lenses. Apply a topical anesthetic to the patient's cornea and a lubricant (e.g., methylcellulose: be sure to avoid bubbles) to the diagnostic contact lens. After positioning the patient comfortably at the slit-lamp, ask the patient to look up and then place the bottom of the lens onto the inferior sclera. Tilt the lens toward the eye until contact is made. Direct the patient to look straight ahead while you center your view, the slit beam, and the pupil under low magnification.

Optimize the location, size, and angle of the slit, the magnification, and the focus for the pathology being photographed. The Goldmann fundus lens requires a medium or high magnification and a slightly decentered slit. Use a slit shape that coincides with the shape of the medium-sized, 67-degree mirror of a Goldmann three-mirror lens for views of the far periphery. A wide, off-center beam and the Panfundoscope lens will expose a large retinal area. Bracket your standard exposures at each magnification. Work quickly to avoid any corneal edema that may cloud your photographs. Your sharpest photographs will be obtained during the first 2 minutes.

Fundus photography using a photo slit-lamp is not a replacement for standard fundus camera procedures but is an alternative technique for experienced photographers. It is more time consuming than retinal photography using a fundus camera, and the results can be less predictable.

Auxiliary lenses can also be used at the fundus camera. A non-contact double aspheric 28-D lens placed between the cornea and the fundus camera objective lens significantly increases the field of view in a wide-angle camera. [25]

Conclusion

Fundus photography is a challenging but rewarding procedure requiring knowledge, skill, repetition, and patience to master. Although we have focused your attention on technique in this chapter, remember that whether you are a novice or an experienced fundus photographer, you should not lose sight of this most important concept: The patient is the most important person in your fundus photography room. Every photographer remembers their first patient, their worst patient, and of course, their greatest fundus photograph. Try this: The next time you sit a patient in front of your fundus camera, take a moment to reflect on the impact your fundus photographs will make on your patient's life and well-being. And then make the pictures as if your eyesight depended on it—because theirs might.

Pediatric Ultra-Wide Angle Imaging

Leslie D. MacKeen

Instrumentation and Software

Historically, the narrow angle of film-based fundus cameras (30- to 60-degree) requires more than a single picture to image the entire retina. Photographers have subsequently montaged their images, either manually or digitally to appreciate a wide field of view.[26,27] With the need for improved documentation of the retinal periphery, various designs of wide-field fundus cameras and contact lens techniques have evolved over the years.[28–30] In pediatrics, the requirement has been not only for wide field but portability as well. An indirect lens held suspended between the patient and the portable camera could achieve a wider field than direct fundus imaging, although it is difficult to capture at a standard magnification. The success of this technique, as with many of the wide-field technologies, has often been dependent on factors such as the operator's skill level, a steady hand, and a compliant subject.

Currently, three systems are available that can provide wide-field fundus imaging: One is still in the research and development phase, the second is a scanning laser ophthalmoscope, and the third is a wide-field pediatric retinal camera. All of these current cameras are digital capture.

The Panoret-1000A (Figure 2-71) is currently under development by Medibell Medical Vision Technologies, Haifa, Israel. The hand-held, 100-degree non-mydriatic contact camera is supported by an articulated arm and uses transscleral illumination. Software includes the production of color and monochrome images, fluorescein and indocyanine green

FIGURE 2-71
The Panoret-1000A 100-degree system. (Image courtesy of Medibell Medical Vision Technologies, Haifa, Israel.)

FIGURE 2-72
The Panoramic200 Non Mydriatic Ophthalmoscope **(A)** and the Optomap Image **(B)**. (Images courtesy of Optos North America, Marlborough, MA.)

angiography, and optical zoom. Image acquisition and focusing takes place using a footswitch. Once the technology becomes available, it may have the capability of imaging adults and children.

The Panoramic200 Non Mydriatic Ophthalmoscope (Figure 2-72) (Optos North America, Marlborough, MA) uses a unique optical system and scanning laser ophthalmoscope technology to produce the Optomap examination. Available commercially on a limited basis since mid-1999, it is non-contact and provides a 200-degree field of view (FOV). (The FOV is measured from the center of the eye [Figure 2-73] which is the appropriate metric for panoramic imaging.) A 2000 × 2000 pixel, color image is displayed on a Windows NT system. Image capture is patient activated and does not require a dilated pupil. The image exposure process takes 0.25 second. It is received as a full-color composite image using red and green laser wavelengths. Because the system is not portable, it is suited for anyone who would be appropriate for standard fundus imaging. Research is under way to assess the value of the Panoramic200 as a tool to be used as part of the comprehensive eye examination and in the possible screening and diagnosis of diabetic retinopathy and macular degeneration.

In 1996, Wei Su, PhD, and Bert Massie, PhD, at Massie Research Laboratories of Dublin, California, developed a hand-held, real-time, digital, wide-field pediatric retinal camera, named the RetCam 120 (Figure 2-74). They worked with pediatric ophthalmologist Dr. A. L. Murphee of Childrens Hospital of Los Angeles for the initial development and testing, especially as related to retinoblastoma, a multifocal pediatric eye cancer. The RetCam was introduced to the market in 1997 as a 120-degree

FIGURE 2-73
The field of view (FOV) as measured from the center of the eye.

wide-angle, hand-held, pediatric, contact, digital camera and has rapidly become the "standard of care" in the treatment of this rare disease.

The RetCam offers many advantages to retinoblastoma management. Its 120-degree FOV provides a reproducible and standardized way to "see the whole picture." By angling the camera, most of the retina can be covered with five images versus at least 30 narrow FOV montaged images. Thus, it facilitates the imaging of large or multiple retinoblastoma tumors, or both, illustrating their spatial relationships to one another (Figure 2-75). With a real-time display and a large depth of focus, physicians can make immediate critical judgments about changes in tumor status between visits. The camera is easy to use and, by applying scleral depression, it is also possible to image out to the ora serrata.

The immediacy and convenience of digital documentation has also opened up the opportunities for exploring the benefits of teleconferencing and telescreening other pediatric ophthalmic diseases. Subsequently, peripheral retinal development in retinopathy of prematurity (ROP) has become a large application for the RetCam (Figure 2-76). Feasibility studies are currently under way internationally to assess its role in ROP screening.[31] Additionally, documentation of the widespread retinal hemorrhages evident in shaken baby syndrome has augmented ophthalmic examinations as an important medical and legal tool (Figure 2-77).

RetCam images are produced through a hand-held image capture unit (ICU) attached to a computer assembly on a mobile cart. The patient is in the supine position for imaging while the lens tip of the RetCam comes into contact with the surface of the cornea after instillation of topical anesthesia. A coupling gel, such as methylcellulose, or a gel formula of artificial tears is applied as a cushion between the cornea and the RetCam. The dry eye gel is a thicker consistency than methylcellulose whereby the camera tip remains coupled within it even if angled slightly and is comfortable to the patient postprocedure. The user controls the illumination and focusing. A footswitch captures the image previewed on the computer screen.

FIGURE 2-74
The RetCam 120 system is comprised of the following devices assembled on a mobile cart:
(a) A high-resolution 17-in. monitor, mouse/trackball and keyboard; (b) image capture unit (ICU)—the hand-held camera handpiece incorporates optics with a 3-CCD video camera; (c) lenses (also known as *nosepieces*, are attached by a bayonet mount); i. = standard children's lens; ii = premature infant lens; iii = high magnification lens; iv = portrait lens. (d) light control unit—contains a halogen illumination source, a 3-CCD camera control unit, and circuitry for the footswitch controls. A fiberoptic cable extends from this unit to the ICU handpiece. A British naval connector at the back of the unit provides the connection of other video devices; (e) image processing unit (IPU)—this is a Windows NT computer system currently equipped with an internal DVD RAM drive employing 5.2 GB double-sided DVD RAM discs for storage media. Older versions of the system have 650 MB PC/CD drives installed. A standard floppy drive, a 100-mb Zip drive, a high-speed modem, and an Ethernet connection provide options for transmission of information; (f) uninterruptable power supply (UPS)—protects against the loss of data caused during power surges or interruption of power and will sustain the monitor and IPU for approximately 5 minutes. This allows the RetCam system to be moved without shutting down the system; (g) footswitch—controls focusing, illumination and image capture; (h) power conditioner—protects the RetCam 120 system from powerline disturbances. Hardware options include (i)—printer: produces small 3.5 × 4.5 dye sublimation prints for the chart or patient teaching; (j) fluorescein system—separate illumination source that provides the excitation light.
(Image courtesy of Massie Research Laboratories, Inc., Dublin, CA.)

FIGURE 2-75
A. Two retinoblastoma tumors in the same fundus: one is active (*asterisk*) and the other has been treated with laser (L). **B.** Large multifocal retinoblastoma tumors showing activity surrounding calcification (*short arrows*). **C, D.** Large cystic exophytic tumor in the right eye causing a retinal detachment. Nasal to the nerve, the scalloped edge of ora (O) can be seen using scleral depression. (ON = optic nerve.)

FIGURE 2-76
Retinopathy of prematurity.

FIGURE 2-77
Multiple hemorrhages in shaken baby syndrome.

FIGURE 2-78
Wide field of view (FOV) of an active retinoblastoma tumor (*arrow*) and laser scars (*asterisk*). The original image illustrates the FOV of the preemie 130-degree lens. The black inside line indicates the FOV of the 120-degree standard baby lens. High-magnification 30-degree lens detailing the active retinoblastoma tumor (*arrow*).

Interchangeable lenses, also known as *nosepiece*s, are attached to the ICU by a bayonet mount. The current assortment of lenses are the 120-degree standard baby lens (Figure 2-78), the 130-degree preemie lens, also known as the *ROP lens*, 30-degree high magnification lens, and a portrait lens. All lenses except for the portrait lens have a smooth concave tip that comes in contact with the cornea. Additionally, the tip of the preemie lens is slightly smaller than the standard baby lens, permitting better camera/cornea contact in small eyes. It can be applied to infants and older children to facilitate a 130-degree FOV, although in these patients there may be an increase in optical haze using this lens. A high-magnification lens (which works on adults as well as children) is optimized for imaging the optic disc or macula, or both. In addition to documenting the face and eyes, the portrait lens can document associated skin lesions and medical procedures, image chart information, and capture computed tomography and magnetic resonance imaging scans (after being placed on a light box).

Many adult retinal diseases could benefit from wide-field photography, but the RetCam is not an ideal instrument for this purpose. To illuminate the periphery of the retina, the camera projects light across the crystalline lens of the eye. This requires the patient to have a clear anatomic lens, a condition usually met only with children. A combination of the optical design of the camera as well as age-related changes in the adult crystalline lens and vitreous produces a hazy view in the older population.

The video camera inside the ICU is a 3-CCD device, producing 72 dpi, 640×480 resolution images. The images are captured directly to the storage media (PD/CDs or DVD Ram) with an associated header (.hdr) file containing the patient and visit information required by the RetCam software. Images are saved in the bitmap (.bmp) format, are more than 900 k in size, and easily importable into standard software programs such as Powerpoint and Photoshop. Once the appropriate information is entered into the patient registration screen, the user moves to the capture mode where a live image of the camera input can be viewed on monitor.

Individual images can be enhanced with contrast, brightness, and color correction in the image processing menu. A limited drawing and measuring palate is available. Images that have been manipulated can be stored elsewhere ("save as"), leaving the original untouched. A delete/transfer function allows the user to view nine images simultaneously, similar to a contact sheet. The user can identify images he or she would like copied elsewhere or those he or she wants to delete. The delete function in this menu does not actually delete images, but only hides them from view, thus no space is actually saved on the storage media using this feature.

RetCam Imaging Procedure

Although the RetCam is an easy device to learn how to use, keeping a few elements in mind may decrease the learning curve. The following is a step-by-step procedure for performing wide-field pediatric fundus photography using the RetCam.

Preparing the System

1. Turn on the system starting first with the power conditioner, followed by the uninterrupted power supply, the computer, and then the light control unit (LCU).
2. Insert the appropriate storage media into the computer.
3. Review chart or notes and select an appropriate lens. Attach it securely to the camera and wipe the tip clean (see Artifacts).
4. Input the patient name to the database and prepare the software to start a new session of image capture.
5. Have anesthetic drops, coupling gel, a lid speculum, scleral depressor and tissues close by.
6. Have extra storage media formatted and ready to use if the software shows that the active one is close to full.

The User

Operator comfort and safety are important in obtaining images.

1. Practice universal precautions of hand washing and using gloves, mask and safety clothing as needed.
2. Sit, if possible, keeping the RetCam unit and footswitch within comfortable reach.
3. Place yourself at the head of the supine patient and position the RetCam system so you are comfortably facing the monitor. Avoid dramatically twisting your back and neck.
4. Minimize distracting glare and reflections on the monitor.

5. After inserting topical anesthetic and a lid speculum, apply a moderate amount of coupling gel to either the tip of the lens or to the cornea of the patient.
6. When applying the camera to the eye, hold it close to the tip of the camera lens to provide maximum maneuverability and control.
7. Gently rest the base of the hand that is holding the camera on the patient for stability.
8. Reduce the weight of the ICU by draping the fiberoptic cable over your shoulders.

Camera Orientation

Maintaining the correct orientation of the ICU is necessary for images that document disease progression. The fiberoptic cable attached to the ICU should be at the 12:00 o'clock position of the supine patient's head. For example, if the photographer is sitting at the head of an operating room bed, the cable should drape from the ICU over the top of the patient's forehead toward the user.

Using the Footswitch

While the user observes the real-time image on the monitor, focusing, illumination and image capture are controlled using a footswitch. It has two rocker-style pedals. The right pedal controls light intensity: The light intensity increases when rocked to the right, and decreases when rocked to the left. The left pedal controls focusing and image capture: When depressed on the left side, an image is captured and stored. The right side of the left pedal controls focusing: When depressed once, focusing travels in one direction. Depressed again, focusing travels in the opposite direction.

Coordinating the focus and image capture requires practice. When beginning, consider asking an assistant to control the buttons on the front of the LCU, which also performs these functions. With practice, you will become better acquainted with the footswitch.

The point of focus varies between each of the auxiliary lenses. When switching between lenses, the focal plane could lie within the crystalline lens in the mid-vitreous or beyond the retina. Sometimes, it is difficult to know in which direction to depress the footswitch to achieve clarity, and the time required to reestablish recognizable ocular structures can seem long. After changing a lens, bring the examination room in focus before re-applying the camera to the eye. This sets the focal plane to the approximate level necessary for fundus imaging. Only minor focusing refinements will be required.

Imaging

Below is a description of four clinical scenarios that require pediatric RetCam imaging. Each situation requires a slightly different approach.

Awake Older Children

Children of any age can be challenging to image when awake. RetCam imaging of children between the ages of 1 and 5 years is usually distressing to the patient and not often successful without sedation. Children older than the age of 4 or 5 years require a great deal of positive reinforcement. Explain the procedure in simple terms to the patient and parents. Topical anesthetic is required, and time must be taken after instillation to let the child settle, as these drops do sting slightly. Sometimes to win their favor you can direct the camera at them or their parents so they can see themselves on the monitor. The imaging proce-

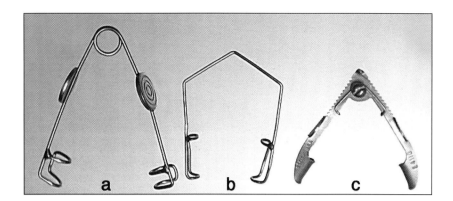

FIGURE 2-79
A variety of pediatric speculi: **(A)** Alfonso, **(B)** Barraquer, **(C)** Sauer. (Image by Cynthia Vandenhoven using the RetCam.)

dure is performed with the patient reclined on a chair or a stretcher. The instillation of a lid speculum may undo the trust you have just gained, so we suggest gently holding the eyelids open. Either the RetCam user or an assistant can hold the lids open. An overhead fixation light or target is helpful in directing the patient's gaze. As the camera comes in contact with the globe, the patient will have the tendency to look away from the bright illumination light and will usually require direction and encouragement to maintain appropriate fixation.

AWAKE INFANTS AND NEONATES

Awake infants and neonates must be bundled or papoosed to restrain their limbs, with their head gently but securely held by an assistant. Parting the lids manually is not possible due to the small size of the eyes combined with moisture from tears and coupling gel. An eyelid speculum is therefore essential after topical anesthetic, but this often causes distress to the child when first inserted. The child's soother may calm him or her during the procedure. Inform the parents of the need for a speculum, and give them the option of observing the procedure or exiting until it is finished.

Based on the size of the child, select a speculum that does not spread the lids too aggressively yet allows for the tip of the camera to come in contact with the cornea (Figure 2-79). Neonates undergoing imaging for ROP have tiny eyelid fissures, so the design of some speculum blades can limit the camera-cornea interface.[31] The RetCam preemie interchangeable lens features a slightly smaller tip and slightly wider FOV, which facilitates better camera/cornea contact.

Insertion of a lid speculum may induce a more pronounced Bell phenomenon, requiring the globe to be rotated down to adequately photograph the posterior pole. Nurseries may require an individually sterilized lid speculum and scleral depressor for each infant's examination to prevent the spread of infection. A neonatal scleral depressor or small squint hook are two instruments used to manipulate the globe of neonates.[32,33] It is introduced into the conjunctival fornix after topical anesthesia is applied. It is important to have your ophthalmologist teach you the finer techniques of this procedure.

When imaging neonates in the nursery, conditions can be warm, brightly lit, and the incubator, infusion lines and ventilation devices may hamper access to the infant. The attending nurse who is aware of the infant's medical status should handle the child.

SEDATION

Topical anesthetic is required for sedated patients. Although asleep, they are still sensitive to sensation and can stir at the instillation of drops, rotating or indenting the globe, and bright light. Periodically their eyes

FIGURE 2-80
Wide-field fluorescein angiogram of a retinoblastoma tumor.

may drift upward or downward, especially as the sedation is wearing off. Instead of manually rotating the eye, which may wake the patient, it sometimes helps to turn their head to the side and back facing upward again in a doll's head maneuver.[33] The eyes will remain centered for a short period after this maneuver.

GENERAL ANESTHESIA

Children under general anesthesia are the easiest group to photograph in terms of compliance. Topical anesthetic is not required for these patients. They can withstand globe manipulations; therefore, images beyond the equator out to the ora are easily achieved by applying scleral indentation and tilting the ICU.

Special Considerations

Minor local complications, such as subconjunctival hemorrhages, may occur during routine manipulation of the globe.[34] Additionally, be aware of and avoid arterial pulsations within the nerve. It is easy to become engrossed in indenting and focus on peripheral pathology and forget about watching for pulsations within the nerve on the other side of the screen. These pulsations indicate that too much pressure is being placed on the eye. The amount and length of time the eyeball is indented can cause the intraocular pressure to rise to the degree that ocular circulation is compromised.

The oculo-cardiac reflex refers to a slowing in cardiac rate (bradycardia), which results from various ocular stimuli, particularly undue pressure on the eye and traction on the extraocular muscles. It has been reported that bradycardias can be elicited in ROP babies by the stimulus of screening examinations that include the instillation of drops, speculum insertion and globe rotation.[34,35] RetCam imaging also requires these elements, therefore it is important to be aware of neonates who are being "too quiet" during the process.

Wide-Field Fluorescein Angiography

It is possible to perform wide-field fluorescein angiography using the RetCam (Figure 2-80). Steps involved are somewhat different than a traditional study.

1. Start a new session on the RetCam and select the fluorescein option.
2. Insert the barrier filter between the lens and the ICU by removing the lens and placing the filter into the hole inside the lighting ring.
3. Replace the lens. Position, focus and capture an image of either eye. The image has a yellow cast when seen live on the monitor. The

software converts stored images to monochromatic for storage and viewing.

4. Set the illumination to maximum using the control knob on the fluorescein light box. The footswitch will not control the fluorescein light intensity, as it is only connected to the standard LCU. It may be required to modify this setting as the fluorescein progresses.

5. Move the fiberoptic cable from the regular LCU to the fluorescein light source. You will see the typical blue glow coming out of the tip of the camera lens. Once the fiberoptic cable is plugged into the fluorescein unit, the view of the fundus is lost until fluorescein appears in the eye. It is helpful to have a second person adjust the cable for you, as it is difficult to check your positioning if you inadvertently move.

6. Begin the test. Have an assistant start the timer button on the screen to time stamp images as the fluorescein is injected. When viewing the live fluorescein sequence on the monitor, the images are green, just as they are through the ocular of a fundus camera. Fluorescein dosage is reduced for children based on body weight. The calculation can be found on the drug information enclosure within a box of fluorescein. Dioptic Laboratories, for example, recommends 35 mg of fluorescein per 10 lb (4.5 kg) body weight as printed on their insert. On young children, instead of a direct injection done simultaneously with the start of a fluorescein, an intravenous line is first established in the back of the hand. This allows the child time to recover from the trauma of a needle puncture, at which point the dye can be pushed into the intravenous line to start the test. You will notice the hand-to-eye circulation may be somewhat longer than the standard arm-to-eye transit unless the arm is elevated.

7. Capture sequential images with the footswitch.

8. If switching RetCam lenses, secure the lens that has been removed to avoid dropping it. Also keep the ICU held in the upright position to avoid dropping the barrier filter before the second lens is fitted.

9. Replace the fiberoptic back into the original light box when the fluorescein session is finished, and turn off the power to conserve the bulb.

10. When reviewing the captured images, the RetCam software converts them from fluorescein green to 24-bit grayscale.

Artifacts

Contact wide-angle imaging shares selected artifacts with traditional fundus imaging but also has a few of its own. Although we try our best to eliminate them, the first step is to recognize them so they are not confused with actual pathology.

Dust

Even in a digital world, photographers have not escaped dust. Dust can collect at any location on the inner surface of RetCam lenses (Figure 2-81). The remedy is usually a very gentle tickle with a dustcloth-wrapped cotton applicator and a slight breeze of compressed air.

Bubbles

Just as in gonio photography, bubbles can degrade and confuse an image (Figure 2-82). Store your methylcellulose cap side down; empty film cans make an ideal storage unit. Try to apply the coupling gel in a bubble-free manner: squeeze the first drop onto a tissue, then, without releasing pressure on the bottle, apply to the cornea. When imaging awake infants,

FIGURE 2-81
Dust (*arrows*) on the inside of the lens.

FIGURE 2-82
A bubble in the coupling gel (*arrow*) can cause confusion with pathology such as retinoblastoma seeds (*asterisk*).

FIGURE 2-83
Persistent embryonal vessels (tunica vasculosa lentis) (*arrows*) and Y-shaped lens sutures (*asterisk*).

bubbles can be easily whipped up due to their rapid eye movements, especially if they are upset. This is often unavoidable, and sometimes the best solution is to keep reapplying the gel.

Poor View

Poor camera/cornea contact will prevent a good peripheral view. In neonates, it may help to change the speculum or use the preemie lens, which has a smaller diameter tip, or both. Inadequate amounts of coupling gel may also reduce the optical clarity of the camera/cornea interface.

Haze

Neonates may have persistent vessels on the lens (tunica vasculosa lentis), hyaloid vascular remnants (Figure 2-83), or corneal and vitreous haze,[34,35] each of which reduces contrast and clarity of images. Due to the camera optics, increased haze is also seen in dark pigmented fundi and in adults. Image clarity can also be compromised in children who are on life support, by the ointment applied to protect the cornea from exposure. Ocular lavage with normal saline may assist in obtaining clearer images.

FIGURE 2-84
A central shadow artifact resulting from poor pupil dilation hides the optic nerve in a patient with retinoblastoma.

FIGURE 2-85
Enlarged image of interlaced **(A)** and deinterlaced **(B)** artifact.

Central Shadow

The camera requires pupil dilation of at least 6 mm to provide optimum results. The preemie lens can see through a slightly smaller pupil aperture. Tiny pupils result in a central shadow artifact that can mask pathology. It may sometimes be possible to move the shadow away from the area of interest (Figure 2-84).

Movement Artifact

The method a video camera uses to show a picture on a screen is that it creates two scans of an image and transmits them consecutively at a rate that the human eye barely perceives. This is called *interlacing*. One scan is the odd-numbered lines of a picture and the other is the even lines.[36] Together, these two fields make up one picture (Figure 2-85). If there is extensive movement of the video subject, these two fields can become slightly separated at the time of image capture by the computer, thereby creating deinterlacing. Because the camera inside the RetCam ICU is a video camera, deinterlacing can occur if there is extensive movement by the patient or the photographer when an image is frozen. This results in images that may look out of focus or out of sync.

Care of the Unit

Like most ophthalmic photography equipment, the RetCam is a hearty investment: The following will help you keep it well maintained. Before moving the system, be sure the hand-held ICU is secure in the holster and that the tip of the lenses are periodically inspected for nicks or scratches. When switching interchangeable lenses, secure the removed lens to avoid dropping it. Optical fibers in the camera umbilical cord can easily break if kinked or bent. Do not wrap the cable tightly when storing the camera or compress the cable in any way. Conserve the bulb in the LCU by switching it off when not in use. It is highly recommended to eject the PD/CD or DVD when shutting down the system, as it reduces the time required for the system to start up. It also prevents the loss of data from bad sectors found on the storage media during system startup. Following these guidelines will decrease the need for expensive repairs, keep the user and the patient safe, and reduce the negative impact on patient care from downtime and the loss of patient data.

Cleaning the RetCam Lens

Because the RetCam 120 is a contact camera, care must be observed to avoid the spread of infection and disease between patients. Protocols for infection control may vary between institutions, therefore it is important to check local requirements. A basic guideline as recommended by the American Academy of Ophthalmology to follow is to wipe the tip with either diluted bleach or alcohol. Mechanical wiping is an essential part of the process and if bleach is used, be absolutely certain that it is removed with sterile water before imaging a patient. Also, periodically wipe down the ICU and cart surfaces with disinfectant.

Conclusion

As the technology of wide-field imaging progresses, it continues to benefit both the patient and the ophthalmologist. It provides a new appreciation of ophthalmic pathology to ophthalmologists and students in training. The digital wide field of view offers screening opportunities and early detection of adult and pediatric disease. Collaborative treatment options are enhanced through telemedicine. Wide-field imaging provides the ophthalmic photographer with a valuable addition to his or her armamentarium of imaging devices, giving him or her a great deal of satisfaction in producing dramatic panoramic images.

References

1. Wilhelm H, Brower C. The Permanence and Care of Color Photographs: Traditional and Digital Color Prints, Color Negatives, Slides, and Motion Pictures. Grinnell, IA: Preservation Publishing, 1993;1.
2. Tyler M. A way to sharper ophthalmic photography through astigmatic correction for the photographer. J Ophthal Photog 1981;4:20.
3. Barry CJ. Angiography chairs allowing cardio-pulmonary resuscitation. J Ophthal Photog 1999;21:48.
4. Fishman M, Waxler M, Sliney DH, et al. Symposium on light toxicity and its meaning to ophthalmic photographers. J Ophthal Photog 1987;10:6.
5. Holladay JT. Optics, Refraction, and Contact Lenses, Basic and Clinical Science Course. San Francisco: American Academy of Ophthalmology, 1988;173.
6. Milder B, Rubin M. The Fine Art of Prescribing Glasses without Making a Spectacle of Yourself. Gainesville, FL: Triad Scientific Publishers, 1978;27.
7. Holladay JT. Optics, Refraction, and Contact Lenses, Basic and Clinical Science Course. San Francisco: American Academy of Ophthalmology, 1988;109.
8. Ducrey NM, Delori FC, Gragoudas ES. Monochromatic ophthalmoscopy and fundus photography. Arch Ophthalmol 1979;97:288.
9. Blaker A. Handbook for Scientific Photography. San Francisco: W.H. Freeman, 1977;97.
10. George TW, D'Anna SA. Comparison of retinal fundus cameras: user's survey results. Ophthalmology Instrument and Book Supplement 1983;90(Suppl):80.
11. Kelly MP. A superior method of achieving high myopic retinal focus. J Ophthal Photog 1995;17:66.
12. Schatz H, Burton T, Yannuzzi L, Rabb M. Interpretation of Fundus Fluorescein Angiography. St. Louis: Mosby, 1978;27.
13. Wong D. Textbook of Ophthalmic Photography. New York: Inter-Optics Publications, 1982;67.

14. Coppinger JM, Maio M, Miller K. Ophthalmic Photography. Thorofare, NJ: Slack, 1987;89.

15. Szirth BC, Murphee AL, McNamara W. Infant fundus photography. J Ophthal Photog 1985;8:30.

16. Montague PR, Weingeist TA. Monitoring AIDS-Related Cytomegalovirus Retinitis in Ganciclovir Therapy for Cytomegalovirus Infection by S.A. Spector. New York: Marcel Dekker, 1991;115–128.

17. Bursell SE, Cavallerano JD, Cavallerano AA, et al. Stereo nonmydriatic digital-video color retinal imaging compared with Early Treatment Diabetic Retinopathy Study seven standard field 35-mm stereo color photos for determining level of diabetic retinopathy. Ophthalmology 2001;108:572.

18. Busse B, Mittelman D. Use of the Astigmatism Correction Device on the Zeiss Fundus Camera for Peripheral Retinal Photography. In J Justice Jr (ed), Ophthalmic Photography. Boston: Little, Brown, 1982;69–76.

19. Chamberlin JA, Bressler NM, Bressler SB, et al. The use of fundus photographs and fluorescein angiograms in the identification and treatment of choroidal neovascularization in the macular photocoagulation study. Ophthalmology 1989;96:1526.

20. Delori FC, Gragoudas ES, Francisco R, Pruett RC. Monochromatic ophthalmoscopy and fundus photography: the normal fundus. Arch Ophthalmol 1977;95:861.

21. Ducrey NM, Delori FC, Gragoudas ES. Monochromatic ophthalmoscopy and fundus photography: the pathological fundus. Arch Ophthalmol 1979;97:288.

22. Barry CJ. Retinal nerve fiber layer photography: how widespread is it? J Ophthal Photog 1994;16:26.

23. Morton GV, Lucchese N, Kushner BJ. The role of funduscopy and fundus photography in strabismus diagnosis. Ophthalmology 1983;90:1186.

24. Martonyi CL, Bahn CF, Meyer RF. Clinical Slit Lamp Biomicroscopy and Photo Slit Lamp Biomicrography. Ann Arbor, MI: Time One Ink, 1985;53–63.

25. Clark T, Ozerdem U, Bartsch DU, et al. A simple non-contact wide angle fundus photography and fluorescein angiography procedure for clinical research. Investigative Opthalmology and Visual Sciences 2000;41(4):S139.

26. Mody CH, Farr R, Ferguson EL. A digital approach to wide field photomontages of the ocular fundus. Br J Ophthalmic Photog 2000;3:12–17.

27. Hackel R. Editor's letter/About the cover. J Ophthalmic Photog 1995;17:53.

28. Szirth BC, Good WV, Zarbin AM. The 35-year journey of the hand-held retinal camera. J Ophthalmic Photog 2000;22:64–68.

29. Pomerantzeff O, Govignon J. Design of a wide-angle ophthalmoscope. Arch Ophthal 1971;86:420–424.

30. Gilman JP. Wide-angle photography of the retinal periphery using the Rodenstock panfundoscope. J Ophthalmic Photog 1989;11:61–63.

31. Roth DB, Morales D, Feuer WJ, et al. Screening for retinopathy of prematurity employing the RetCam 120. Arch Ophthalmol 2001;119:268–272.

32. Lawes DE, Morton C, Weindling M, Clark D. Systemic effects of screening for retinopathy of prematurity. Br J Ophthalmol 1996:80:425–428.

33. Flynn JF, Tasman W. Retinopathy of Prematurity: A Clinician's Guide. New York: Springer-Verlag, 1992;39.

34. Dhillon B, Wright E, Fleck BW. Screening for retinopathy of prematurity: are a lid speculum and scleral indentation necessary? J Pediatr Ophthalmol Strabismus 1993:30:377–381.

35. Clarke WN, Hodges E, Noel LP, et al. The oculocardiac reflex during ophthalmoscopy in premature infants. Am Ophthalmol 1985; 99:649–651.

36. Saine PJ, Tyler ME. Ophthalmic Photography: A Textbook of Fundus Photography, Angiography and Electronic Imaging. Butterworth–Heinemann, 1997;219.

Chapter 3

Stereo Fundus Photography: Principles and Technique

Marshall E. Tyler

Introduction:
Stereo Fundus Imaging in Ophthalmic Photography

The ophthalmic photographer's ability to record accurate three-dimensional images is one of the most exciting capabilities in our profession. Stereo fundus photography permits clinical examination of the patient's pathology beyond the ordinary two-dimensional view of a conventional photograph. It is fascinating to be able to study an image of an optic nerve or a tumor, leaking fluorescein dye in the retina or staining indocyanine green in the choroid, without patient movement, and in three dimensions!

In stereo fundus photography, two slightly different images are created photographically and, when viewed, are fused by the brain. When you view the images, your left eye is presented with the left image, your right eye is presented with the right image, and your brain then recreates the depth relationships that were observed at the time of photography. If you

Terminology Note

The phrases used to describe a stereo image can be confusing. At times, a "stereo pair" is used to discuss two images that comprise a stereo image, whereas at other times you will see "a single stereo image" used to discuss the two images that make up the "stereo pair." Thus, though it may seem a bit confusing, "stereo pair" and "a (single) stereo image" mean the same thing.

have created the stereo photographs by a reproducible technique, they may also permit comparison of three-dimensional changes over time.

Many ophthalmologic photographers routinely expose all fundus images in stereo. Obtaining two exposures is a good idea in case a single image is not perfect. Therefore, why not provide extra information by taking them as a stereo pair? Accept the challenge: Photograph every fundus in stereo and you will find—literally—a new dimension in fundus photography.

First, the history of stereo ophthalmic photography is reviewed. Although some stereo history is just plain fun, some of it is important to fully understanding how to create excellent stereo images. To start our adventure in stereo imaging, Timothy Martin, MD, discusses Stereo Perception—how we see in stereo. Next, the two methods of stereo fundus photography—sequential and simultaneous—are discussed. This is followed by an exploration of stereo viewing techniques and then a short discussion of the future of stereo imaging.

Historical Review of Stereoscopic Fundus Photography

Although stereoscopic vision was first described by the Greek mathematician Euclid (280 BC), it was not until the 1830s that Charles Wheatstone (inventor of the linear motor and concertina) described a device for the stereoscopic display of visual information (Figure 3-1).[1] Wheatstone's first experiments were limited to drawings, as the photographic media of his time, daguerreotypes, were difficult to illuminate evenly. In 1850, David Brewster developed a more practical stereoscope, one that used lenses for the direct viewing of photographs placed in a darkened box (Figure 3-2).[2] Stereo viewing became a popular parlor pastime in Victorian England after Brewster introduced his lenticular stereoscope at the Great Exhibition of 1851.[3] It was popularized in the United States after Oliver Wendell Holmes, Sr. (physician, poet, and essayist) described (but did not patent) the familiar Holmes stereoscope (Figure 3-3).[1] Among the many types of stereo cards that were published was an elaborate set of fundus paintings in stereo.[4]

Early fundus photography (see Chapter 1) was such a technical challenge that the first stereoscopic photographs (by Thorner[5]) were not published until 1909 (Figure 3-4). Thorner's stereo technique included an elaborate scheme for flipping the camera upside down between exposures. A more practical sequential technique involving side-to-side shifting was described by Metzger in 1926.[6] Better stereoscopic fundus photographs (but without technical explanation) are contained in Bedell's 1929 atlas, the first atlas to include stereoscopic images.[7]

In 1939, a physician and a photographer, Louis Bothman, MD, and Reuel W. Bennett, created a fundus atlas, *Stereoscopic Photographs of the Fundus Oculi*.[8] It included 50 stereo cards printed on photographic paper. The images had been taken with the Nordensen fundus camera. In 1954, Blodi and Allen published a stereoscopic atlas using View-Master reels.[9]

Other methods for sequential stereo imaging were attempted in the early 1960s. Stenstrom described the rotation of the fundus camera about the pivot point,[10] but this technique ignored cornea-induced parallax, which, by itself, optically creates a "convergence view" of the fundus and resulted in non-stereo images that were difficult to fuse. Allen used the technique of shifting the fundus camera laterally and later created a stereo separator using a solenoid to control the angling of an optical flat (plano-lens): As the glass flipped between two positions, the optical axis

A

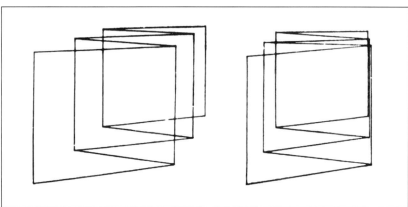

B

FIGURE 3-1
This diagram of Wheatstone's stereoscope **(A)** illustrates his use of mirrors to view stereoscopic drawings **(B)**. (Reprinted with permission from J Jones. Wonders of the Stereoscope. New York: Knopf, 1976.)

FIGURE 3-2
A variation of Brewster's stereoscope is used daily by ophthalmic photographers on light tables around the world. (Reprinted with permission from J Jones. Wonders of the Stereoscope. New York: Knopf, 1976.)

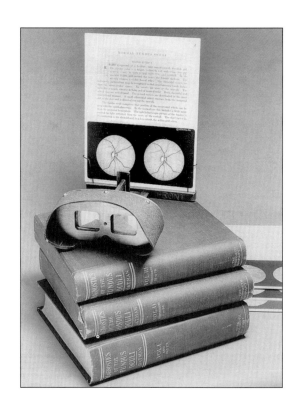

FIGURE 3-3
The inexpensive Holmes stereoscope used "half-lenses" and displayed 80-mm–wide photographs. It is shown here with a card from the collection "Diagnostics of the Fundus Oculi."

A

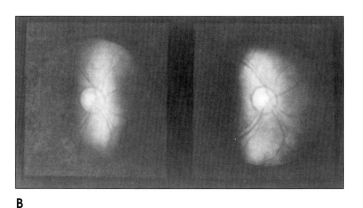

B

FIGURE 3-4
Thorner's sequential stereo fundus camera **(A)**. Thorner published the first stereoscopic fundus photographs **(B)** in 1909. Illumination is uneven, as with most Thorner fundus photographs. (Reprinted with permission from W Thorner. Die stereoskopische photographie des augenhintesgrundes. Klin Monatsbl f Augenh 1927;78:338.)

of the fundus camera was displaced laterally by a fixed amount.[11] The next section describes the use of this device.

Norton's 1953 fundus camera, based on the indirect ophthalmoscope, introduced simultaneous stereo fundus photography[12,13] but never became commercially available. A more practical design was developed by David Donaldson and Harold Edgerton (Massachusetts Institute of Technology optical engineer and photographer who perfected the modern stroboscope) in 1964. Their stereo fundus camera used two prisms, which split the light from a single front lens element and directed it to two different frames of film (Figure 3-5).[14] Variations of this design remain in use today. Simultaneous stereo imaging is an important factor for visually or electronically comparing and analyzing stereo photographs.

A

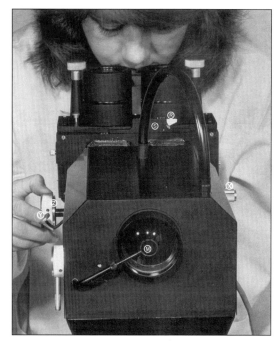

B

FIGURE 3-5
Donaldson's simultaneous stereo fundus camera.
A. Dr. Donaldson with his stereo fundus camera.
B. Front/top view of camera. **C.** Cross section of
camera optics. (Reprinted with permission from the
Operating Instructions for the Donaldson
Simultaneous Stereoscopic Fundus Camera.)

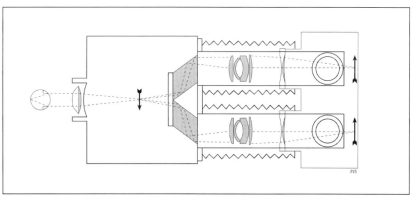

C

Stereo Perception

Timothy J. Martin

The eye, not unlike a camera, is equipped to focus light rays on a light-sensitive substrate. The retina plays the role of the film and is responsible for mapping the formed images. Otherwise, the dynamic, interactive characteristics of the living eye, coupled with the complexities of retinal and cortical visual processing, are quite different from the static interpretation offered by even the finest cameras. Even so, the retina and photographic film share a common limitation: They can only provide a two-dimensional map of the three-dimensional world. Photographers, artists, and one-eyed people will be quick to add that there are many depth clues encoded in a single, flat image (Table 3-1), but the most immediate and elaborate sense of depth requires both images from two different vantage points (i.e., two eyes) but also the neural processing that produces stereopsis.

Stereopsis (from the Greek word *stereos* meaning "solid," hence "solid vision") is the ability of the brain to reconstruct a true sense of depth from

Table 3-1. Monocular Depth Clues

Apparent size: The known size of an ordinary object can be compared to its apparent size (if it appears smaller, it must be farther away).

Interposition: An object must be forward if it blocks the view of others.

Aerial perspective: Distant objects appear more hazy, less distinct.

Shading: Objects farther from the light source may be shaded by those nearer.

Geometric perspective: Just as parallel railroad tracks seem to converge to a vanishing point the distance spacing appears closer, more crowded in the distance.

Relative velocity: Distant objects appear to move slower than near objects at the same speed.

Motion parallax: Movement of the observer produces greater apparent motion of near rather than distant objects.

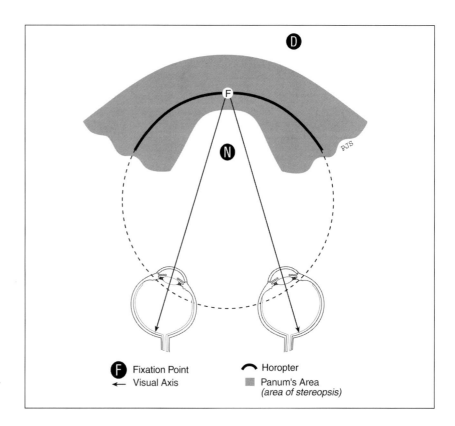

FIGURE 3-6
Schematic representation of Panum's area and its relationship to important components in the physiology of stereopsis. Physiologic diplopia would be present for objects D and N, both lying outside Panum's area (not to scale).

the flat images transmitted from the two eyes. The physiology of depth perception is extraordinarily complex. This discussion provides an understanding of the basic physiologic tenets and provides a foundation for many practical aspects of stereo photography and stereo viewing.

When the eyes are directed at an object in space, the fovea of each eye is trained on that object (Figure 3-6). If the object is at infinity, the visual axes of the two eyes are parallel. For a near object, the eyes (separated horizontally in the adult face by approximately 65 mm) must turn in, or converge, in order to place the object on each fovea. At the same time, the shape of the lens in each eye must change to produce a shorter focal length (accommodation) to focus the near object. This neural linkage of convergence and accommodation, along with miosis (which is a decrease in the pupillary aperture) make up the synkinetic near triad. However, the "effort" required to focus an object provides only a coarse estimate of distance and thus contributes little to stereopsis.

Through a common fixation point (the intersection of the two visual axes), one can construct a curved surface on which any point would be

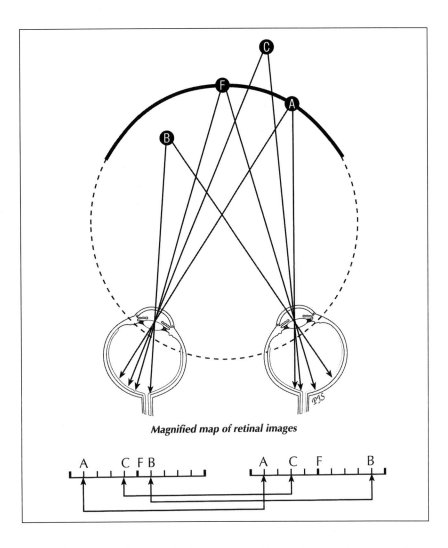

Magnified map of retinal images

FIGURE 3-7
Retinal images of objects on and around the horopter (not to scale). F is the fixation object; lines connecting this object to the fovea of each eye represent the visual axis. The retinal images formed by objects A, B, and C are mapped on a scale to show their position on each retina (relative to the fovea), with the resultant interpretation of retinal disparity as depth. Point A maps precisely to corresponding points on each retina. Thus, A is on the horopter and is the same distance from the observer as the fixation point F. Point B is shifted temporally and thus is perceived as being closer to the first viewer. Point C also maps to different locations; as it is shifted nasally, it is perceived as being farther away from the observer than F (not to scale).

focused or mapped to precisely corresponding points on the two retinas. This surface is the horopter, often simplified as a curved line in the horizontal plane (Figure 3-7). For example, a point 4 degrees to the right of fixation on the horopter would be imaged on each retina precisely 4 degrees to the left of each fovea (point A in Figure 3-7). Any points lying in front of this surface would not fall the same distance from each fovea, but would be shifted temporally on each retina. Any points beyond the horopter would be shifted nasally, again to noncorresponding retinal points. The further from the horopter, the greater is the retinal disparity. The complex neural circuitry associated with vision is capable of synthesizing depth information from these disparate images, giving the sensation of stereopsis.

However, beyond a certain distance on either side of the horopter, the brain cannot cope with the disparity, and an image becomes double rather than being perceived as a single object in three-dimensional space. This limit of stereopsis defines a curved space, represented for simplicity in the horizontal plane as Panum's area (see Figure 3-6). The shape and size of the horopter and Panum's area vary with the viewing distance, the distance between the two eyes (or cameras), the firmness of fixation, and an individual's own stereoscopic abilities. Given the constraints of Panum's area, we are subjected to many objects in virtually every view of our environment, which results in "physiologic diplopia." (Physiologic diplopia can be experienced by focusing on the thumb of an outstretched arm, while noticing an object more distant, and vice versa.) Cortical processing is very effective in suppressing the awareness of this ever-present diplopia.[15]

Because this sense of depth is essentially resynthesized from disparate two-dimensional maps from each eye, one can understand how a synthetic sense of depth can be created by appropriately produced two-dimensional images presented simultaneously but independently to each eye. To achieve fusion, there must be enough similarity in the two images for the eyes to "agree" on fixation points, and to achieve stereopsis; the disparity of image components must not exceed the limits of Panum's area, because the parameters of the horopter and Panum's area are dependent on apparent nearness (via the synkinetic triad), and the amount of convergence and accommodation required to view these images should also be within the normal physiologic range.

Not everyone can synthesize depth. An obvious exception would be the observer who has only one seeing eye. The mechanism responsible for this complex phenomenon forms during early childhood and is not always entirely successful. The developing visual system must meet a number of challenges for success: clear, equal vision in both eyes, with both eyes capable of being pointed precisely at the object of regard. Keeping one's eyes properly aligned (orthophoric) requires precise feedback (clear images), as well as intact machinery (working muscles and nerves) to make appropriate adjustments in eye position. Fusion is achieved when the brain can successfully use the images from the two eyes to "lock" the visual axis of each eye onto the object of interest. A poorly seeing eye that cannot achieve fusion has trouble keeping alignment, causing a "sensory" strabismus, as no feedback is available to check the eye's position in space. Poorly seeing eyes tend to drift, often becoming exotropic (turned out). On the other hand, nerve or muscle deficiencies in eye positioning ("motor" strabismus) make fusion difficult and cause two completely different images to be presented to the brain; because the machinery cannot move the eyes to eliminate this disparity, diplopia and confusion may result. The visual system in young children may overcome this intolerable state by "turning off" one eye. If the inactivation becomes chronic, the neglected eye never develops normal vision and becomes amblyopic.

Profound amblyopia or overt strabismus precludes stereopsis, but stereopsis is not an all-or-none phenomenon. The power of an individual's stereopsis can be estimated by noting the minimal retinal disparity required for that individual to perceive depth. A common clinical assessment uses polarized glasses and the Titmus stereo test (see Figure 3-37). The subject is required to identify which of four circles appears elevated, using nine images of increasing difficulty. Mild amblyopia or small-angle strabismus may allow good fusion, but crippled stereopsis.[16] In short, many people (including some photographers and ophthalmologists) may not be able to appreciate the full sense of the depth conveyed in stereo photographs.

Stereo photography—no matter how cleverly performed—cannot convey the same visual experience as the "real thing." If the photographs are high quality, taken from ideally disparate positions, and viewed with a device that creates the optimal amount of physiologic accommodation and convergence, then what is missing? First, in viewing a real three-dimensional object, the fixation point is not confined to a specific plane as defined by a photograph but is dynamically varied by the viewer in all three dimensions of space. Also, the viewer can vary the viewing distance, which will alter convergence and accommodation factors and dynamically optimize Panum's space, giving additional depth clues. As in monocular parallax, stereopsis may be greatly enhanced by side-to-side movements of the viewer's head, and this full stereo effect can only be approximated photographically with holography. However, despite these shortcomings, creating a stereo photograph often provides visual information the sum of which is far greater than its parts.

Instrumentation and Technique

Stereo fundus photography and angiography are specialized forms of stereo photography. The understanding of typical stereo photography and special considerations of macro-stereo-photography is addressed first. The methods of achieving optimal sequential stereo images are covered next. Then specialized timing techniques for stereo angiography as well as advanced stereo techniques are discussed. Finally, the advantages of simultaneous stereo imaging are extolled.

Stereo Photography—Basic Principles

Stereo photography creates two images of the same subject taken from two positions—that of the photographer's left eye and that of the photographer's right eye. After being processed, the images are then presented to the appropriate eye for viewing, and the viewer's brain re-creates the three-dimensional view. The goal of this process is to re-create the image as if the viewer were at the site of the photography. Images should be viewed parallel to the visual plane (Figure 3-8) to introduce the least amount of distortion in the film.

In conventional stereo photographs, the optical systems are kept parallel to each other and perpendicular to the plane of the subject. The horizontal distance between the two optical systems is the stereo base (Figure 3-9). The greater the stereo base, the greater is the stereo effect. The stereo base for realistic stereo images focused at infinity is 70 mm, the average intraocular distance.

Distortion of (deviation from) the subject's original dimensions occurs when the subject is photographed from different positions (Figure 3-10). A photographic subject that is relatively flat in elevation is sometimes photographed with cameras in which the lenses and film planes are rotated and aimed at a single point on the subject (Figure 3-10B). Flatness, or elevation, is the relative distance from the near-point of the subject to the far-point anywhere in the picture. This technique creates some image distortion, which makes the stereo image pairs more difficult to fuse and thus to view (Figure 3-11). This disparity can be minimal if the subject is relatively flat, and the center of the image is the prime

FIGURE 3-8
Conventional stereo photographic technique has all of the optics and imaging planes parallel to the subject. The stereo base, the separation between the optics, is held constant throughout the optical system.

A

B

C

FIGURE 3-9
Nonophthalmic stereo cameras. **A.** Realist stereo camera. **B.** Optical system of Realist stereo camera. **C.** Stereo slide in a Realist mount.

FIGURE 3-10
In stereo macro-photography, the subject will not be imaged squarely on the film **(A)** as the subject is very close in relationship to the stereo base distance between the optical center of the lenses. To compensate for the closeness of the subject, the lenses are sometimes rotated **(B)**, minimally, to have the same subject imaged on the film.

A

B

A

B

FIGURE 3-11
Image distortion is created when the camera is rotated to look at the same subject. These photographs (*upper pairs*) show **(A)** a block photographed with a lateral shift of the camera—keeping the film parallel to the subject plane of focus. In the second set of images **(B)**, the camera is rotated about the subject—keeping the subject centered in the frame. The lower pairs of images show the cropped results of these two techniques. Note that in the lateral shift photographs **(A)** the top and bottom line of the block are parallel and, in the image with camera rotation **(B)**, the horizontal lines of the block are closer together in the image where the block is further from the camera. This rotation technique makes the stereo of a deep image harder to fuse. This, however, is the photographic technique that we use in corneal-induced parallax photography.

point of interest. This technique also can be used to increase the stereo effect (increased stereo base). When photographing close-up subjects, any detail in the background produces a double image and makes the stereo pair hard to fuse. However, there is no part of the ophthalmic fundus "subject" visible in the far distance.

Stereo Fundus Photography

The technique used in fundus photography takes advantage of the smallness of the subject, the flatness of the subject, the lack of a distant subject, and, most important, the anatomy of the normal human eye. This close-up macro-photography technique is easily accomplished by using the optics of the human eye (Figure 3-12).

Most modern mydriatic fundus cameras are capable of producing sequential stereo images—that is, taking one image of a stereo pair and then the other. Precise techniques are needed to create clinical image pairs of the highest quality with the least stress to the patient.

The requirements for camera positioning are evaluated from the perspective of the optical systems that are in front of the subject—that is, cornea, lens, and retina. Understanding the optical systems makes it easier for the photographer to achieve consistent stereo images. Light rays traced from a single point on the human fundus are imaged by the eye's optical components at a distant point, perhaps even at infinity. It is this phenomenon that permits corneal-induced parallax stereo photography to image the same point of the fundus from two vantage points.

Convergence (rotation of the camera viewpoint) around the subject occurs inside the patient's eye, because the optics of the eye is being used when taking the fundus photographs. Convergence is permitted in macro-photography (typical magnification of 1–25×) with a subject of a limited depth, such as the eye.

Sequential Stereo Fundus Photography

ALLEN STEREO TECHNIQUE

Lee Allen,[11] in 1964, described the technique that most ophthalmic photographers now use for achieving sequential stereo fundus photographs. Positioning of the camera for stereo fundus photography starts in the same manner as for monocular fundus photography. The camera is first shifted slightly to the left and then to the right of the central position, the stereo pair being thus exposed at each position (Fig. 3-13).

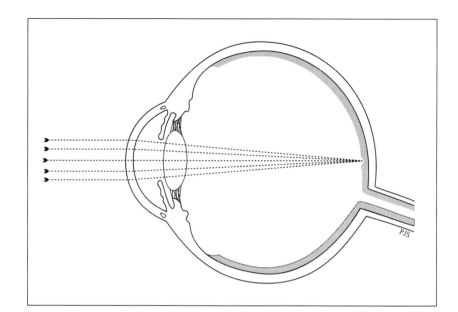

FIGURE 3-12
The eye in cross section showing parallel light (focused at infinity) converging on a single point on the fundus. Imaging rays coming from the patient's fundus also produce similar parallel rays of light. A fundus camera pointed at any portion of the pupil records an image of the same part of the fundus. Sliding the camera simply records the fundus from a different vantage point.

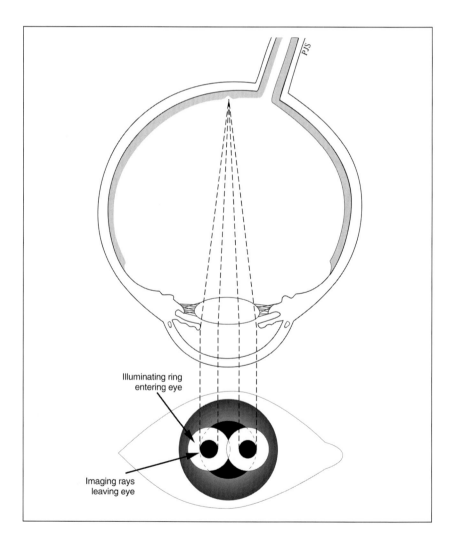

FIGURE 3-13
Stereo fundus imaging. Two fundus photographs are required to make a stereo pair. The diagram shows the pupillary positioning of the two image areas (*small dark circles*) and the fundus camera's doughnut of illuminating light for stereo fundus photography.

FIGURE 3-14
Illumination positions through a dilated pupil. A monocular photograph results when you center the illuminating ring in the pupil **(A)**. A small stereo separation **(B)** reproduces a minimal stereo effect (hypostereo) in the final photographs and, with images, will be evenly illuminated. Shifting each view slightly to each respective side **(C)** creates a crescent-shaped artifact. Further shifting to each side, past the crescent artifact, produces a wide-based stereo pair **(D)**. Notice that the images are unevenly illuminated due to amputation of the illuminating ring. Further sideways camera movement reduces both the illuminating and imaging light rays, resulting in an underexposed image that cannot be used **(E)**.

There are multiple locations where the fundus camera's doughnut of light (see Figure 2-21) can be positioned for stereo fundus photography. Factors influencing the choice of positioning include pupillary dilation, the desired stereo base, and media opacities.

Photographers with 30-degree cameras have found that another view of the fundus can be seen after going beyond (side-to-side) the area where iris reflections form a bright yellow–light colored, crescent-shaped, artifact. By sliding the camera laterally, you can see the bright crescent reflex followed by another clear image. Because the latter image is taken through the peripheral cornea, its quality (sharpness and evenness of illumination) may not be as good as that of the images obtained centrally, but it will greatly increase the stereo base of your photographs. The peripheral cornea may introduce corneal-induced astigmatism into the optical system, but this can be compensated for with astigmatic correction.[17] Illumination may also be decreased or uneven, or both, because part of the illuminating doughnut of light does not enter the pupil (Figure 3-14).

FIGURE 3-15
Three positioning methods for stereo fundus photography. Positioning both illuminating beams inside the dilated pupil results in minimal stereo **(A)** but may be necessary in patients with peripheral opacities of the media. Central camera placement maximizes image quality: The central and a right or a left partner **(B)** can create your stereo pair. This choice provides a minimal stereo base but may permit stereo photography when there is a localized opacity of the media that would interfere with an image pair taken with the desired stereo **(C)**.

Media opacities in the peripheral lens may limit your stereo base (Figure 3-15), but a stereo pair with minimal stereo information is often preferable to a single good monocular image.

If your images are exposed in a consistent order for each patient, then editing is easier. For a glaucoma patient, a routine photographic sequence might be the following—Right eye: disc-left image, disc-right image, repeat this pair, macula-left image, macula-right image; left eye: repeat for left disc and macula. This provides a backup set of stereo disc images in case of a patient blink.

REPRODUCIBILITY OF STEREO BASE

The stereo base, the distance to the subject, and the relative depth of the subject are all important factors when photographing in stereo. To produce realistic stereo, the stereo base should be approximately one-thirtieth of the distance from the lens to the near-point of the subject. This rule is founded on the assumption that the photograph has a far-point at infinity, but it is not applicable to fundus photography, as the far-point in fundus photography is only approximately 25 mm away. For example, patients with high elevations of neovascular complexes that extend into the vitreous may have images with relatively distant far-points. Also, retinal detachments are often located anterior to the normal fundus location and therefore may need to decrease the stereo base to create fusible stereo images.

The stereo base (the horizontal displacement of the optical center of the fundus camera lens between stereo pairs) of sequential stereo frames, and therefore the three-dimensional effect, may be inconsistent between

A

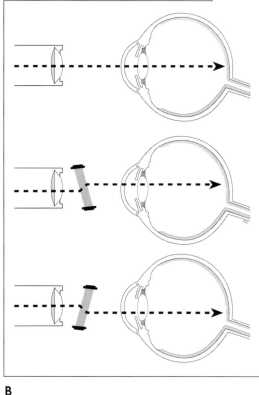

B

FIGURE 3-16
Allen Stereo Separator. **A.** Photograph of the solenoid-activated plano glass plate mounted in front of the Zeiss fundus camera. **B.** Optical path using the Allen Stereo Separator shows how the camera is optically shifted in front of the patient's eye.

photographic pairs taken at the same session, as well as at different patient visits. When interpreting visit-to-visit photographs, then, the physician should judge only relative changes in position of various anatomic structures and should not attempt to determine absolute depth perception information between stereo images. Measurements are also invalid because of this potential variability of stereo bases.

ALLEN STEREO SEPARATOR

In an effort to increase the repeatability of the stereo base, Lee Allen[11] developed a solenoid-controlled plano-glass lens in front of the front objective lens of the fundus camera (Figure 3-16A); this attachment is named the Allen Stereo Separator (manufactured by Zeiss). When the angle of the optical flat is changed, the optical position of the fundus camera is displaced horizontally left to right (L–R)—that is, slide the camera sideways (Figure 3-16B). The amount of stereo separation (stereo-base) is adjustable from 2.25 mm to 3.50 mm. With a test switch, the photographer alternates the two positions of the separator to preview the camera's optical position. To use the Allen Stereo Separator, first line up the left image and then flip the separator and see if the right image is clear. Adjust and repeat until you think that you have two clear images. Finally, return the separator to the first position, and then take the two images. With a cooperative patient, a good photographer will expose both images without the patient's eye moving. The Allen Stereo Separator automatically alternates positions after each photograph is taken.

While the separator improves the repeatability of the stereo base between stereo pairs, there is still no guarantee of a consistent stereo base, as there may be patient movement. The quality of the image pairs may be reduced because the predetermined stereo base cannot be optimized for each patient. Additional record keeping is required to note the stereo base and which pairs were unsuccessful due to poor patient cooperation.

The glass plate is another surface for children's fingerprints and adult nose-prints. Some photographers think that it is an advantage to have the "lens protector" in place for pediatric patients, whereas others prefer to use a true lens cap whenever the camera is not in use.

Some fundus camera manufacturers have a small locking knob that limits the camera's lateral movement to a stereo base of approximately 3 mm. The steps needed to take a stereo pair using this method are the same as for any other sequential stereo pair, and the patient movement problems are the same. Only stereo photographs obtained simultaneously can guarantee a repeatable stereo base.

Remember that a photographer who sees with only one eye can still take excellent stereo photographs with standard monocular cameras, as both eyes are not required to use a monocular camera.

Fluorescein Angiograms in Stereo

The same techniques to align the camera in color fundus photography are used in stereo fluorescein angiography. The final viewing method determines whether the angiogram is shot R–L or L–R order. The film in most fundus cameras travels from left to right (photographer's point of view). Don't forget that the fundus image is, at the film plane, inverted. If film fluorescein angiography studies are cut into strips of five or six frames to have the first image at the upper right corner of the contact sheet so that the images are right side up, then the first image is to the right of the second image. In this situation, you would expose the right side of the stereo pair first: right side, left side, etc. If the order is not correct, then the pairs of images may produce stereo images in which the stereo depth information is reversed (depressions may seem to be elevations and retinal vessels will appear to lie beneath the choroid). Alternatively, if negatives are stripped with the first image in the upper left corner, the image will be upside down, but the first image will be on the left. If the negatives are mounted in slide mounts, then the standard L–R stereo technique should be used.

Timing of the Stereo Images

The interval between the stereo pairs in angiography is important because the fluorescein sodium dye is moving during the study. Just as it is desirable to have as little patient movement as possible between stereo pairs, it is also important to have as little movement of dye between the two images that comprise the stereo image. Reducing the time interval between stereo fluorescein images reduces the image discrepancy within stereo pairs. By increasing the time between each set of stereo pairs, the patient may have time to blink, and less film is used. A typical sequence would be as follows: Take the right image and pause for 0.8 seconds; take the left image and pause for 2.2 seconds; then repeat (Figure 3-17). This timing uses the same amount of film as taking one image every 1.5 seconds but reduces the image disparity by almost one-half.[18] The total time per pair of images remains 3 seconds. In digital angiography, even with unlimited number of images, the reduction of dye-flow induced image disparity produces images that are easier to fuse. Simultaneous stereo systems completely overcome this problem.

FIGURE 3-17
Optimal timing for stereo pairs during angiography. Visual disparity among stereo pairs reduces the appreciation of stereopsis. Angiography is a dynamic process: The visual representation of blood vessels may change rapidly throughout the process. Expose your stereo pairs with little time between the pictures to reduce the visual differences between the individual pictures in a pair.

Advanced Stereo Techniques

INCREASING DEPTH-OF-FIELD

Ocular pathology may exceed the depth-of-field of fundus cameras. Sequential stereo photography can be used to increase the depth-of-field by combining two images that are focused at slightly different planes of focus [19]. This is known as *high-low* or *differential focusing* (Figure 3-18).

When working with a subject that is concave, like the cupping of a deep optic nerve, select one view to be focused high and one view to be focused low. Decide whether the right or left image will have the best "view" of the bottom of the optic nerve. That image should be focused deep. The other image should be focused at the rim of the cup. An elevated subject (e.g., tumor) may have a better side to show with the lower focused image.

There is a limit to the amount of image blur that can be fused to create a clear stereo image. Stereo image pairs with large out-of-focus zones between the two images are difficult to fuse. There must be enough clear common points-of-image information for image fusion to take place.

STEREO ORIENTATION—VERTICAL STEREO

The shape of the pathology is important when determining the appropriate stereo orientation for the photograph. If all of the elevation is in the vertical cross section (Figure 3-19A), little stereo information will be gained if the images are taken with the conventional L–R stereo orientation. If for the best stereo view through an indirect ophthalmoscope you would tilt your head 90 degrees in either direction, then using this vertical stereo technique would be beneficial. This same stereo view can be photographed by modifying your stereo technique.

Rather than shifting the camera laterally, shift it in the up-down direction using the camera elevation control. The photographs can then be rotated 90 degrees and viewed as if you had rotated your head when examining the patient. Slides should be labeled to reflect the stereo technique that you used (Figure 3-19B, C).

STEREO WITH HIGH MAGNIFICATION AND WIDE-FIELD FUNDUS CAMERAS

High-magnification and wide-field fundus images can be taken in stereo, but the wide-field fundus images may show less depth effect, due to the lower subject-to-film magnification.

The green alignment dots on some Canon or Topcon wide-field fundus cameras can simplify camera positioning for stereo photography. These dots are located at nine and three o'clock and are normally used

FIGURE 3-18
Differential focusing. Less visual information is conveyed when the focus is adjusted for a single plane **(A)** than when two different planes are in focus **(B)**. This technique is less effective when the focusing planes are far apart and without commonality **(C)**.

for monocular camera alignment. The basic principle is that the green dots replace the crescent reflections that are seen on 30-degree cameras. First align the dots for a standard monocular fundus photograph with both dots showing. Move the camera left until the nine o'clock dot disappears and then shoot. Then shift right until you see both dots, continue until you just see the three o'clock dot, and shoot again. This will give the maximal stereo base while maintaining evenly illuminated fields.

Simultaneous Stereo Fundus Photography

Simultaneous stereo cameras (Figure 3-20) have the distinct advantage of providing the physician with images guaranteed to be of constant stereo base. This technique allows both subjective and analytical analysis to be made with a greater degree of accuracy, as the stereo photographs are exposed with an identical image magnification and stereo base at the exact same moment in time.

Photographing stereo images simultaneously offers other additional advantages. Patient cooperation is not needed while taking two photographs, and there is only one flash for each stereo pair of images! The disadvantage is the difficulty of simultaneously finding two clear, sharp, and evenly illuminated images through a potentially small pupil.

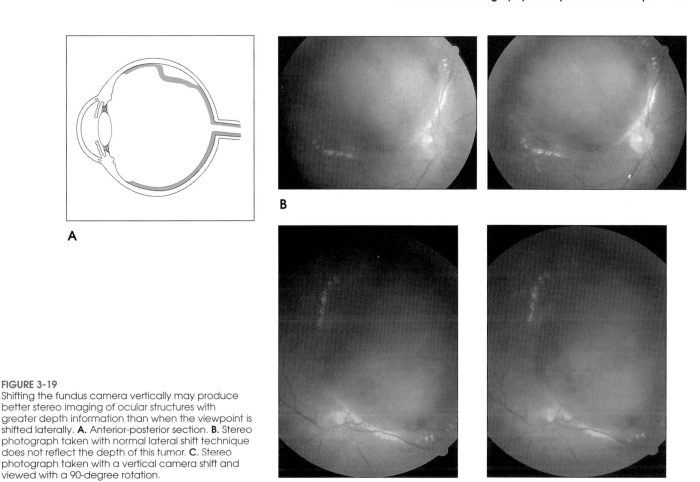

FIGURE 3-19
Shifting the fundus camera vertically may produce better stereo imaging of ocular structures with greater depth information than when the viewpoint is shifted laterally. **A.** Anterior-posterior section. **B.** Stereo photograph taken with normal lateral shift technique does not reflect the depth of this tumor. **C.** Stereo photograph taken with a vertical camera shift and viewed with a 90-degree rotation.

The starting point for alignment of simultaneous stereo fundus photography is the same as that for monocular photography; however, you must have two images aligned simultaneously. Aligning these cameras properly requires a modified technique because you are recording two images with a single exposure. Check the quality of each image by alternately closing each of your eyes to ensure that both images are sharp and evenly illuminated.

Although all fundus cameras have external fixation devices, some stereo cameras have an internal fixation light that, when the patient fixates, attempts to center the optic nerve in the image frame. Keep in mind that these split frame stereo images are vertical, with each image area being 18-mm wide and 24-mm high. The view through the oculars of these cameras is round. If they do not indicate the outside margins of the rectangular photographic field, then you will have to estimate what part of the view will be included in your photograph.

If a photographer has vision in both eyes, but still lacks stereopsis, he or she may successfully use a simultaneous stereo camera. As for all photographers using simultaneous stereo cameras, alternately close each eye to check the quality of both images.

Although the magnification, and often the stereo base, of these cameras are fixed, the position of the camera at successive visits may not be identical for each image. Obviously, the centering of the subject—the optic nerve, for example—must be achieved with consistency to permit optimal analysis. The optical position of the camera in the pupillary aperture should also be precisely located to achieve greater consistency for

A

C

B

FIGURE 3-20
Simultaneous stereo fundus cameras. **A.** Nidek 3Dx. **B.** Topcon TRC-SS2. **C.** Zeiss-Humphrey RC-310. (Courtesy of the manufacturers.)

visit-to-visit repeatability. If this is not done, the photograph may not be taken from the same viewpoint, and therefore image comparison becomes less useful. However, because the pupil can only be so large, the potential amount of change in the vantage point is a maximum of approximately 9 degrees (Figure 3-21). Use good photographic technique and line up the camera on the corneal reflex to reduce this variability.

Rotation of the eye is another variable that can compromise stereo consistency. Check to ensure that your patient's head is not tilted. Camera enhancements to improve the ease with which the photographer can achieve consistent and repeatable optical alignment will make these cameras an even more uniform diagnostic tool.

One simultaneous stereo fundus camera permits adjustment of the stereo base. This may be an advantage if a wider stereo base is required to avoid lens opacities (e.g., cataracts) or if there is limited dilation, as might be encountered with a patient taking glaucoma medications. Make sure that the stereo base is recorded so that the same stereo base is used for photography on subsequent visits.

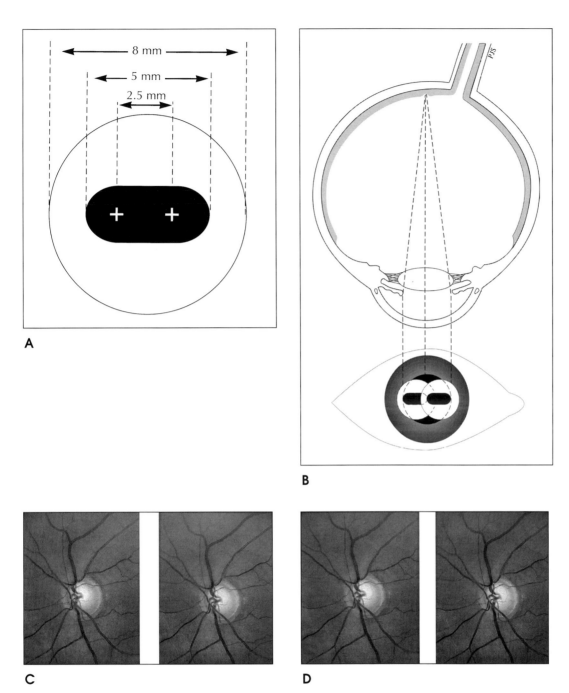

FIGURE 3-21
Variation of simultaneous stereo camera viewpoint. Cross section of eye being photographed with a stereo camera that uses a stereo base of 2.5 mm and an illumination circle that is 1 mm beyond the image aperture. Camera position at the extreme left of the pupil **(A)** versus camera position at the extreme right of the pupil **(B)** shows a maximal change in vantage point of approximately 9 degrees. **C.** Stereo pair taken from the left side of the pupil and a second stereo pair **(D)** taken from the right side of the pupil. Note the different viewpoint of the same subject.

Once the film is processed and returned, it is very important that you review your work. During alignment and photography, the brain does a marvelous job of registering even a marginal stereo image, and you may be astonished to find, on occasion, that one-half of your image pair is of low quality. Constantly check your work and refine your technique.

Table 3-2. Camera Formats and Some of the Ophthalmic Cameras That Use Them

Format	Image Size (Width × Height)	Fundus Camera
6 perf.	28.5 mm × 23.0 mm	Donaldson*
5 perf.	23.5 mm × 23.0 mm	Realist
Full-frame 35 mm	24 mm × 36 mm (22-mm diameter active image)	Zeiss 30-degree
Split-frame 35 mm	18 mm × 24 mm	Nidek, Topcon, Zeiss

perf. = perforation.
*41 × 101 mm (1⅝ in. × 4 in.) mounts.

Advanced techniques, such as high-low focusing or up-down/90-degree stereo technique, have not yet been incorporated into simultaneous stereo cameras. Astigmatic adjustments are presently unavailable. It may be difficult for the photographer who does not have stereopsis to take full advantage of this technology.

Assessing Stereo Images

Once stereo images are exposed and processed, they are prepared for viewing. This section describes how stereo image pairs are identified, the various stereo formats and how they are mounted and labeled for viewing.

Editing for Quality

Selecting only the best quality images of each view helps maintain a medical record of the highest quality. Selecting appropriate images is easier when stereo images are photographed using a standard sequence. The slides can simply be placed in a standard slide page with the stereo images paired together. All processed stereo images should be checked by the photographer to ensure that the images are properly aligned and the stereo-depth relationships are correct (i.e., the retinal blood vessels are seen in front of the choroid and optic nerve cupping is seen as a depression [not as an elevation]). It is important to be familiar with the normal and abnormal retinal pathology, because it is relatively easy to trick an inexperienced viewer into perceiving a depression where there is in fact an elevation, or vice versa. Only the best pairs should be saved and labeled as stereo. Monocular images may also be kept, but not marked as stereo.

Stereo Slide Formats

In the pictorial stereo (or three-dimensional) photography world, there are many stereo slide formats.[20] Fortunately, only a few transparency (slide) formats are used in ophthalmology. Formats include two full frames (two 2 × 2 mounts), split-frame 35 mm (two half-frame images a single 2 × 2 mount), Realist formats, and, finally, the View-Master disks (Table 3-2 and Figure 3-22). There are many other stereo slide formats, including those for 6-cm × 7-cm format cameras, but the 2 × 2 formats are most commonly used in ophthalmology. For more information about other stereo formats, see the reference section at the end of this chapter.[20]

2 × 2 SLIDE MOUNTS
Except for photographic competition entries and specially designed stereo projection systems, we suggest using 2 × 2 mounts to store, view, and project your clinical stereo slides. This choice permits the easy projection of a single monocular frame for conventional (non-stereo) projection. Realist

FIGURE 3-22
Photograph of various stereo slide formats. **A.** Two 2 ×
2 35-mm slides. **B.** Split-frame 35-mm slide mount.
C. Realist stereo slide mount. **D.** View-Master disk.

mounts require labor-intensive mounting procedures, and there are no split-frame 35-mm stereo projectors currently being commercially manufactured. Separate 2 × 2 slides are easy to reposition if alignment is not optimal.

SPLIT-FRAME 35 MM
These are ready-to-go stereo pairs. The easiest filing solution is to use split-frame stereo pairs mounted in conventional 2 × 2 slide mounts. Make sure that the film-processing laboratory understands that these are stereo images and that two similar images are to be mounted in one standard mount. Occasionally, a laboratory will mount 36 stereo images as 72 half-frame 2 × 2 slide mounts. Send a correctly mounted sample slide or explanatory note with the unprocessed film to avoid confusion.

DONALDSON FORMAT
Donaldson fundus[14] and anterior segment cameras use a variation of the Realist mounting system. The frame width of the images from the Donaldson stereo fundus camera is less than the standard 36-mm frame width of standard 35-mm slides, 28.5 mm. Realist mounts are known as the "6-P" or "6-perf." (6-perforation). This format is named after the width of the image, which is six perforations on the 35-mm film. The "standard" Realist mount is an image with a width of five perforations. This common five-perforation size of Realist mount obscures a bit of the left and right sides of the actual image area from a 30-degree Zeiss fundus camera. If you wish to calculate the frame width for any of these standards, you may use ANSI Standard PH 1.14-1990, which shows a perforation-to-perforation distance of 4.75 mm.

The Donaldson camera images are exposed in groups of two stereo pairs (four images). The film is wound a short distance after the first pair of images and a long distance after the second pair of images. They are laid out in the following order: #2-R, #1-R, #2-L, #1-L (remember the camera inverts the image). If you wish to use 2 × 2 mounts, please note that these cameras require special 2 × 2 slide mounts, which have a narrower aperture than full-frame, 35-mm slides (6-perf.: 28.5-mm wide × 23-mm high).

VIEW-MASTER

An interesting stereo format from the 1950s was the ubiquitous View-Master reel. These disks held seven stereo pairs of transparencies (10.5-mm × 11.7-mm image area). Hand-held viewers and projectors are still available in toy stores. They permit viewing one pair of images at a time when you hold the viewer up to a light source. These disks are still used as a distribution format for ophthalmic books that include stereo images.[9, 21]

Monocular Sorting of Stereo Slides

There is no substitution for binocular vision when studying stereo images. It is necessary to have two images fused into one for you to actually see in three dimensions. This does not mean, however, that binocular vision is required to shoot stereo, nor to identify stereo pairs. Although it is not possible to "see" stereopsis if you have monocular vision, it is possible to predict with some reliability whether two slides will constitute a stereo pair. With some knowledge of the anatomy, the left and right images may be identified. Working at a light box and using a loupe (magnifier), lay the two slides on top of each other. Look for lateral deviation of structures (typically vessels) in the superimposed images. If there is a deviation, then the two images will form a stereo pair. Usually, the greater the degree of deviation that is seen, the greater is the amount of stereopsis that is achieved.

The following procedure is based on a L–R stereo technique (shooting the left image first, then shifting laterally to shoot the right image). When using this L–R technique, the left image takes the left position in the slide sheet, and the right image takes the right position in the slide sheet. This technique is not essential, but establishing a routine when shooting stereo adds to the predictability factor and eases the identification process. Also, when superimposing the image by overlaying slides, the slide mounts must be lined up precisely over each other without overlap.

First, lay the presumed left image (slide) of an attempted stereo pair on a light box. Take the presumed right image (slide) of the pair and lay it precisely over the left image so that the slide mounts line up exactly on all four sides. Second, using a loupe, carefully observe the superimposed image—see if the top image deviates to the right of the bottom image.

When elevation has been documented, lay the right image (right half of the pair) over the left image (left half of the pair) and look for a deviation of the top image to the right. When cupping or depression has been documented, the top image should deviate to the left. If you orient the slides so that the right deviating image is the top image and place it in the "right half" position of the slide sheet, the depression or cupping will actually look as if it is coming toward you, instead of falling away! To determine which is the left image, try to identify a structure that is deep (posterior) in the image. This "deep" structure will be laterally to the left on the left slide.

This monocular technique for identifying stereo pairs may seem tedious and time consuming. It will, however, enable the photographer who is monocular and unable to see stereo to orient the slides properly into stereo pairs.

Slide Mounting and Labeling

If stereo pairs are projected, the photographer mounting the slides has a responsibility to the audience. The audience members do not have the option of repositioning the slides to permit fusing of the images. For audience comfort and ease of stereo fusion, you should ensure that the images are aligned perfectly in the slide mounts. You do not need to view this in stereo. You will need a light table with a grid for checking similar image

64mm

FIGURE 3-23
Grid for aligning stereo images into Realist slide mounts using 64-mm spacing.

points on two images. The grid must have like points under each of the stereo images (Figure 3-23). Position the mounts so that the slides are aligned on the grid horizontally. Use the grids to ensure that identical points in both images are positioned similarly on the grid. Obviously, the two images are slightly different as they are stereo images, but aligning central image points works well. Tape the properly positioned slide film in place to finish the slide mounting.

If you are mounting stereo image pairs into Realist, or other special stereo mounts, take advantage of special stereo slide mounting guides that have numerous horizontal lines for checking the vertical placement of the slide frames. They are also useful for checking for any rotation that has occurred between exposures. Note that there are vertical lines for adjusting the stereo window. Place corresponding parts of each slide over the same horizontal line and the vertical lines. Place the "far line" under the most distant subject in your slides.

If stereo pairs of slides are taken with the vertical stereo technique—that is, with an up-down photographic technique—you must rotate each slide 90 degrees for proper viewing. The stereo pair should be oriented so that the view would be the same as if the clinician had tilted his or her head to the right. The top slide would be placed as the left slide of the pair and both of the slides would be rotated 90 degrees clockwise for viewing (see Figure 3-19C). Stereo slides should be edited, marked, and placed into the chart so that they are easily identifiable.

Marking of the stereo pairs can be accomplished using a variety of methods. Pairs for a particular patient from each visit can be numbered sequentially and identified as to whether the individual image is the left or the right image (Figure 3-24). If the slides are not to be removed from the plastic slide pages, then a simple line or a pair of lines may be used to indicate stereo pairs. The word "stereo" can be written or rubber-stamped between the two slides. [22]

Viewing Stereo Images

Stereo images may be viewed by an individual or by a group. First we address the newest technology, computer-based stereo image presentation,

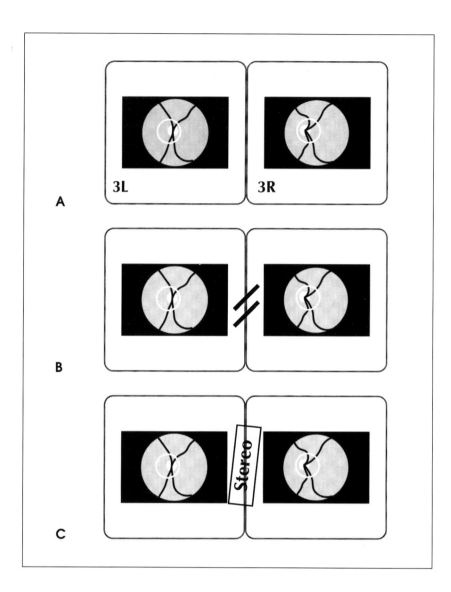

FIGURE 3-24
Labeling conventions for indicating stereo on the pairs of 2 × 2 slides. Slide pairs labeled with sequential pair numbers and "L" and "R" **(A)**, a simple set of lines **(B)**, or a rubber stamp with the word "stereo" **(C)**.

as it works for both individual viewers and groups. The section on individual viewing discusses dual 2 × 2 transparencies; split-frame, 35-mm transparencies; Realist stereo formats; View-Master transparencies; and lenticular images. Several methods of viewing paper prints, lenticular prints, and Vect-O-Grams are covered. The section on group viewing outlines various non-computer projection systems, equipment requirements, and their use.

Viewing Electronic Stereo Images

All of the imaging systems for viewing small images will work with images displayed on computer monitors. Use viewing aids the same as you would for stereo images that are printed on paper or film transparency material. Side-by-side (small), side-by-side (larger than 60 mm), and anaglyph images are useful viewing methods. Although you can free-view small images, the granularity of the screen limits fine detail. The dynamic range and color saturation is very good on computer screens. Stereo images can be displayed on the monitor or printed on paper (from the computer image file), the same as for the standard viewing systems. However, monitor resolution is a limitation, as it is less than one-tenth that of 35-mm slide pairs. Zooming the image on the monitor may help to overcome the limits of screen resolution. Larger side-by-

A

B

C

FIGURE 3-25
A. Schematic drawing of a Wheatstone stereoscope.
B. Modern four-mirror view being used to increase the viewer's inter-pupillary distance for larger images. **C.** Top view—note that one of the outer mirrors has an adjustable angle to permit viewing images of slightly different sizes.

side images viewed with a 4-mirror stereoscope provide good detail (Figure 3-25).

Stereo viewing hoods with mirrors can be used to cover the monitor and provide the appropriate optics to aid in seeing side-by-side images (Figure 3-26). Over-under image pairs are viewed with a different mirror configuration.

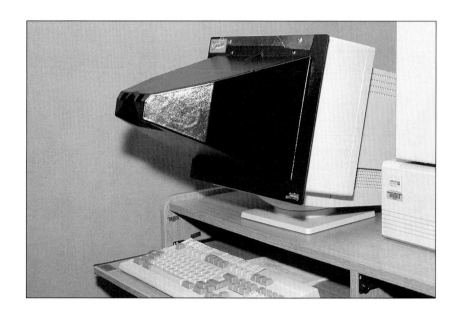

FIGURE 3-26
Mirrored stereo viewing hood for a computer monitor.

A

B

FIGURE 3-27
A. Over-under "squished" stereo images for use with liquid crystal device (LCD) glasses. **B.** LCD glasses used with a computer-controlled monitor to display color stereo images. (Courtesy of StereoGraphics Inc.)

Computers can be used to present stereo images either on a monitor or to a larger audience via a liquid crystal device (LCD) computer projector. Some type of stereo glasses are required for each system. There are also methodologies that are not possible with either prints or slides.

One system requires electronically synchronized glasses. The computer alternately displays the images comprising the stereo pair at a rate of at least 30 images per second. The image is viewed, on a single screen, by a person wearing computer-controlled LCD glasses. To ready the images, each of the two images of the stereo pair is first processed to reduce its height by one-half. The two images are then placed into a single image, with the left image of the stereo pair in the top half of the image and the right image in the bottom. The new single image is then saved as a single file (Figure 3-27A). An electronic device is inserted between the computer and the monitor and displays the two images alternately. This control box sends out an infrared timing signal to the LCD glasses to synchronize the opacity of the lenses. The LCDs have the ability to turn opacity on and off and therefore permit the two stereo images to be alternately displayed and thus viewed through the appropriate eye (Figure 3-27B). This system works well for both monochromatic (angiographic) and color images.

Another system uses a polarized LCD panel placed over the computer monitor screen while the person viewing it wears standard polarized stereo glasses. With this system, the viewing glasses must be horizontal to create maximal image extinction, the same as for stereo slide projection. If this system is used for computer projection, then a lenticular projection screen is required. The glasses are inexpensive, so this system is useful if a large audience is involved.

Red-cyan stereo glasses may bring back memories of comic books and grade-B movies, but in ophthalmic photography, they have some very good applications. Because angiographic images are usually viewed as monochrome (gray-scale) images, it is possible to color one of the two stereo images red and the other cyan, display them on a color computer screen, then view them through red-cyan glasses. The left image is typically colored red and is viewed through a red lens in front of your left eye. The right eye has a cyan (and sometimes green or even blue) filter, and, as such a filter does not pass very much red light, your right eye will not see the left image (and vice versa).

Anaglyph images work well using computer image projectors, individual computer monitors, photographic slides, and prints.

Color stereo images may be combined into a single color image that is viewed with red-cyan glasses. This technique works well for images that have a full spectrum of colors as well as monochromatic images (e.g., angiograms). The stereo effect on the mostly red fundus image is not useful, as there is minimal information in the cyan (blue and green) colors of the image. Software to create anaglyph images should not only store the aligned stereo images, but also permit the printing of these images as paper prints or onto slide film.

Personal Viewing of Stereo Slides and Prints

Personal viewing techniques fall into two categories, based on image size: images that are smaller and images that are larger than the average pupillary distance (PD) of approximately 60 mm.[24] Of the two techniques that allow you to perceive stereo images without viewing paraphernalia, one requires that you accommodate your focus but not to converge your eyes, called *parallel viewing*, and the other requires that you overconverge your eyes (cross-eye) to achieve stereopsis. All other techniques require optical devices to assist you in seeing the stereo images.[23]

Stereo Slides

The most commonly used stereo viewing techniques in ophthalmology utilize two full-frame, 35-mm stereo slides. The slide exposed through the left side of the pupil is positioned in the viewer so that it is viewed by your left eye, and the right image is positioned so that it can be viewed by your right eye. Most stereo slide viewers contain a pair of +4-D to +12-D lenses (see Appendix C). This permits you to relax your accommodation and avoid convergence. The best stereo viewers use compound lenses to reduce distortion and increase sharpness. Once the two images are seen as one, you can adjust the focus with either a focusing adjustment or by physically changing the distance between the slides and the lenses (Figure 3-28). For extensive viewing, you might consider having an optical shop make you some +8 to +10 glasses.[23]

If you have a large amount of accommodation or are myopic, or both, you may not need a viewer. Simply place the slides, side by side (or with a space between the slide mounts up to 10 mm) on a light table and orient

A   **B**

FIGURE 3-28
A. 2 × 2 slide viewer. Standard 2 × 2 stereo viewers allow you to lay two 35-mm slides side by side on a light table to view them in stereo **(B)**. The best viewers have high-quality, two-element glass lenses, a comfortable interpupillary distance, and ample space for your nose.

your eyes exactly perpendicular to the center of the slides. Using a sloping light box may make it easier to position your head and eyes properly. Place your face very close to the slides and relax your convergence by imagining that you are looking far into space. Allow both images to overlap and then become one image. Do not be concerned about image sharpness at this point. Rather, keep your eyes perpendicular to the two slides and slowly move your head away from the slides to a distance of 6–8 in. while attempting to focus on the slides without losing the single image and having it become two images. If you see two separate images, you are moving back from the slides too quickly, and your eyes are converging. Relax and try again. Viewing stereo slides cannot be practiced in a rush!

With time, you may be able to grab a slide page out of a chart, hold it up to a light source, and view the images in stereo. The key phrase is, "with practice."

Split-frame (sometimes mistakenly called *half-frame*) stereo images have two vertical images displayed on a single 35-mm slide frame (Figure 3-29). Most camera systems produce slides with the left image on the left, but a few systems produce slides with the image that is to be viewed with the left eye placed on the right side of the slide. Consequently, there are two types of split-frame stereo viewers. If you get a viewer with the wrong configuration of optics for the slides you are producing, you will get stereoscopically reversed image (e.g., disc cupping will be presented as an elevation).

Realist stereo slide mounts can be viewed with a set of plus lenses, in a simple stereo viewer (Figure 3-30), or a drum viewer that holds 18 stereo pairs.

View-Master reels are often used to illustrate ophthalmic textbooks, usually with foldout viewers. Purchasing a higher quality viewer is well worth the investment. Even a toystore viewer will outperform most folding viewers (Figure 3-31).

Prints and Publications—Special Considerations

Prints are more commonly used to view stereo images in a clinical setting since the introduction of digital color fundus photography. There are several viewing methods that you may use to see stereo images both in photographic prints and in publications.[23] An understanding of these viewing methods will assist you in selecting the appropriate printing or publishing method for stereo images and to instruct the person how to view the stereo images. It is important to be able to inform the publication's editor and printer of size requirements for easy viewing.

A

B

C

FIGURE 3-29
A. Split-frame 35-mm stereo slide. **B.** Schematic drawing showing the optical paths. **C.** Photograph of split-frame stereo viewer.

A commonly used stereo printing method involves two images printed just less than 2 in. in width with a small space between them. It is important to make sure that the distance between common points on the stereo images is not greater than the average PD of 60 mm. A good working rule is that each of the images should be no wider than 55 mm. If you have a narrow PD or the printer has made the prints too large for convenient viewing, then you can use base-out prisms, one for each eye to assist in viewing (Figure 3-32A).

Some stereo magazines print larger images to increase the total resolution of the image. To assist in viewing, they often include a set of +4.0, 8-D base-out prism viewing glasses with each subscription. These glasses are also useful for viewing stereo images that are each 60- to 90-mm wide. Larger images, viewed with a prism, will exhibit some distortion unless the images are pre-distorted to compensate for the difference in distances from the viewer to the center of the image versus the outside edge (horizontal) of the image.

Usually, the left image is on the left and the right on the right. If the images have been printed in reverse, you must cross your eyes to see

FIGURE 3-30
A. Realist battery-operated viewer. **B.** Schematic drawing of the viewer. (L = light source.)

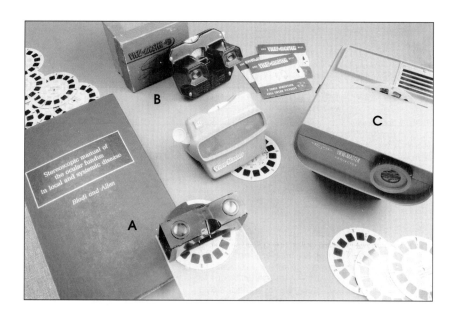

FIGURE 3-31
Viewers for View-Master reels showing a foldout-type supplied in textbooks **(A)**, two commercial viewers **(B)**, and a non-stereo projector **(C)**.

stereo with the proper depth relationships. The cross-eyed method prohibits the easy use of magnifying lenses and makes it difficult for some individuals to fuse the images. There also is some image distortion, as some parts of the image are farther away from the eye than the center of the image. If you cannot cross your eyes sufficiently for free viewing, try base-in prisms to imitate cross-eyed viewing of large prints (Figure 3-32B).

In the clinical setting, often four images are printed on 8 1/2-in. × 11-in. paper. This permits, for example, a stereo pair of the right optic nerve and a stereo pair of the left optic nerve on a single sheet of paper. The images

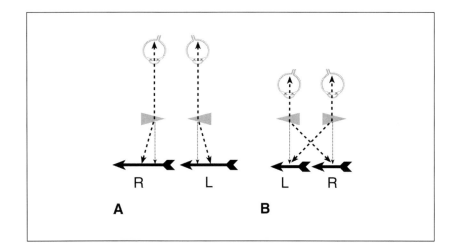

FIGURE 3-32
Print viewing with pairs of prisms. Prisms can be helpful when viewing stereo print pairs. **A.** Use base-out prisms, 4 D, when viewing prints wider than 60 mm. **B.** Use base-in prisms to assist in cross-eyed viewing.

FIGURE 3-33
Set of three images for stereo viewing. Images **A** and **B** may be viewed using the parallel technique; images **B** and **C** may be viewed using the cross-eyed technique to show an elevated optic nerve.

Stereo in Publications

Below are sample instructions that you might use to convey your stereo reproduction needs to the publisher and your explanatory text for the viewer:

INSTRUCTIONS TO THE PUBLISHER:
This figure is a stereo pair. The two images, although they may appear similar, are different. The figure has been submitted to you precisely and correctly aligned so that the readers can view the image in stereo (three-dimension). Exact sizing must be followed to have the image viewable by the greatest number of readers. The image must be run at 100%, so that the final images will be reproduced as two 55-mm–wide (2-in. or 12-pica) squares with a 4-mm (¹⁄₆-in. or 1-pica) gap between the images. Please include the two black dots that are positioned directly over the exact center of each image. These are important aids to assist readers in viewing this image. **Caution:** Under no circumstances should you strip the two images separately or reverse their placement, as that will destroy the scientific integrity of the image.

INSTRUCTIONS TO THE READER:
These two images comprise a stereo pair. When viewed properly, you will see a three-dimensional view of the subject. To do this, you must look at the left image with your left eye and the right image with your right eye. The following steps may assist you in viewing this stereo image:

1. Use stereo viewing glasses of +5 to +8 D.
2. Situate yourself in a comfortable viewing position with good lighting on the stereo image.
3. With both the print and your eyes level, place the image very close (2 in.) to your face with the left image in front of your left eye and the right image in front of your right eye. You should see a single out-of-focus image, with a single dot over it.
4. Slowly increase the distance between your eyes and the image until you see a sharp stereo image.

can be enlarged to show more detail. These larger prints must be viewed with a mirrored viewer (see Figure 3-25A).

An interesting approach is to provide three images: L, R, and L. The first two images are paired for "parallel" viewing, and the second and third images are paired for cross-eyed viewing (Figure 3-33).

It is important that you purchase the proper equipment to view large-print stereo images (see Appendix C). I know of one experienced ophthalmic photographer who prided himself on being able to free-view large prints using the cross-eyed method. He did this for many years and later in life acquired double vision whenever he was tired.

Printing monochromatic stereo images as a single color image lets most viewers perceive stereo image with anaglyph (red-cyan) glasses (Figure 3-34). The left image is printed in red and the right in cyan. Red-cyan stereo allows images to be printed large, presenting more information than small side-by-side images. They may appear to be a black and white image with poor printing registration—you will see red or cyan "ghosts" to the left or right of the main image. Computer programs can be used to create red-cyan images (see previous discussion on computer images). This technique is useful for the printed page, computer screens, computer projection, and slide projection (see the sidebar Stereo in Publications). Anaglyphs were prepared on the computer for the *Stereo Atlas of Fluorescein and Indocyanine Green Angiography*.[25]

Lenticular prints require no viewing aids: no mirrors, lenses, or glasses! The two stereo images are "sliced" vertically and then re-created

A

FIGURE 3-34
Anaglyph (Bi-color) stereo image viewing. **A.** Red-cyan anaglyph glasses. **B.** A stereo fluorescein angiogram (central serous chorioretinopathy) to be viewed with red-cyan anaglyph glasses.

B

A

B

FIGURE 3-35
Microphotograph (75×) of a lenticular print. Front view **(A)**. Cross section **(B)**.

in alternating thin vertical strips, which are positioned, in pairs, behind a series of vertical lenticular lenses. The lenticular lens permits both of your eyes to see the many small vertical slices of an image. Your left eye sees the left image, and your right eye sees the right image (Figure 3-35). The width of each individual lenticular lens determines the horizontal resolution of the image. The image resolution on one system of small lenticular prints is 180 lenses per inch. Each lens has an image pair behind it. A 4-in. × 3-in. print of an optic nerve will not provide as much information as a stereo pair of 35-mm slides due to the resolution limitation of the number of lenses used to create the image.

Lenticular prints and transparencies can be printed as poster-size images. One lenticular print has been used on the cover of the *Journal of Ophthalmic Photography*. [26] The image was created using a Nidek 3-Dx

A   B

FIGURE 3-36
A. Use a single, small mirror for viewing an image pair when one of the images is left-right reversed. **B.** The right image has been printed in a "mirrored" version. For correct viewing of the print, a mirror must be used to interrupt the vision of your right eye.

FIGURE 3-37
Vectographs are viewed using polarized glasses. A common vectograph is the Titmus fly test.

simultaneous stereo camera, and the split-frame stereo image was reproduced by Lentec, Inc (Lentec—see Appendix C).

A unique stereo viewing technique requires just a single mirror to view the stereo image (Figure 3-36). As usual, the image for the left eye is on the left and that for the right eye is on the right, but the right image is printed as a left-right reversed image. Follow this viewing technique: The right image is reversed with a mirror that is placed vertically in front of your nose, with the reflecting side toward the right. Look directly at the left image with your left eye and with your right eye also try to view the left image. If the mirror is aligned properly, you will view the reversed right image through the mirror. Fusing these two views reveals a stereo image. The only catch is that either the right image must be printed slightly larger, or you must lean your head to the right so that both image paths are the same length.

Vectographs are single prints that can be viewed without lenses or mirrors, making viewing easier for people who have difficulty fusing images that may not be optimally aligned. The Titmus stereo fly test is an example of the Vectograph viewing system. It uses two superimposed, polarized images viewed through polarized glasses (Figure 3-37).

The over-under-print method allows you to perceive stereo with two vertically stacked horizontal images. The viewer contains multiple mirrors that are precisely set for a specific print size and a specific stereo separation. If you are interested in this format, obtain the viewer first and then create your images to fit.

Group Viewing

The key principle of stereo projection is the same as other stereo viewing strategies. As with all stereo viewing systems, each eye must be presented with an individual image.

Anaglyph images can easily be projected via computer projector or standard 35-mm projector onto any type of projection screen. Color fundus images may be computer projected and viewed through LCD glasses. This is currently the best way to see projected color fundus stereo images. Stereo projection in ophthalmology can be performed with two polarized images projected on a single lenticular screen. Other alternatives include projecting two separate side-by-side images, as well as projecting two black-and-white images through red-cyan filters, or projecting digitally created red-cyan anaglyphs.

POLARIZED STEREO PROJECTION

Polarized image projection can be performed either with two standard 2 × 2 slide projectors with polarizing filters over the lenses, specialized stereo projectors (requiring Realist mounted slides), or with split-frame stereo images and a custom stereo projection lens (Figure 3-38).

Satisfactory stereo projection can be obtained with two standard 2 × 2 slide projectors, polarizing filters, proper screens, and polarizing lenses. Polarizing filters reduce the amount of projected light. The light level is further reduced by the polarizing glasses, making it important to use bright projectors for stereo projection. We prefer the optics in the Kodak Ektagraphic projectors, because (1) they deliver more light than the equivalent Carousel models, (2) their light sources can be modified to further increase the screen brightness, and (3) they precisely align the slides horizontally, whereas the Carousel models do not.

Polarizing filters (e.g., Polaroid #HN38) are mounted in front of the projection lenses of standard 2 × 2 slide projectors. The rotational orientation of these filters is crucial to successful stereo projection. These filters, like stereo glasses, must be oriented 90 degrees from each other.

Because the projection screen must not disrupt the orientation of the polarized light from the projectors, silverized screens are used. Lenticular silverized screens reflect brighter images for audience members who are seated to the side of the projection axis (Figure 3-39). Glass-beaded screens, the most common type of projection screen, will reorient the polarized nature of the light from the projectors, and thus will produce poor stereo images.

Position the projectors next to each other (side-by-side or stacked) and "on axis" with the projection screen. Use two identical, non-stereo slides for preliminary alignment. The edges of the mount should be projected clearly, with an image of a grid of vertical and horizontal lines. A pair of slides of an Amsler grid is an ideal subject. Photographing each grid through different colored filters will help you keep track of each image while you are aligning the projectors. Align the images on top of each other. Adjust the zoom for identical image size. Align the slides horizontally with the projector feet. Fine-tune the vertical and horizontal adjustments. Finally, recheck the magnification.

To align the polarizing filters, first put on a pair of polarized stereo viewing glasses. While projecting the right image on the screen, view the image with your left (wrong) eye. The glasses should be square on your face, and your head should be held level. Why view the right image with

A

B

C

FIGURE 3-38
Two-stereo slide projection with internal polarizing filters. **A.** Realist dual lens projector (no longer manufactured). TDC stereo projector (no longer manufactured). **B.** RBT stereo projector (Aichwald, Germany). **C.** Custom-made, split-frame, 35-mm stereo projector (courtesy of Chris Barry, CRA). **D.** One of the two 35-mm projectors with polarizing filters used for stereo projection.

D

the left eye? Because it creates the minimal amount of light for the wrong image to reach an eye. Rotate the filter for maximal extinction. It is important to get maximal reduction of image brightness for the image that is not to be seen. Repeat the procedure for the other filter with the other eye. Double-check your work by viewing the right image with your left eye and vice versa. Recheck for maximal extinction. The filters in the glasses are typically set at 45 degrees to each side of vertical.

The projectionist plays an important role in ensuring that the audience will have a great viewing experience. A good projectionist can make a great

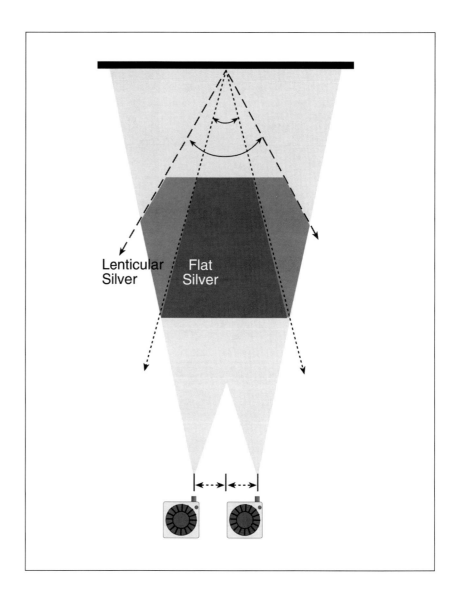

FIGURE 3-39
Lenticular silver screens provide a wider angle of acceptable stereo viewing when compared to flat silver screens. Projector lenses should be equidistant from the center of the screen and equidistant from the front of the screen surface.

session; a poor projectionist can ruin the show. All stereo images are not created equal; camera-subject alignment, camera rotation, and slide mounting are just a few of the variables. The projectionist is like an airplane pilot. The pilot can safely navigate a pleasant trip around a storm, at the same time presenting the passengers with a great view. Or the pilot can fly straight through the storm and hope that not too many people get sick. Poor stereo projection and motion sickness are similar—neither is very pleasant.

The projectionist may need to do some touch-up alignment with each pair of projected images. If the projectors are mounted in multimedia racks, the adjustments will be smooth. Marks on the adjustment knobs will permit you to return the projector to its primary calibrated position while switching to the next stereo image. A good projectionist will remind the audience to take a few-seconds' break between images to permit him or her to check the alignment of the next pair of images.

Remove your stereo glasses when you align the images. You will need to see both images to position one on top of the other. The central portions of the subject should overlap. If mounting is imperfect, ignore the frame edges and adjust the projectors for maximal subject overlap. Vertical alignment is critical. The audience can, to a greater degree, overcome horizontal alignment, so set the vertical first and then bring the images together horizontally.

The horizontal position of the images will place the image in space—that is, at the screen, in front of the screen, or behind the screen. Review the information in the stereo mounting section about positioning the stereo window.

SPECIALIZED STEREO PROJECTORS

Slide projectors made specifically for stereo projection use a built-in two-lens configuration and Realist stereo slide mount. The projector permits horizontal and vertical image positioning, as well as focusing adjustments. The Realist and TDC projectors are no longer manufactured but are available on the used market (see Figure 3-38A, B). A pair of standard 35-mm projectors can be used with individual polarizing filters attached (see Figure 3-38D).

Split-frame stereo images can be projected through a specially equipped "dual lens" 2 × 2 projector. This lens assembly produces two overlapping images, which are filtered with polarizing filters (see Figure 3-38C).

A pair of standard 35-mm projectors can be used with individual polarizing filters attached (see Figure 3-38D). Two images can be projected side by side, either in a split-frame format or by two separate 2 × 2 slide projectors. These are the same techniques used to look at side-by-side images in print or on a computer screen. Viewing these images can be accomplished in one of two ways. If the images are placed with the image for the right eye on the left screen, and vice versa, then those viewing them must cross their eyes while maintaining focus in the distance. A pair of base-in prisms or viewing the images from the back of the room, or both, may help. If the images are oriented with the image for the right eye on the right and so forth, then base-out prisms are used to assist in viewing the images. These images are referred to as being for "wall-eyed" viewing.

Future Stereo Imaging in Ophthalmology

The value of the two images that comprise a stereo pair is truly greater than the sum of the parts. The additional information that stereo imaging provides the clinician should not be underestimated.

Stereo images in telemedicine increases the diagnostic capabilities of the consulting physician. In the changing medical community, the ability to obtain multilevel and high-level consults without the patient needing physically to see each and every consultant will play an important role in the future of ophthalmic photography. With computer network capabilities, the ability to access a stereo view of the fundus of a patient in a remote location may become an accepted practice.

Simultaneous stereo camera images taken with reproducible stereo techniques permit high-quality image computer analysis of these images. Through disc analysis, the diagnosis of glaucoma may become possible even before functional field loss manifests itself. Thus, the ability to photograph stereo images is a crucial skill. The ophthalmic photographer must have complete understanding and control of the theories and practices of ophthalmic stereo photography to ensure the ultimate care for the patient.

References

1. Jones J. Wonders of the Stereoscope. New York: Knopf, 1976;14.
2. Darrah WC. The World of Stereographs. Gettysburg, PA: W. C. Hannah, 1977;2.
3. Morgan H, Symmes D. Amazing 3D. Boston: Little, Brown, 1982;10.
4. Oatman EL. Diagnostics of the Fundus Oculi. Troy, NY: Southworth, 1913;1.

5. Thorner W. Die stereoskopische photographie des Augenhintesgrundes. Klin Monatsbl f Augenh 1909;47:481.
6. Metzger E. Die stereophotographie des Augenhintesgrundes. Klin Monatsbl f Augenh 1927;78:338.
7. Bedell AJ. Photographs of the Fundus Oculi. Philadelphia: Davis, 1929;1.
8. Bothman L, Bennett RW. Fundus Atlas—Stereoscopic Photographs of the Fundus Oculi. Chicago: Year Book, 1939;1.
9. Blodi FC, Allen L, Braley AE. Stereoscopic Manual of the Ocular Fundus in Local and Systemic Disease. St. Louis: Mosby, 1964.
10. Stenstrom WJ. A modification of the new Zeiss fundus camera. Arch Ophthalmol 1960;64:935.
11. Allen L. Ocular fundus photography. Am J Ophthalmol 1964;57:13.
12. Norton HJ. Absolute three dimensional colored retinal photographs. Trans Am Acad Ophthalmol 1953;57:612.
13. Norton HJ. Absolute electronic retinal stereophotography. Am J Ophthalmol 1947;40: 808.
14. Donaldson D. A new camera for stereoscopic fundus photography. Trans Am Acad Ophthalmol 1964;62:429.
15. Tychsen L. Binocular Vision. In W Hart Jr (ed), Adler's Physiology of the Eye: Clinical Application (9th ed). St. Louis: Mosby–Year Book, 1992;773–853.
16. Von Noorden GK. Binocular Vision and Ocular Motility: Theory and Management of Strabismus (4th ed). St. Louis: Mosby, 1990.
17. Bussy BJ, Mittelman D. Use of the astigmatism correction device on the Zeiss fundus camera for peripheral retinal photography. Int Ophthalmol Clin 1976;16:2.
18. Tyler ME. Stereo sequence programmer for retinal fluorescein angiography. J Biol Photographic Assoc 1977;45:19.
19. Tyler ME. High-low focusing to increase depth of field. Ophthalmic Photographers' Society annual meeting, 1977.
20. 3D-Web. 3D Frequently Asked Questions, 1996. http://www.stereoscopy.com
21. Gass JM. Stereoscopic Atlas of Macular Diseases: Diagnosis and Treatment (3rd ed). Vol 1. St. Louis: Mosby, 1987;1.
22. Walker BP. Photographic filing systems. Int Ophthalmol Clin 1976;16:2.
23. Merin L. Construction and use of stereo viewers. J Ophthal Photog 1981;4:39.
24. Ferwerda JG. The World of 3-D: A Practical Guide to Stereo Photography. Borger, Netherlands: 3-D Book Productions, 1987.
25. Stevens RA, Saine PJ, Tyler ME. Stereo Atlas of Fluorescein and Indocyanine Green Angiography. Boston: Butterworth–Heinemann, 1999.
26. Tyler M. Cover: lenticular print of optic disk edema. J Ophthal Photog 1993;15:1.

Chapter 4

Fluorescein Sodium and Indocyanine Green: Uses and Side Effects

Paula F. Morris

A. Introduction
B. Angiography as a Diagnostic Tool
   1. Nonocular Angiography
   2. Ocular Angiography
C. Dyes Used in Ocular Angiography
   1. Fluorescein Sodium (Resorcinolphthalein Sodium)
   2. Fluorescein Sodium Angiography
   3. Indocyanine Green
   4. Indocyanine Green Angiography

Introduction

Angiography is a diagnostic tool used to reveal circulation characteristics. Ocular angiography documents certain ocular pathologies using either of the biological stains, fluorescein sodium and indocyanine green (ICG). To better understand the different types of ocular angiography, this chapter discusses these two dyes—their origins and mechanisms, how they are used, and the consequences of their use.

Angiography as a Diagnostic Tool

Angiography has had a place in the diagnosis and treatment of pathologies involving circulation since 1919, when Heuser first performed an angiogram on a living person.[1] Before the discovery of x-rays by Wilhelm Roentgen in November 1895, studies of the circulatory system had been done without being able to observe the actual pattern of blood flow. In January 1896, Haschek and Lindenthal performed an angiogram on a cadaver hand by injecting a chalk-like substance into a vein. It took 57 minutes of x-ray exposure to produce the picture.[1]

By injecting a marker (an indicator) into the bloodstream and using appropriate equipment to image it, the presence or absence of blood flow and its pattern can be determined. This is helpful in determining the caliber of vessels, detecting circulation blockage, and observing circulation patterns in ischemia or neovascularization.

As angiography is a study of circulation, it can be performed anywhere there are vessels to be imaged. Fortunately for ophthalmic patients, angiography of the eye is less physically invasive and uses simpler equipment than angiography of the rest of the body, which requires x-rays and radio-opaque agents.

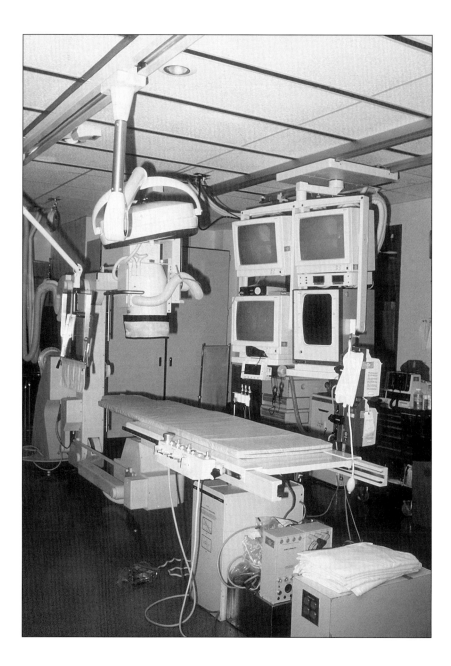

FIGURE 4-1
Nonocular angiography. The imaging chain needed to record nonocular angiographic images consists of a generator/cine pulse system, an x-ray tube, an image intensifier and optical distributor, a cine camera, a television camera, a monitor, a gantry, and a table. (Courtesy of Michael Palczynski, Virginia Eye Institute, Richmond, Virginia.)

Nonocular Angiography

Usually, nonocular angiography is performed as the patient lies down on a support table, using cardiac monitoring equipment and an imaging chain.[2] The imaging chain consists of a generator/cine pulse system, an x-ray tube, an image intensifier, an optical distributor, a 35-mm cine camera, a television camera and monitor, and a gantry. Also, most x-ray imaging room walls must be shielded with 1 mm of lead up to a height of 7 ft and must have windows of lead-treated glass to protect personnel (Figure 4-1).[2]

In contrast, an ocular angiography patient routinely sits on a stool or chair. Retinal angiography requires a fundus camera with a 35-mm film camera back or a digital camera, whereas choroidal angiography requires a fundus camera with an infra-red digital imaging system. In either case, special shielding of personnel and patient is unnecessary because no x-ray radiation is involved, and the procedures can be performed in any area of reasonable size to accommodate the patient, the camera, and the photographer.

In nonocular angiography, the radio-opaque agents, called *contrast agents*, are based on iodine. Organic iodine is an excellent opaque medium because of its high atomic number and chemical versatility and because it is less toxic than inorganic iodine. Currently, nonionic iodine–based agents with medium osmolality characteristics and low-osmolality contrast materials are gaining in popularity because they improve patient comfort and lower the incidence of side effects.[2] (*Osmolality* refers to the number of particles in a given volume of solution, which affects the ability of a solution to permeate through membranes to equalize its concentration.)

Nonocular angiography is accomplished radiologically by generating x-rays and directing them through the area of the body being studied. It exposes patients and operators to the highest radiation levels of any x-ray studies.[2] For this reason, the number of radio-opaque angiograms a patient can receive may be limited. A maximum number of procedures per patient is being investigated. Most of the incident radiation is absorbed by the patient, with less than 1% of the radiation passing through the body to the image intensifier. The rest of the incident radiation scatters back into the room where the people conducting the test may be exposed. Because the x-ray tube is located beneath the support table, most of the scatter radiation is directed back to the floor. Shielding methods are used to protect parts of the patient's anatomy and to reduce the operator's scatter dose of radiation.

When a radio-opaque agent is present in the bloodstream, it blocks the transmission of the x-rays to the image recording system and provides the contrast that delineates the vessels. Materials that are dense are less transparent, and radio-opaque agents are very dense because of their high molecular weight.

In nonocular angiography, the contrast agent can be introduced to the bloodstream in various ways, depending on what part of the anatomy needs to be studied and the patient's physical condition. Some techniques are more invasive than others, but all involve exposing arteries and veins so that catheters can be inserted and the introduction of the contrast agent can be controlled and directed to the study area. The large branches of the circulatory tree—the femoral artery or the brachial artery—are most frequently used.[3]

To produce a nonocular angiogram, a catheter is threaded to the appropriate site and the contrast material is released in a bolus. The agent circulates through the vessels to be studied and then moves on, quickly becoming dilute and losing its ability to be imaged. Many boli of the contrast agent are introduced in the course of a nonocular angiogram, resulting in a large amount of dye being used, sometimes exceeding volumes of 100 ml.

Ocular Angiography

Ocular angiography is accomplished photographically through a dilated pupil, recording fluorescent light waves emitted from the dye present in the bloodstream. Fluorescence is one of two kinds of light emission called *luminescence*, the other being phosphorescence (Figure 4-2). Photoluminescence occurs when certain substances are exposed to short-wave electromagnetic radiation, and the substances absorb energy. This excites the molecules of the substance to a higher energy state. As the molecules return to their original state, they emit a longer wave length radiation, or they luminesce.[4] Fluorescence is short-lived, occurring during excitation and ending 10^{-8} seconds after the exciting stimulus is removed. Phosphorescence is a delayed light emission that continues for periods after the exciting stimulus is removed, as in a child's "glow-in-the-dark"

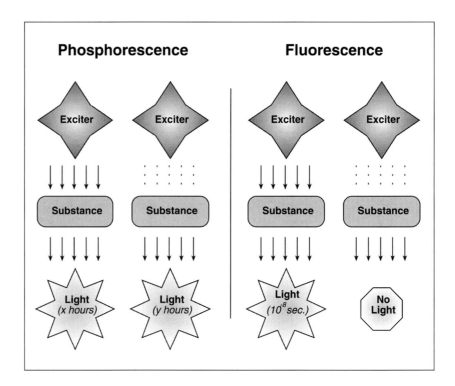

FIGURE 4-2
Types and durations of luminescence. Luminescent materials may be categorized as either phosphorescent or fluorescent. A properly exposed substance with phosphorescent properties continues to emit light for hours after the exciter is taken away. A properly exposed substance with fluorescent properties only emits light in the presence of the exciter.

toy. Fluorescein sodium and ICG both have fluorescent properties, and their emissions can be recorded on photographic film or electronic sensors. Excitation is supplied by light from the flash tube passing through an excitation filter.

In a normal eye, no tissues obscure the view of the posterior pole vascular system. Because of the unique anatomy of the eye, light from the camera can be directed through the transparent cornea, through the pupil and lens, to shine directly on the retina. The light then travels back along the same pathway to the camera's film plane. The dye can be injected into the bloodstream via any vein and travels along the venous system to the heart, flows through the cardiopulmonary circuit, then up the carotid arteries to the ophthalmic arteries, where some circulate through the choroid and some course through the central retinal artery to the retina.

Dyes Used in Ocular Angiography

Fluorescein sodium and ICG are the primary dyes used to perform ocular angiography (Figure 4-3). They do not have similar chemical configurations and are not of the same chemical "families." Although they both have fluorescent properties, fluorescein sodium has much stronger fluorescence abilities. ICG contains a small amount of sodium iodide, but it is not radio-opaque. It is used in ocular angiography because of its fluorescent properties.

Although the retina and choroid of the eye are intimately associated, their circulatory characteristics are very different, as are methods for performing angiography of each. It is not surprising, then, that the dyes used to accomplish these studies are very different as well. Because of these differences, this chapter discusses each of these dyes individually.

Before describing the unique characteristics of these dyes and clearing up some misconceptions, it is valuable to explain some basics about biological stains.

FIGURE 4-3
Types of ocular angiographic dyes. Vials of fluorescein sodium and indocyanine green dye as prepared by the manufacturers. The fluorescein sodium is ready for use, but the indocyanine green must be combined with the accompanying saline solution before injection. Both dyes have fluorescent properties.

Biological dyes are colored substances used to help reveal the gross and microscopic structure and nature of plant and animal tissue.[5] Manufacturers of dyes give them two classifications: natural and synthetic. Natural dyes are mineral or plant products. Because of their natural impurities, which cannot be controlled, they are decreasing in use because they cannot be certified for use in drugs and cosmetics. Synthetic dyes are manufactured dyes produced through chemical reactions. The first synthetic dyes were derived from aniline, a derivative of coal tar. Synthetic dyes used in drugs, cosmetics, and food are assigned identifying food, drugs, and cosmetics (F, D, & C) and color index (CI) numbers by the Federal Color Standards Directory.

The color of a dye is determined by its chemical configuration in combination with its chromophore. Chromophores are carbon rings with double bonds involving carbon, oxygen, and nitrogen that are associated with color. Dye groups based on their color are classified by similar chemical structure. Chromophores alone do not dictate color, as identical chromophores can be found in all the colors of the rainbow.[5]

Fluorescein Sodium (Resorcinolphthalein Sodium)

Fluorescein sodium ($C_{20}H_{10}Na_2O_5$) (Figure 4-4), or resorcinolphthalein sodium, is the biological dye used to perform retinal angiography. In drug supply catalogs, it is called *uranin* or *uranine yellow*. It is the disodium salt of the biological dye fluorescein ($C_{20}H_{12}O_5$), also called *eosin*.

There are some misconceptions associated with the dye fluorescein (eosin), including the mislabeling of retinal angiography. Fluorescein is not the dye used in retinal angiography. We use the salt fluorescein sodium.

According to its chemical structure, fluorescein is in the xanthene dye group. There are three classes of xanthene dyes: fluorenes, rhodols, and fluorones. Fluorones (hydroxyxanthenes) are called the *fluorescein derivatives* as fluorescein has the simplest chemical structure of the group. Other members of the fluorone group used in medicine are rose bengal and mercurochrome.[5]

Fluorescein was first synthesized by Adolf Baeyer in 1871 as a derivative of the dye gallein.[6] It produced a bright yellow color and was

FIGURE 4-4
Molecular diagram of fluorescein sodium.

Table 4-1. Comparing Fluorescein and Fluorescein Sodium

	Fluorescein	Fluorescein Sodium
Chemical name	Resorcinolphthalein	Resorcinolphthalein sodium
Common name	Eosine	Uranine yellow
Chemical formula	$C_{20}H_{12}O_5$	$C_{20}H_{10}Na_2O_5$
Dye description	C.I. SOLVENT yellow 94 C.I. 45340 F, D & C yellow #7	C.I. ACID yellow 73 C.I. 45340 F, D & C yellow #8
Physical characteristics	Yellowish red–red powder Insoluble in water, benzene, chloroform, ether Soluble in hot alcohol, glacial acetic acid, alkali derivatives	Orange–red powder Freely soluble in water

Note: Although the term *fluorescein* is generally used as shorthand for the chemical fluorescein sodium, there is a difference between the two compounds.

intended for use in dying wool and silk. As fluorescein is insoluble in water, benzene, chloroform, and ether, Baeyer used hot alcohol to make the textile dye.

Because fluorescein cannot dissolve in water, it cannot be used in a solution that is compatible with injection into the human body. Fluorescein sodium, however, is freely soluble in water—thus, its use in retinal angiography. Because of the practically universal use of the term "fluorescein angiography," it is not reasonable to try to correct the mislabeling, but it is valuable to know that there is a difference (Table 4-1).

WHAT IS FLUORESCEIN SODIUM?

Another misconception about fluorescein sodium is its origin. It has been mistakenly described to patients as a "sugar-based" dye, a vegetable dye, and a seaweed extract, and in some of the ophthalmic literature it is listed as a plant resin.[7,8] Actually, it comes from a mineral. Its primary component is naphthalene or tar camphor, which is the most abundant component of the carbolic acid fraction of distilled coal tar.[9] Naphthalene's most famous use is as the odor for moth balls! It is also used to manufacture indigo dye, solvents, lamp black, and celluloids. That fluorescein sodium does not occur naturally but is actually a synthetic is reinforced by its assigned F, D, & C, and CI color standard numbers.

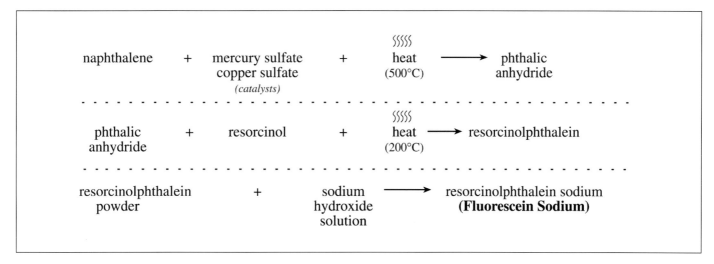

FIGURE 4-5
Fluorescein sodium synthesis.

To synthesize fluorescein sodium (Figure 4-5), naphthalene is oxidized in the presence of the catalysts mercury sulfate and copper sulfate (used to stabilize the reaction) at 400–500°C to produce phthalic anhydride. Phthalic anhydride is then heated with resorcinol to 200°C to make resorcinolphthalein. Phthalic anhydride is used in producing benzoic acid, phthaleins, synthetic indigo, and artificial resins. Resorcinol is used in manufacturing resins, adhesives, explosives, and cosmetics.

Finally, the yellowish-red powder resorcinolphthalein is dissolved in sodium hydroxide solution, which yields resorcinolphthalein sodium, another name for fluorescein sodium. The drug companies that prepare the fluorescein sodium used in ophthalmology purchase it from chemical supply houses as an orange-red powder that comes in jugs. They purify the powder with heat by autoclaving the jugs with 15 lb of pressure at 250°C. The fluorescein is precipitated out, redissolved in sodium hydroxide solution to make fluorescein sodium, standardized for color and concentration, and adjusted to a pH of 8+, which maximizes its fluorescence.

The color of the fluorescein sodium dye is often described as dark or light. Some photographers prefer the light-colored dye, because it is easier to distinguish its color from that of the patient's blood when it is drawn back into the butterfly needle's tubing.

Several times in the past, manufactured "lots" of intravenous (i.v.) fluorescein sodium have been recalled by drug companies because of contamination by mercury, which can be traced back to improper purification of the fluorescein sodium powder. Remember that the mercury is used in the initial synthesis of phthalic anhydride. Elevated mercury levels in fluorescein are not necessarily an issue in manufacturing industrial products, but they are of critical importance if found in medical supplies.

Fluorescein sodium is highly fluorescent. Its fluorescence is easily visible even in low dilutions. The maximum light absorption and fluorescent excitation of fluorescein sodium is 485–500 nm. Its maximum fluorescence emission is 520–530 nm (Figure 4-6).[10]

When injected into the bloodstream, fluorescein sodium is absorbed by the plasma proteins, particularly the albumins. It is also absorbed by hemoglobin. As this occurs, the intensity of the fluorescence is significantly decreased.[10] The suppression of fluorescence is referred to as *extinction*, and the absorption of fluorescein sodium and resulting loss of

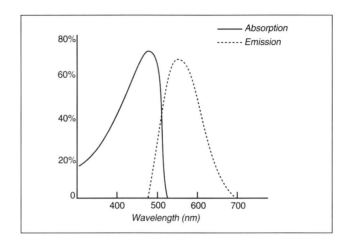

FIGURE 4-6
The absorption and emission spectra of in vitro fluorescein sodium.

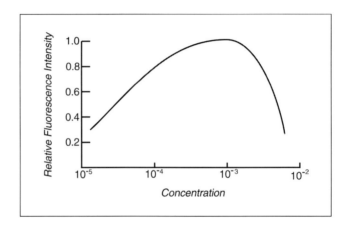

FIGURE 4-7
Fluorescence extinction by concentration. Fluorescence ability can be diminished if too much dye is injected over a short period and concentration builds up. (Adapted from A Wessing. Fluorescein Angiography of the Retina. St. Louis: Mosby, 1969.)

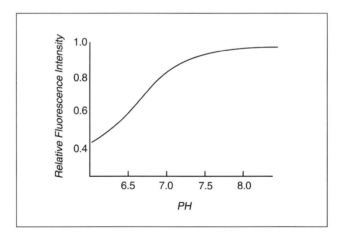

FIGURE 4-8
Fluorescence ability depends on pH value. Fluorescein sodium reaches a maximum fluorescence at pH of 8+. (Adapted from A Wessing. Fluorescein Angiography of the Retina. St. Louis: Mosby, 1969.)

fluorescence in the bloodstream is called *extinction by contamination*. This can also occur in the presence of the pyrazolone derivative drugs, such as butazolidin (an anti-inflammatory), and with some iodine compounds.[10] Concentration affects extinction; if a fluorescent material becomes too concentrated, the molecules begin to interact with each other, suppressing electron excitation. In fluorescein sodium, increasing the concentration of dye to an excess of 25% results in loss of fluorescence, which is called *extinction by concentration* (Figure 4-7).[10]

Fluorescence is dependent on pH values. The normal blood pH of 7.38–7.44 allows for almost maximal fluorescence (Figure 4-8).

Table 4-2. Fluorescein Sodium Availability and Distribution

Trade Name (Manufacturer)	Form
Injectable 10%	
AK-Fluor (Akorn)	5-ml amp and vial
Fluorescite (Alcon)	5-ml amp and syringe
Funduscein-10 (Ciba Vision)	5-ml amp
Ophthifluor (Deklerht)	5-ml amp
Injectable 25%	
AK-Fluor (Akorn)	2-ml amp and vial
Fluorescite (Alcon)	2-ml amp

amp = ampule.
Note: Fluorescein sodium is available for intravenous injection from multiple pharmaceutical companies in vials, ampules, and, in one instance, a ready-to-use disposable syringe.
Source: Reprinted with permission from T Burnham (ed). Drug Facts and Comparisons. St. Louis: Facts and Comparisons, 2000.

USES OF FLUORESCEIN SODIUM

The Merck Index lists the primary use of fluorescein sodium as examining subterranean waters.[9] It is used to determine the source and volume of springs, to find connections between springs and seas, to detect drinking water contamination sites, and to determine soil contamination by factory waste waters. Fluorescein sodium is the dye used to color the Chicago River green during the annual St. Patrick's Day observance in Chicago (as seen in the 1993 motion picture, "The Fugitive").

Fluorescein sodium has also been approved by the U.S. Food and Drug Administration (FDA) for use in manufacturing topical drugs and cosmetics as CI Acid Yellow 73, or D&C Yellow Dye #8. It is used in analytic and clinical reagents for laboratories as a protein label, an immunohistologic stain, and an immunofluorescent label.[9]

Fluorescein sodium was first used in ophthalmology by Erlich in 1881 when he injected the dye into rabbit eyes to observe aqueous flow.[11] Currently, fluorescein sodium's primary use in ophthalmology is as an external diagnostic aid, combined with topical anesthesia for use in applanation tonometry. It is also used topically to detect corneal epithelial defects and to assess contact lens fit. Fluorescein sodium for external use is available in a 2% solution form. It is instilled in the cul-de-sac of the lower lid or dried and heat-sterilized on paper strips, which are moistened with sterile water and applied to the conjunctiva in the lower cul-de-sac.[12]

Fluorescein sodium use for retinal angiography is reported last in the frequency of use list. The injectable dye comes in sterile vials or syringes in concentrations of 10% or 25%. The 10% solution comes in a 5-ml ampule (500 mg), and the 25% solution comes in a 2-ml ampule (500 mg).[13] The dye is not currently available specifically for oral administration. Several pharmaceutical companies prepare fluorescein sodium for ophthalmic use. Table 4-2 lists fluorescein distributors and availability.

Fluorescein Sodium Angiography

Retinal angiography allows the ophthalmologist to study the entire retinal vasculature, not just the larger veins and arteries observable by ophthalmoscopy. The properly filtered fundus camera records fluorescence wherever it is present, including the tiny retinal capillaries. Because the fluorescein sodium reaches the choroidal vasculature (choriocapillaris) approximately 1 second before it reaches the central retinal artery, the field of view brightens or lights up before dye can be seen in the retinal arteries. This effect is known as *choroidal flush*. The fluorescence from the retinal vessels is much brighter than the choroidal fluorescence, which is partially blocked by the retinal pigment epithelium. In cases in which the retinal pigment epithelium is thinned or absent or if something (such as drusen) is present that will transmit choroidal fluorescence to the retina, choroidal fluorescence can be as bright as retinal vessel fluorescence. If retinal vessel fluorescence cannot be seen, either the dye is not present in that area or the fluorescence is being blocked by something between the retina and the camera. The presence of fluorescein sodium can also be documented in vessels in the iris.

To obtain a good retinal angiogram with distinct circulation phases and adequate dye concentration, the dye is injected into the bloodstream in a good bolus (a concentrated mass). The most common injection site is the antecubital space on the medial side (inside) of the arm, in front of the elbow joint. The median cephalic vein, the median basilic vein, and the median cubital veins all run through this area. These are large, superficial veins that are usually visible, palpable, and sufficiently large to handle the injection of a bolus of fluid. A disadvantage of this area is that in some people, the brachial artery may rise just behind the median cephalic vein and run superficially. This increases the possibility of an accidental intra-arterial injection. If it is known ahead of time that the i.v. line needs to stay in for more than just a few minutes, the antecubital veins should not be used because the patient's arm movement will have to be restricted.

There is a short delay from the time that dye is injected and circulates through the heart and lungs to the time it finally appears in the choroidal and retinal vasculature. This time, referred to as the *arm-to-retina* time, is usually 8–16 seconds, assuming an antecubital injection. Injections made further down the arm or in the hand take a second or two longer to reach the retina. If the physician is interested in the arm-to-retina time, he or she should be informed of the location of the injection site.

When an antecubital injection is not possible, usually the dorsum (or back) of the hand is the next site considered. The metacarpal veins found there are easily accessible and lie flat on the back of the hand. However, the metacarpal veins are more fragile than the antecubital veins, they may have a smaller caliber, and insertion is more painful because of the large number of nerve endings in the hand.

Another possibility is the accessory cephalic vein, which runs along the radius and is most readily found in close proximity to the bend of the wrist. The vein is usually large and insertion is less painful than in the hand, but it rolls easily and can be difficult to stabilize. Also, any movement in the wrist can cause discomfort or cause the needle to be dislodged, which can result in extravasation of dye.

Sometimes, an i.v. injection is not possible in the arms or hands, as in patients with impaired circulation, scarring due to burns, damaged vessels due to diabetes, or other extenuating circumstances. Alternate injection sites may include the great saphenous vein of the leg, which is superficial at the internal malleolus (inside ankle bone), or the dorsal veins on the top of the foot. Injection at either site slightly increases the possibility of deep vein thrombosis. Elevating the foot after injection may decrease the delay of dye to the eye if the patient has impaired circulation, but it also may cause undue discomfort to the patient as he or she tries to maintain the position at the camera. Most often, unless the patient is a contortionist, the early phases of the angiogram are sacrificed if the foot is used as an injection site.

Before performing ocular angiography, properly educate your patient about the procedure and also take an appropriate history. Obtaining a history of the patient's previous fluorescein sodium angiographic experiences is of primary importance. Patients who have had previous adverse reactions to fluorescein sodium injections are especially likely to experience them again,[14] and some extra precautions or first aid supplies may be indicated.

Besides reviewing the patient's chart and determining the previous angiographic history, you should ask about general health, drug allergies, and recent episodes of chest pain or respiratory problems. In reference to the impending i.v. injection, questions should include asking the patients if their veins are easy to find, if they have experienced previous difficulty during blood draws, or if they have ever had surgery to their lymphatic system, as happens with a mastectomy. There have been reports of tissue damage when arms without intact lymphatic systems have been injected with fluorescein sodium. Asking the patient to indicate a "favorite" injection site is usually a good idea—the patients know their own history, and it gives them a sense of some control, which lessens their anxiety.

INJECTION TECHNIQUES

Proper injection technique is a learned behavior requiring thorough education. There is controversy in the field of ophthalmic photography over who should inject the fluorescein sodium when performing ocular angiography. Several surveys have been performed, with different results. One survey indicated that of the physicians responding, the majority performed the injections, whereas others used nurses or other physicians. Few indicated that a photographer performed the injection.[15] However, in a survey of ophthalmic photographers, 24 of 86 respondents reported that they performed the fluorescein sodium injection.[16] In most states, it is illegal for anyone who is not a licensed physician or physician assistant or registered nurse to administer drugs intravenously. In some states, it is legal for an unlicensed medical professional to perform venipuncture (insert the needle into the vein) but not push the plunger of the syringe and introduce the dye into the bloodstream.[16] However, some hospitals have policies that are contrary to this finding, and unlicensed personnel are allowed to administer i.v. injections. There are no official universal guidelines that dictate who should perform the injections. Ophthalmic photographers are not licensed as medical professionals and therefore do not meet the specifications stated in the study mentioned above. Some physicians request that their photographers perform i.v. injections anyway. In any scenario, the issue of liability should be considered.

In 1998, the Ophthalmic Photographers' Society (OPS), issued the following policy statement on performing venipuncture and i.v. injections[17]:

The OPS wishes to make its members aware that OPS has no legal authority to determine who may perform venipuncture or intravenous injections. The current position of OPS, taken through its Board of Directors, is that OPS neither advocates nor opposes venipuncture or the administration of intravenous injections, such as dyes, by photographers. The OPS also wishes to inform its members that: OPS is unaware of any federal laws which address who may perform venipuncture or intravenous injections; and the scope of practice of medical professionals has been established traditionally on the state level, meaning that the states determine the activities each medical specialty is allowed to perform under their state license. Accordingly, OPS recommends that each individual photographer check with the appropriate agency or agencies in the state in which they practice to determine whether the performance of venipuncture or the administration of intravenous injections falls within their scope of practice.

You should find out what the legal ramifications of intravenous injection are in your community and discuss it with your employer. No matter what decision is made, no one should perform venipuncture or intravenous administrations without being IV-certified by a reputable medical education facility. The best scenario allows the photographer to concentrate on the photography while a second person performs the injection and monitors the patient.

The following discussion of i.v. injection technique is intended to offer basic knowledge of the procedure and not to replace i.v. certification training. Whether you perform i.v. injections or not, you should be very familiar with injection protocols and the equipment needed. You should also be knowledgeable about first aid for failed injections, dye side effects, and adverse reactions to the dye. Cardiopulmonary resuscitation (CPR) training is essential for anyone performing ocular angiograms. Ocular angiography is not a benign event. It is a very valuable diagnostic procedure but is invasive and carries risks for patients. The risk of possible adverse reactions and complications should be taken seriously by the physicians ordering the procedure, the person administering the drug and the photographers performing the study. That the procedure is performed frequently or routinely does not justify a cavalier attitude by the medical personnel involved.

The risks associated with ocular angiography are not limited to the patient. Any time you are exposed to blood or other potentially infectious materials, as in performing venipuncture, you are at risk. The Occupational Safety and Health Administration (OSHA), which is part of the U.S. Department of Labor, is charged with protecting the health and safety of personnel in the workplace. The Occupational Health and Safety Act, Title 29, Chapter XVII, Part 1910, Subpart Z "Toxic and Hazardous Substances," a1910.1030, "Bloodborne Pathogens" (Dec. 6, 1991), requires that specific precautions be taken to ensure against occupational exposure to and inadequate disposal of potentially infectious materials.[18] This act requires by law that employers provide employees with adequate protection from occupational exposure by providing handwashing facilities, personal protection equipment, engineering controls ("sharps" containers, disposable gloves, etc.), exposure control plans, employee education, and exposure-incident follow-up. The act also mandates that employees follow strict protocols and methods of compliance for "universal precautions," which include proper handwashing, proper use and disposal of needles, appropriate use and disposal of gloves and other protective equipment, proper sterile technique, and other precautions in the workplace. Each health care facility, whether a major medical center or private physician's office, must have written procedures for carrying out the OSHA mandates regarding bloodborne pathogens. You should check with your clinic or office manager to get a copy of those procedures and guidelines and then follow them to protect yourself, your coworkers, and your patients.

Injection techniques can vary greatly among facilities, as can the brands and designs of the equipment used. Specific supplies should be dictated by the individual facility, following established i.v. protocols and procedures. If the facility does not have an existing i.v. protocol, as may be the case in private offices, state nursing associations or the hospital or surgical center where your ophthalmologist is affiliated can help you obtain copies of i.v. protocols.

In most cases, supplies are chosen by the trained professional performing the injection. In any case, patient safety and comfort should be the first priority in choosing supplies. Table 4-3 lists the supplies needed to perform an efficient, safe i.v. injection. In thinking through the procedure step-by-step, you can understand the need for each of these items.

As in any medical procedure, sterile technique should be followed. This includes handwashing before assembling the injection supplies, again before donning gloves, and after the procedure is complete. The

Table 4-3. Intravenous Injection Supplies for Fluorescein Angiography

Arm board
To stabilize patient's arm and hand

Tape
For securing needle at injection site

Alcohol swabs
To cleanse the skin around the injection site
3×3 gauze pads: Apply to the injection site after the needle is removed or protect a site that is already prepared

Tourniquet
To restrict venous flow, causing veins to become more prominent; blood pressure cuff may be used

Gloves
An Occupational Safety and Health Administration requirement whenever there is potential exposure to blood

Syringe and filter needle/filter straw
To extract fluorescein sodium from vial/ampule

Butterfly infusion set of 21- or 23-gauge needles
To inject fluorescein sodium into antecubital vein; 3-in. or 12-in. tubing connects the needle to the syringe; tubing allows greater flexibility when positioning needle; tubing less intimidating to patient than a rigid needle/syringe unit

Stopcock
For injecting more than one substance (i.e., fluorescein sodium and indocyanine green or fluorescein sodium and saline)

Sharps container
For proper disposal of needle and syringe, always observe universal precautions

Adhesive bandage
To cover the venipuncture site

Portable lined receptacle
Should a patient become nauseated

Emergency kit
Minimal: oxygen, cardiopulmonary equipment, antihistamine, smelling salts
Ideal: Standard "crash cart" with above and full complement of injection supplies and emergency medications

arm board and the tourniquet or blood pressure cuff that are used should be kept clean as well. All injection supplies should be disposable, and an OSHA-approved sharps container should be within easy reach of the injector for proper disposal of the contaminated needle assembly.

Fluorescein sodium is available in two different concentrations, 500 mg of 10%, and 500 mg of 25%. Which concentration to use is decided by the ophthalmologist and the photographer. The 10% concentration requires that a larger volume of solution be injected (5 cc), but the dye is more dilute. The 25% solution is a smaller volume (2 cc), but because the dye is more concentrated, it is theorized that there may be more potential for tissue damage if extravasated. Preparation of the syringe by transferring the dye from the ampule is done when the injection supplies are assembled.

The usual adult dosages are the volumes and concentrations listed above. The usual pediatric dosage is 3.5 mg per lb of body weight, as a 10% solution.[13] Any pediatric dosage should be calculated and approved by a physician or pharmacist.

The chosen syringe should hold 5 ml or greater to accommodate the volume of dye drawn up from the vial. A straight needle of small gauge, a filter needle with a small bevel, or a filter straw should be used to ensure that no small glass shards, which may have fallen into the vial when the neck was broken, will be drawn up into the injection. The filter needle is not needed if the dye comes in a rubber-stopped vial. One pharmaceutical company supplies fluorescein sodium in a specially prepared syringe, ready for injection.[13]

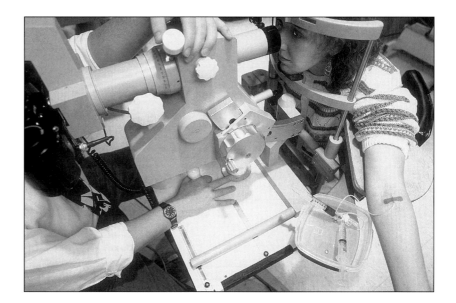

FIGURE 4-9
Multiple-syringe technique. When performing both retinal and choroidal angiography in the same procedure, syringes of each dye can be connected by a stopcock, allowing injection of both dyes via one needle. (Courtesy of William Nyberg, Scheie Eye Institute, Philadelphia, Pennsylvania.)

A butterfly infusion set with a needle of 21 or 23 gauge and a cannula of 3–12 in. is then attached to the fluorescein sodium syringe. A straight needle or angiocath of the same gauge are alternatives. The size of the needle used depends on the caliber and condition of the patient's veins. You should take care to protect the patient and avoid extravasation, but also ensure that you will have an adequate bolus for good early phase photographs.

To help ensure that the dye travels through the bloodstream to the ocular circulation in the greatest concentration possible, the bolus of fluorescein sodium can be followed immediately with the injection of 5 ml of normal saline. If this technique is chosen, an i.v. lock (or stopcock), a sterile adapter that attaches to the butterfly cannula and facilitates additional ports, is used. By using this attachment, several syringes can be added to the line, and several fluids, such as fluorescein sodium, saline, ICG, or heparin, can be injected at different times via the needle inserted in the arm (Figure 4-9).[19] This saves the patient from the discomfort of multiple needlesticks and saves time.

Efficient ocular angiography technique requires that the patient be positioned properly and comfortably at the fundus camera, with the camera and the target eye properly aligned before the needle is inserted. This avoids moving the patient's arm after i.v. insertion, which may result in dislodging the needle, possibly perforating the vessel. Also, in the case of the Zeiss fundus camera, this eliminates the camera table movement, which may be necessary for proper alignment.

Performing an i.v. injection is a logical, step-by-step process. First, the injection site is selected and then the site is stabilized using an arm rest. Next, a tourniquet (used as a restricting band) or blood pressure cuff is attached and pressure is applied to restrict the flow of blood from the veins, which makes them more prominent and eases the injection. Sometimes when the veins are small or scarred, they can become more prominent by having the patient make a fist and pump the hand, or hang the arm down by the side and swing the arm back and forth. Patting the vein firmly with the fingers or applying hot packs can assist with vasodilation. These extra efforts may be helpful or even required when the patient cannot offer an easy injection target because of diabetes or other circulatory problems. When the target vein has been chosen, the skin is cleansed with several alcohol preps, using a circular movement around the injection site, which moves from the center out, or in a "clean skin to dirty skin" pattern.

The needle is then inserted into the target vein with the bevel up, taking care to keep the angle of entry low so the needle does not go completely through the vein. Once the injector feels that the needle is positioned well within the caliber of the vessel, he or she should draw back on the syringe plunger gently to look for the presence of blood in the cannula. Once assured of proper positioning, the blood pressure cuff or tourniquet pressure is released. Injection should not be attempted until the pressure is released.

The photographer should signal the start of the injection. The injection should not begin unless the patient is properly aligned to the camera, or the early phases of the angiogram may be lost. However, the injection should start quickly before the needle can be moved accidentally or the needle bevel clots off. In some patients with poor circulation, as the vessel becomes irritated by the presence of the needle, it may collapse, resulting in a failed injection. Any attempt to inject fluid into a collapsed vessel may result in extravasation of dye into the surrounding tissue, with little dye actually getting into the bloodstream.

In an uncomplicated procedure in which the patient has good target vessels and no history of previous complications with fluorescein sodium angiography, the needle is removed as soon as the injection is finished. Removing the needle relieves the patient's discomfort and anxiety. However, if there is a chance that a second i.v. medication might be needed, such as diphenhydramine (Benadryl) or epinephrine, it is useful to keep the needle in place to avoid a second needle insertion.

If the needle needs to stay in the vein, the injection of 1 ml of heparin or a gradual infusion of saline can ensure against blood clotting at the end of the needle. This step is performed when an already in-dwelling i.v. line is used for the injection of fluorescein sodium. Using a saline flush will clean remaining fluorescein sodium out of the in-dwelling line but will not give the same assurance against clotting that heparin will. Heparin, of course, should not be used if the patient has clotting problems. The decision to use heparin should be made by a physician before the injection is started.

The speed with which the dye is injected is a source of controversy in the field of ocular angiography. There is little disagreement that the quicker the injection, the more concentrated the dye bolus will be and the better the contrast in the early phases of the study. The differences of opinion lie in whether the speed and pressure of the injection affect the incidence of adverse reactions to the dye. A study indicated that there was a higher incidence of adverse reactions in all fluorescein sodium angiographic patients who receive slower injections (greater than 6 seconds) than with faster injections (2–5 seconds).[14] Although this study was not designed specifically to address speed of injection, a formalized, repeatable technique was used by the angiographers participating in the study, and adverse reactions occurred 12 times more frequently with slow injections than with fast injections. Currently, no study has been conducted that specifically addresses all the implications of injection speed. Until such a study has been designed and implemented, the best procedure is to let the patient's physical condition and vessel tolerance dictate the speed of the injection while considering the patient's previous angiographic history and aiming to achieve the best photographic results. Some photographers prefer having an injection of a smaller volume of dye by using 2 cc of 25% fluorescein sodium.

Anecdotally, some angiographers believe that the added volume of the post-dye saline flush may also contribute to nausea. This has not been documented. Others think that the flush is essential to good dye concentration in the early angiogram phases, because it flushes the dye remaining in the butterfly cannula into the bloodstream. Some think that it is an unnecessary step that adds expense and time to the procedure. Whether or not the saline flush is used during routine angiography should be a mutual decision between the physician and the angiographer.

Any time the i.v. line will be used for more than one type of injection, however, a saline flush should be used to clean out the cannula. There has been a case report regarding a potentially serious reaction between two different drugs in an i.v. cannula.[20] After injection of fluorescein sodium during an angiogram, the patient rapidly developed hives (urticaria) as an allergic response. Promethazine (Phenergan), an antihistaminic drug, was introduced into the i.v. syringe, but the remaining fluorescein sodium had not been flushed out. The result was a chemical reaction between the promethazine, which has an acid pH, and the fluorescein sodium, which has a basic pH. The combination resulted in the precipitation of crystals in the syringe, which blocked the cannula. However, the crystals were not injected. A new i.v. line was established at another site to treat the patient's allergic reaction.

Once the injection has been successfully completed and there is no further need for access to the vein, the needle should be removed and the entire injection apparatus immediately discarded into an OSHA-approved sharps container. The needle should be discarded only by the injector to reduce possible exposure of additional personnel to a contaminated needle. Usually, an adhesive strip or bandage is all that is necessary to cover the puncture wound. Any excess dye or blood should be wiped off the skin surface. The history taken before the angiogram should alert you to whether the patient is on anticoagulants or has clotting problems. If so, apply pressure to the injection site to aid in clotting and puncture sealing. Any other injection supplies that have been contaminated with blood, such as alcohol preps or gauze sponges, must also be disposed of properly.

SIDE EFFECTS AND REACTIONS TO FLUORESCEIN SODIUM INJECTIONS

Drugs and dyes have predictable actions on which we base their use. Fluorescein sodium is used in retinal angiography because of its ability to reveal retinal vasculature with fluorescence and because it is relatively safe to inject into the human body. The fluorescent light emitted by the dye from the retinal and choroidal vessels can be easily documented, then interpreted to determine the presence and possible treatment of ocular pathologies.

Drugs and dyes can have other actions that may not be predictable or desirable. Some of these actions are labeled *side effects*; some are called *adverse reactions*. Several studies have been conducted to try to determine the incidence of various adverse reactions to fluorescein sodium, with a wide diversity of results reported. Both retrospective studies, which analyze past occurrences, and prospective studies, which follow a set protocol that looks for specific responses, have been conducted. Because of the difference in their design, it is difficult to compare the results of these studies, and it is of little value to state all the percentages reported in each study. What is of value is that all the studies concur in ranking the incidence of these reactions.

Side Effects.   A drug side effect is a bodily response that is usually predictable and may have a negative impact on the patient. Side effects are transient and do not require follow-up treatment. Fluorescein sodium has several side effects that are very predictable and a few that occur randomly. The product information inserts in each box of fluorescein sodium ampules list common side effects of the drug under the "patient information" heading. As part of the informed consent process, you should educate patients about the predictable side effects of fluorescein sodium.

Some side effects of fluorescein sodium happen 100% of the time. Staining of the skin, sclera, and mucous membranes is the first noticeable side effect. The dye becomes visible as it circulates through the capillaries of those tissues. The discoloration fades within 2–6 hours of the injection and in deeply pigmented individuals may not be very noticeable. Various secretions, including tears and saliva, may also be stained. The patient's urine will be colored orange-yellow and will fluoresce for 24–36 hours after injection. Fluorescein sodium is metabolized in the liver to become fluorescein monoglucuronide, which, along with the excess fluorescein sodium, is excreted exclusively in the urine.[21] Nevertheless, there is no increased frequency of adverse reactions in patients with renal insufficiency or who are on hemodialysis.[22]

The presence of fluorescein sodium in the bloodstream interferes with some clinical laboratory tests because of its serum concentration.[23] What tests are affected, how long the interference persists, and how to deal with this side effect are discussed later in this chapter.

Other side effects that occur with far less regularity are a "flushing" sensation in the skin, a strong metallic taste in the mouth, tingling of the lips, and sneezing, all of which are transient.

Adverse Reactions.   Adverse reactions are consequences of drug administration that have a negative impact on the patient, may be transient, may require medical intervention, and may lead to death. They have been classified as mild, moderate, severe, and death.[24] These classifications were based on the duration of the reaction, whether medical intervention was required, and whether there were any enduring consequences to the reaction. Also, an attempt was made to determine the frequency of adverse reactions among all patients receiving fluorescein sodium angiography.

MILD ADVERSE REACTIONS.   Mild adverse reactions include nausea, vomiting, and a vasovagal response resulting in dizziness and lightheadedness. Of all adverse reactions, nausea occurs most frequently. This condition is often accompanied by hypersalivation and gagging, which occurs more frequently than vomiting. The reaction is transient and clears rapidly. It usually begins 30 seconds after the start of the injection and usually only lasts 30–90 seconds. Some photographers instruct their patients to breathe slowly and deeply if they start to feel nauseated, which helps them relax and lessens their anxiety. Some photographers advocate having patients rinse their mouths out with cool water just before the injection. In patients who have experienced more prolonged nausea or vomiting, or both, with previous fluorescein sodium angiograms, prochlorperazine (Compazine) or promethazine (Phenergan) can be administered either orally or intramuscularly at least 45 minutes before the procedure. In the unusual instance in which nausea is more prolonged, either of the above medications may be helpful.

Vasovagal responses, which are usually evoked by stress or pain, are actions of the vagus nerve that can reduce heart rate and blood pressure. These attacks can respond favorably to the deep breathing technique, too. No one knows exactly why nausea occurs, but there is speculation that because fluorescein sodium is very soluble and permeable and has a high pH (8+), it easily crosses the blood-brain barrier and triggers the nausea response through the hypothalamus gland. Some patients who have experienced significant vasovagal response previously may do well with a small dose of diazepam (Valium) given at least 30 minutes before the angiogram. The decision to premedicate patients should be made by the physician, with input from the photographer.

MODERATE ADVERSE REACTIONS.   Moderate adverse reactions include urticaria (hives), syncope (fainting), phlebitis (vascular inflammation), local skin necrosis (skin death), and localized nerve palsy (paralysis). Urticaria is the second most common adverse reaction, after nausea or vomiting. It is most often a histaminic (allergic) response and should be treated with an antihistamine, such as diphenhydramine (Benadryl) or promethazine. The severity of an allergic reaction is difficult to predict, so medical intervention should be undertaken any time allergic symptoms appear. Although it is unusual for a patient to exhibit an allergic response to fluorescein sodium during his or her first ocular angiogram, some patients may be exposed and become sensitized to the dye when it is used topically during ophthalmic examinations. Any time a patient reports an allergic reaction experienced during a previous fluorescein sodium angiogram, consider medicating with an antihistamine at least 40 minutes before he or she is injected with the dye. Always report a history of fluorescein sodium allergy to the ophthalmologist so he or she can decide what prophylactic measures should be taken to protect the patient, or decide if it is advisable to perform the procedure.

Syncope (fainting) is a strong vasovagal response that is self-limiting and requires first aid, but not necessarily medical intervention. Precautions should be made to protect the patients from injury, lying them in a position that is optimal for good circulation, monitoring their blood pressure, and reassuring them. Depending on their recovery, rescheduling the angiogram for another time when they can be premedicated might be the best option. A physician should assess the patient's general condition before he or she is released from the clinic.

Phlebitis is an inflammation of blood vessels that may occur as a response to the presence of an irritating injection or because the inner wall of the vein has been injured. The symptoms of phlebitis are localized pain at the injection site, redness following the course of the vessel, and pain along the course of the vessel. Phlebitis is usually not diagnosed until at least 24 hours after the injection. Suspicion of phlebitis should be reported to the physician immediately. Phlebitis can be self-limiting, but it also can lead to thrombophlebitis, in which a blood clot is formed in the inflamed vessel. This complication can have far more serious ramifications and requires medical intervention.

Local skin necrosis can occur after extravasation of fluorescein sodium into the skin during an i.v. injection. The high pH of the dye may contribute to the tissue damage. A physician should assess the site any time an extravasation of fluorescein sodium occurs. Have the patient report back the next day after an extravasation so that the condition can be assessed. Any report of edema, redness, or pain should prompt a physical examination of the extravasation site. Medical intervention is required if there is evidence of tissue damage or deterioration.

Nerve palsy can occur if a nerve receives trauma during an i.v. injection. The nerve can be damaged by the needle, or it can be damaged by increased pressure caused by extravasation of dye or blood, resulting in ischemia. Nerve palsies are usually self-limiting, but assessment must be made by a physician about whether medical intervention is indicated.

SEVERE ADVERSE REACTIONS.   Severe adverse reactions involve the respiratory, neurologic, and cardiac systems. All require immediate intervention, all threaten the patient's safety, and all can ultimately result in death. Respiratory reactions include laryngeal edema, bronchospasm, and anaphylaxis. Neurologic reactions are tonic-clonic seizures, and cardiac reactions include circulatory shock, myocardial infarction, and cardiac arrest.

Respiratory reactions may present as difficulty breathing or talking or loss of consciousness. A tonic-clonic seizure is characterized by involuntary movements, heightened muscle tone and muscle spasm, respiratory distress, increased blood pressure, and loss of consciousness. Cardiac symptoms may include chest and radiating arm pain, sweating, increased blood pressure, decreased blood pressure, difficulty breathing, cardiac arrhythmias, loss of consciousness, cessation of breathing, and cardiac arrest.

Although severe adverse reactions are rare, emergency medical supplies, including oxygen, drugs, injection supplies, and CPR equipment should be immediately available anywhere fluorescein sodium angiography is performed (Figure 4-10 and Table 4-4). Everyone performing fluorescein angiography should be trained in basic CPR, and emergency medical personnel should be available immediately. These precautions argue that fluorescein sodium angiography should not be performed unless medical personnel are readily available. In a hospital setting, an emergency code should be called in the event of a severe adverse reaction. In a private office that is free-standing from an emergency response facility, strict protocols for how an emergency team can be summoned must be established. You should never perform a fluorescein sodium angiogram unless there are additional people present who can summon help in case you have to perform CPR.

In the classification of adverse reactions, death was attributed to i.v. fluorescein sodium if it occurred within 48 hours of the injection. The Fluorescein Angiography Complication Survey reported death occurring in 1 of 222,000 ocular angiograms.

COMPLICATIONS OF FAILED INJECTIONS
There are complications arising from failed i.v. injection attempts that are not considered to be adverse reactions caused by the presence of the dye in the bloodstream. They can occur when proper i.v. technique is not followed, or if the target vessel is compromised and cannot facilitate the infusion of the injection. In any case, care must be taken to ensure that a failed attempt does not result in a complication.

The most common complication of failed injection is the extravasation of blood or dye out of the vein and into the surrounding tissue. The extravasation of blood can occur when too large a needle is used and it penetrates completely through the vessel, or if compression to the site is not applied after the needle is removed. The resulting hematoma (bruise) can be painful and may also exert pressure on surrounding nerves, causing nerve palsy. Patients taking anticoagulants, including aspirin, or who have clotting problems are at increased risk of hematoma.

A related complication of failed injection is the extravasation of fluorescein sodium. Because of its high pH, the dye is very irritating to surrounding tissues, and, as stated above, can result in skin necrosis. All of the precautions mentioned in the i.v. injection discussion should be followed. Increased resistance to the plunger of the syringe should signal the injector to stop the infusion and assess the needle position. Although it is helpful for the photographer to have the lights lowered when visualizing the fundus during the early phases of the angiogram, there

A

B

FIGURE 4-10
Medical emergency and first aid supplies. Adverse reactions to fluorescein sodium can range from severe life or death medical emergencies to mild discomfort. **A.** A "crash cart" containing basic life support supplies should be kept in close proximity to where angiography is performed. **B.** This drawer containing drugs used in performing ocular photography or first aid has been arranged for easy access and easy identification. (Courtesy of Michael Palczynski, Virginia Eye Institute, Richmond, Virginia.)

should be sufficient light to adequately assess how the injection is going. Some offices use "mini" lights or flashlights to illuminate the injection site. When you orient the patient before the injection, tell the patient to inform you immediately if he or she begins to experience any stinging or burning around the injection site. Watching the injection site is particularly important with diabetic patients, because they may have reduced sensitivity to pain, and therefore may fail to alert you to dye extravasation. If there is a question of extravasation, needle placement should be assessed, and, most often, the needle should be removed and a new injection site selected.

Table 4-4. Emergency Supplies for Fluorescein Angiography

General medical equipment
  Stethoscope
  Sphygmomanometer (blood pressure cuff)
  Portable oxygen
  Tourniquet
  Alcohol wipes
  Adhesive tape
  Engineering-controlled receptacle
  Ambubag
  Oxygen masks (adult and pediatric)
  Resuscitation mask (cushioned)
  1-cc tuberculin syringes
  5-cc syringes
  Adhesive bandages
  Gloves
Drugs
  Acetaminophen, 500 mg, for analgesia
  Aromatic ammonia inhalants ("smelling salts") for fainting
  Diphenhydramine, 25-mg capsules, and diphenhydramine, 50-mg injection,
    for allergic reactions
  Epinephrine, 1-mg/ml injection, for allergic reactions
  Promethazine, 25-mg capsules, for nausea
  Nitroglycerin, 0.4-mg (1/150 g) sublingual tablets, for angina
  Hyaluronidase, 150-units injection, for subcutaneous injections around extrava-
    sations
  Heparin, 100-units/ml injection, for maintaining in-dwelling lines
  Sterile water for preparing injections
Food supplies for blood sugar imbalances
  Unsweetened fruit juice
  Graham crackers
  Saltine crackers
  Granulated sugar
  Hard candy

If the dye is extravasated out of the target vein, the needle should be removed, and some of the offending dye may be coaxed out of the needle puncture wound by applying light pressure around the puncture, in much the same way that blood is coaxed out after a digital (finger) blood draw. Although cold packs applied to the extravasation site offer pain relief, warm packs are suggested. The heat may slightly increase the immediate pain, but it will also dilate the capillaries and allow the extravasated dye to diffuse out and become less concentrated. This may be especially important in patients with poor circulation or fragile skin, such as the elderly. The warm packs should be applied for 3–5 minutes. After the dye has diffused, cold packs can be applied for pain relief. The use of multiple small injections of the enzyme hyaluronidase (Wydase) around the injection site to improve absorption of the dye has also been recommended. Analgesia may be indicated to relieve discomfort. The patient's status should be checked 24 hours after the extravasation.

A less frequent but potentially serious complication of a failed injection attempt is accidental intra-arterial injection.[24] Injection of fluorescein sodium into an artery results in the dye circulating away from the heart, into the distal peripheral capillaries of the arm. This results in increased pressure sensation and, in some patients, intense pain. The arm below the injection site becomes intensely yellow in patches where the undiluted dye has been circulated (Figure 4-11).

Although arteries usually lie deeper in the arm and pulsate, 10–13% of the population have ulnar arteries that are unusually placed and run superficially next to the basilic vein.[9] When a needle has been placed in

FIGURE 4-11
An intra-arterial injection. Dye has been accidentally injected into an artery, and the bolus has flowed away from the heart, into the hand. The dye stays concentrated in the lower arm and hand, which can result in intense pain. (Courtesy of Csaba Martonyi, University of Michigan, Ann Arbor, Michigan.)

a vessel, the plunger of the syringe should be drawn back, and the blood in the cannula should be checked. Venous blood is dark red in appearance, but arterial blood is bright red because of its oxygen content.

First aid for intra-arterial injection may include plunging the affected area into cold water for pain relief, as well as administering analgesics. A physician should be summoned immediately to assess the patient's condition and determine what analgesia is appropriate. A successful retinal angiogram with concentrated, observable dye in early phases is not possible, as the dye has been deposited in tissues fed by the injected artery. The patient should be closely followed for several days after the injection.

SPECIAL CONSIDERATIONS

Patients who require special caution during i.v. injections include elderly patients with senile skin changes (thin skin due to loss of collagen and adipose tissue); patients with impaired circulation such as diabetics; patients with blood abnormalities; patients with impaired or absent lymphatic systems, such as mastectomy patients; and patients who are dehydrated or underweight.

Fluorescein sodium angiography is contraindicated in patients who are pregnant and in juvenile asthmatics and should be used with caution in patients with a previous history of severe adverse reactions to the dye and patients who have a recent history of chest pain or cardiac irregularities. It is not contraindicated in nursing mothers, although the dye has been found in mother's milk, nor is it contraindicated in patients on hemodialysis or in renal failure.

There have been reports of patients developing skin photosensitivity resulting in increased risk of sunburn after injection of fluorescein sodium. This may be a photoallergic reaction enhanced by sunlight.[25,26] It does not appear to be a common reaction.

EFFECT OF FLUORESCEIN SODIUM ON LABORATORY TESTS

Bloom studied the effect of fluorescein sodium with certain serum laboratory tests.[22] Serum and urine samples were checked. No interference was found in the urine samples, but of 27 serum analyte tests, six were affected by the presence of fluorescein sodium in the blood. Those tests affected by fluorescein sodium were levels of creatinine, cortisol, digoxin, quinidine, thyroxine, and total protein. The interference may persist for

FIGURE 4-12
A molecular diagram of indocyanine green.

as long as 24 hours after injection. These tests can be performed on various analytical systems, and not all tests on all systems were affected.

To avoid false test results, when you orient your patients before fluorescein sodium angiography, they should be informed that the dye may affect some test results. If they are scheduled for tests within 24 hours of the angiogram, either they should have their blood drawn before the injection of the dye or you should give them a list of which tests by which analytical system are affected. They can then take the list to the laboratory where alternatives may be found.

Indocyanine Green

ICG ($C_{43} H_{47} N_2 NaO_6 S_2$) is a tricarbocyanine dye used to perform choroidal angiography (Figure 4-12). According to its chemical structure, it is in the polymethine group of biological stains. It is marketed under the brand name Indocyanine-Green and is also known as Fox Green.

A relatively safe synthetic dye, ICG is the result of a complex synthesis of a derivative of glutaconic aldehyde with an indolium hydroxide compound.[27] Sodium iodide is added as a dipolar ion and is necessary to achieve solubility. There is a misconception that iodine is a major component of ICG, when actually, it is not even part of the empirical chemical formula of the dye. The iodide ion is added to make ICG soluble and safe for human use. The dye comes as a dark green, blue-green, or green-black powder that must be mixed with sterile water to form an aqueous solution for injection.

ICG was first used by the Eastman-Kodak company in the manufacture of Wratten filters and in infrared photography.[27] In the 1950s, after satisfactory treatment by Dr. Fox of the Mayo Clinic, an official of Kodak offered him an array of dyes from their photochemical shelves for possible medical applications; ICG was one of the dyes offered. Eventually, ICG was turned over to the Hynson, Westcott, and Dunning pharmaceutical firm for further development for medical use and received U.S. Food and Drug Administration approval in 1956. It was determined that ICG was appropriate for use in cardiac output studies, then later proved to be applicable for liver function studies and choroidal angiography.

WHAT IS INDOCYANINE GREEN?
ICG is a very complex synthetic that is soluble in water and methanol but is practically insoluble in other organic solvents. Even when dissolved in sterile saline, it is unstable, and the solution must be used within 10 hours.[13] The dye comes as a freeze-dried powder from the manufacturers, which sometimes clumps up or clings to the sides of the vial. This clump-

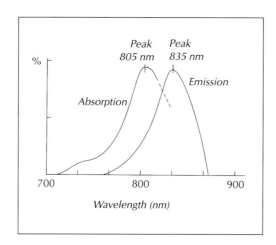

FIGURE 4-13
The absorption and emission spectra of in vitro indo-cyanine green.

ing, however, is not indicative of contamination by moisture because water content is very carefully controlled. It is recommended that ICG powder be mixed only with the aqueous solvent that comes with it from the manufacturer, as there have been reports of incompatibility with some other sterile water for injection preparations.[13] Of course, sterile technique should always be used when mixing the solution for injection.

Currently, only one pharmaceutical company is listed in the drug literature as a source of medical-grade ICG, which is known as Cardio-Green. Other pharmaceutical companies package angiography kits that contain vials of ICG, but the dye is manufactured by only one company. The synthesis of the dye is protected by two U.S. patents.

ICG is not as fluorescent as fluorescein sodium. In fact, it has approximately only $1/25$ the fluorescence efficiency of fluorescein sodium, and its fluorescence is not seen in the visible spectrum of light.[9] Its peak absorption is 800–810 nm, and its emission peak is 835 nm within the infrared spectrum (Figure 4-13).[27] The drug heparin contains sodium bisulfite, which affects the absorption peak of ICG and should not be used in conjunction with injection of the dye. Significant concentrations of heparin in the blood before injection may affect the quality of an ICG study. ICG has a pH of 6 and is mixed with sterile water with a pH of 5.5–6.5.

When injected into the bloodstream, ICG is 98% absorbed by the plasma proteins, especially the albumins.[27] For this reason, the dye does not extravasate freely from retinal vessels or from the highly fenestrated vessels of the choriocapillaris. This characteristic is in sharp contrast to the free-leaking characteristics of fluorescein sodium and makes possible infrared angiography to delineate choroidal vessels. ICG is not metabolized after injection but is taken up completely by the parenchymal cells of the liver and excreted in the bile. It is not excreted by the kidneys as is fluorescein sodium. Patients should be informed that the dye does not cause any of the characteristic staining of their mucous membranes and secretions that happens with fluorescein sodium, but their stools will be discolored for several days.

USES OF INDOCYANINE GREEN

As mentioned earlier, ICG was first used medically in cardiac outflow studies. The dye is used as an indicator, and its concentration in arterial blood flow is determined with the use of an oximeter or earpiece densitometer attached to a needle or catheter. The catheter is threaded to the part of the anatomy to be studied, and a specific amount of the dye is delivered in a single bolus.[28] Dye concentration in arterial blood is then sampled, and the efficiency of blood moving through the heart can be calculated.

Because ICG is exclusively excreted in the bile, it is useful in determining liver function and blood flow. Bile duct obstructions affect the excretion of the dye. To study liver function, blood samples are taken at routine intervals of up to 20 minutes, the samples are centrifuged and coagulated, and densitometry is used to determine the rate of dye retention or dye disappearance in the blood serum.[27] Dye levels exceeding 4% are indicative of impaired hepatic function.[12]

Kogure et al. were the first to use ICG in ophthalmology as ICG absorption angiography of monkey retinas.[29] They performed the procedure in 1970 using a 35-mm fundus camera and color film.[30] In 1971, Hochheimer modified the technique by using black and white infrared film. Then Flower introduced fluorescence angiography using ICG.[31] This new procedure called for improved filters to record the fluorescence with infrared film. Remember that ICG has only 4% of the fluorescence efficiency of fluorescein.

After determining that infrared film was unable to record the presence and location of the poorly fluorescent ICG in the choroidal circulation for long periods, Hayashi introduced videography for recording the ICG images. Although all of these modifications improved the efficiency of ICG angiography, poor image resolution and the potential for infrared radiation toxicity and possible increase of retinal temperature because of infrared radiation exposure hampered the acceptance of ICG angiography as a common clinical diagnostic tool.

Multiple technological advances have modified ICG angiography, however, resolving many of the previous problems, and the procedure is rapidly growing in clinical use and acceptance. The procedure is done using either a scanning laser ophthalmoscope or an electronic digital imaging system. New digital systems include a fundus camera with an infrared radiation source, a video camera, possibly several monitors, a personal computer with accompanying customized imaging software, a video cassette recorder, and an optical disk drive for data storage. In addition, the cameras have 35-mm film capabilities with synchronized flash, enlarged apertures to increase the amount of light that can be used for imaging, and appropriate excitatory and barrier filters with special infrared coatings.

Indocyanine Green Angiography

The circulation dynamics of choroidal angiography are the same as in retinal angiography: Dye injected intravenously in the arm flows in the same pattern to reach the choroidal and retinal circulation, as described in the section on retinal angiography. However, the characteristics of the dyes used to document the two separate vascular systems and the imaging systems used to record the circulation patterns are different. ICG is clearly seen in the retinal vasculature as well as in the choroidal vasculature, but because of its almost complete binding to the albumins in the blood, ICG does not "leak" or extravasate out of the choriocapillaris as does fluorescein sodium. Because ICG stays in both the retinal and choroidal vessels, the distinct outlines of the vessels of the choroid can be seen and identified and are not obscured. Because infrared radiation is much more efficient in penetrating the pigmented layers of the retina, serous exudates, thin layers of subretinal blood, or even medial opacities, ICG can be seen more readily in the choroidal vasculature than can fluorescein sodium despite ocular pathology.

Because ICG angiography is still not widely used and its applications and efficacy are still being investigated, there is some variation in sequencing and technique for performing these studies. Sometimes ICG angiography is performed simultaneously with fluorescein sodium angiography, sometimes sequentially, and sometimes alone.[32] In cases in which ICG angiography is performed solely, a fluorescein sodium angiogram has usually been done within the previous few days, although sometimes ICG angiography is performed specifically because a patient has a known allergy to fluorescein sodium.

The two studies are not interchangeable, as different information is derived from each, but they are commonly used to complement or enhance each other. Whether fluorescein sodium and ICG angiography should be performed sequentially or simultaneously should be decided by the referring physician and the photographer.

For simultaneous fluorescein sodium and ICG procedures, dosages of the two dyes are combined in the same syringe. The dyes are compatible and can be combined for injection safely. During simultaneous procedures, the early fluorescein sodium phase is recorded, then the infrared filters are put in place, and ICG images are captured. Images of the two dyes are taken alternately, switching the camera setting appropriately.

For sequential procedures, one dye or the other is injected first, and the early phase of that study is completed. Then, the second dye is injected after the appropriate filters and flash settings are arranged, and the early phase of that study is completed. As mentioned above in the section on i.v. injections, a single-needle, two-way stopcock arrangement is easiest on the patient.[19] Remember that heparin contains sodium bisulfite and therefore should not be used as an anticoagulant in conjunction with an ICG injection. The sodium bisulfite reduces the absorption peak of ICG in the blood and diminishes the fluorescence abilities of the dye. Any post-injection flush of the butterfly-syringe set should only be done with normal saline.

The sequencing and time intervals for ICG angiography differ with the pathology to be studied. Images are recorded at approximately 10 seconds after injection and continue at several-second intervals. These images are recorded even before an image is visible on the monitor. As ICG fills the retinal and choroidal vessels, the image to the camera deteriorates as "blooming" occurs—the dye concentration in both vascular systems is too intense and the image deteriorates. The flash setting is turned down to avoid overexposed images; then, after this initial phase, the flash setting is turned back up. The images are recorded at approximately 3 minutes, 5–7 minutes, 10–12 minutes, and 25+ minutes. The later phases of an ICG angiogram may yield the most information, depending on the pathology being studied. ICG can remain in neovascular tissue after the dye has left the retinal and choroidal vessels. Sometimes, to assist in photocoagulation of neovascular membranes, reinjection of 1 mg of ICG can help redefine retinal and choroidal vessels, providing landmarks for the physician.[33]

According to the literature, the usual adult dosage for ICG is 40 mg in 2 ml of aqueous solvent.[13] Sometimes a lesser dosage of dye yields good images, and 25 mg in 3 ml is suggested. In simultaneous fluorescein sodium/ICG injections, 50 mg of ICG in 3 ml is mixed with 2 ml of 25% fluorescein sodium.[32]

Because of its characteristic insolubility, ICG is hard to dissolve and prepare for injection. Even when it appears superficially that the dye is dissolved, great care must be taken to ensure that it is actually in complete solution. Because of its instability in solution form, the liquid should be used within 10 hours. These are the chemical characteristics of ICG and are problems that are not easily solved by its manufacturers. Theoretically, other dipolar ions may make ICG more soluble and stable but may not be safe for human use. The manufacturer's instructions for the dissolving and preparation of ICG should be strictly followed.

SIDE EFFECTS AND REACTIONS TO INDOCYANINE GREEN

Unlike fluorescein sodium, ICG does not have multiple side effects and adverse reactions. One possible explanation is that ICG is so bound to the proteins in the blood, it does not extravasate easily out of vessels. The result is that ICG is a relatively benign dye, and patients usually tolerate it well.

The common side effect of ICG is the staining of stools. ICG does not color the skin or the mucous secretions. As it is excreted exclusively by the liver, ICG does not show up in urine. It does not pass to the placenta but has not been proved safe for use in pregnancy.

When adverse reactions occur in a patient during ICG angiography, the first aid and supplies suggested in previous sections of this chapter apply.

Mild Adverse Reactions.   Reported mild adverse reactions include infrequent nausea and vomiting and lightheadedness. The frequency of mild adverse reactions has been reported as 0.5%.[34]

Moderate Adverse Reactions.   Moderate adverse reactions reported have included urticaria, fainting, and vasovagal responses. Possibly, the vasovagal responses are due to the invasive nature of the injection, not to the dye itself. The frequency rate of moderate reactions has been reported as 0.2%.

Pharmaceutical literature states that anyone with an allergy to iodine should not be injected with ICG. Other literature suggests that patients at risk for allergic reactions are only those with a history of iodide ion allergy.[13] The concentration of sodium iodide in ICG is only 5%. It seems that some patients who report iodine allergy do not experience allergic response reactions to ICG. Some reactions to ICG are pseudoallergic, with a nonimmunologic release of histamine.[34] The University of Paris has reported the synthesis of ICG with a dipolar ion different from sodium iodide, which may not carry the same potential for iodine allergy reactions.[35]

Severe Adverse Reactions.   In all the literature, including the cardiac and hepatic specialty literature, there have been 16 severe reactions reported. In each case, the adverse reactions did not seem typical and were not dependent on the dose of ICG. Most of the reactions seemed to be allergic in nature but with no previous histories of allergy. Almost one-half of the patients experiencing adverse reactions had end-stage renal disease and were on hemodialysis. It may be that patients with uremia respond to ICG with allergic hypersensitivity, but no one is sure of the exact response mechanism. Overall, the adverse reaction rate is 0.05%. Two deaths have been reported in the literature, both due to anaphylaxis followed by cardiac arrest.

COMPLICATIONS OF FAILED INJECTIONS

The proper i.v. techniques and precautions mentioned earlier apply to injections of ICG. Extravasation of ICG does not seem to cause the same degree of pain caused with extravasated fluorescein sodium, and tissue necrosis has not been reported. This may be due to the lower pH of ICG, and because it is not easily diffused through tissues. ICG is not hyperosmolar, and there is no specific recommendation that hyaluronidase injections be applied around ICG extravasations.

Instances of intra-arterial injections of ICG seem to have few complications.[36]

SPECIAL CONSIDERATIONS

The same caution used in screening patients for fluorescein sodium angiography should be used for ICG angiography, although fluorescein sodium has a higher adverse reaction rate, and the complications with failed injections are also higher. In a survey of ophthalmic specialists in the year 2001, most would not perform ICG angiography on a pregnant woman.[37] ICG is also contraindicated in patients who have had a previous allergic reaction to it. It seems that allergy to iodine does not always result in an allergic reaction to ICG, but great caution should be taken when using the dye on these patients. First aid and emergency supplies should be immediately available. Nothing has been reported to suggest that juvenile asthmatics are at risk with ICG as they are with fluorescein sodium. There is evidence that patients with uremia on hemodialysis are at increased risk of allergic reaction to ICG.

EFFECT OF INDOCYANINE GREEN ON LABORATORY TESTS

Because of the presence of iodine in ICG, radioactive iodine uptake studies and results can be affected by the dye. As a result, iodine uptake studies should not be performed for at least a week after the injection of ICG.[38]

References

1. Miller S. Cardiac Angiography. Boston: Little, Brown, 1984;4.
2. Grossman W, Baim D. Cardiac Catheterization and Intervention. Philadelphia: Lea & Febiger, 1991;15, 16, 23, 26.
3. Friesinger GC, Adams DF, Bourassa MG, et al. Optimal resources for examination of the heart and lungs. Circulation 1983;68:893A.
4. Wong D. Textbook of Ophthalmic Photography. New York: Inter-optics Publications, 1982;83.
5. Lillie RD. HJ Conn's Biological Stains: A Handbook on the Nature and Uses of the Dyes Employed in the Biological Library. Baltimore: Williams & Wilkins, 1977;19, 21,3:35.
6. Baeyer A. Ueber einen neue klasse von farbstoffen. Ber Dtch Chem Gzellshaft 1871;4:555.
7. Federman J, Maguire J. Intravenous Fluorescein Angiography. In W Tasman (ed), Duane's Clinical Ophthalmology. Philadelphia: Harper & Row, 1991;1.
8. Anand R. Fluorescein angiography. Part 1. Technique and normal study. J Ophthal Nursing Technol 1989;8:50.
9. Budavari S (ed). The Merck Index: An Encyclopedia of Chemicals, Drugs and Biologicals (11th ed). Rahway, NJ: Merck & Co, 1989;786;6287.
10. Wessing A. Fluorescein Angiography of the Retina. St. Louis: Mosby, 1969;12–14.
11. Erlich P. Ueber provocirte fluorescenzerscheinungen am augen. Dtsch Med Wochenschr 1882;8:21.
12. Gennaro A (ed). Remington's Pharmaceutical Sciences. Easton, PA: Mack Publishing, 1990;1271,1275.
13. Olin BR (ed). Drug Facts and Comparisons. St. Louis: Facts & Comparisons, 1993;514–515.
14. Kwiterovitch K, Maguire M, Murphy R, et al. Frequency of adverse reactions after fluorescein angiography. Ophthalmology 1991;98:1141–1142.
15. Yanuzzi L, Rohrer K, Tindel L, et al. Fluorescein angiography complication survey. Ophthalmology 1986;93:613.
16. Szirth B, Wong D, Bate R, Bartlett D. Legal ramifications of intravenous administration of sodium fluorescein. J Ophthal Photog 1989;11:70, 77.
17. Ophthalmic Photographers' Society. OPS position on performing venipuncture and intravenous injections. OPS Newsletter 28:6, November 1998.
18. U.S. Government. The occupational health and safety act. Federal Register 1991;56(235):64175.
19. Bullock JD, Fezza AJ. A double syringe and three-way stopcock for fluorescein injection. Am J Ophthalmol 1974;77:270.
20. Myers P. Case report: a potentially serious reaction between sodium fluorescein and promethazine solutions: flush the cannula before injecting. Arch Ophthalmol 1994;112:734.

21. Chahal PS, Neal MJ, Kohner EM. Metabolism of fluorescein after intravenous injection. Invest Ophthalmol Vis Sci 1985;26:764.
22. Bloom J, Herman D, Elin R, et al. Intravenous fluorescein interference with clinical laboratory tests. Am J Ophthalmol 1989;108:375.
23. Yanuzzi L, Rohrer K, Tindel L, et al. Fluorescein angiography complication survey. Ophthalmology 1986;93:612.
24. Bovino JA, Marcus DF. Accidental intra-arterial injection of fluorescein dye. Ophthalmic Surg 1984;15:983.
25. Hochsattel R, Gall H, Weber L, Kaufmann R. Photoallergic reactions to fluorescein. Contact Dermatitis 1990;22:42.
26. Danis RP, Stephens T. Phototoxic reactions caused by sodium fluorescein. Am J Ophthalmol 1997;123:694–696.
27. Cardio-Green. Cockeysville, MD: Becton Dickinson Microbiology Systems, 1990;5–6.
28. Indocyanine Green: History, Chemistry, Pharmacology, Indications, Adverse Reactions, Investigations, and Prognosis—An Investigator's Brochure. Hunt Valley, MD: Becton Dickinson & Co., 1994;6.
29. Choromokos E, David N, Justice J. The beginnings of indocyanine green angiography. J Ophthal Photog 1994:16:70.
30. Yanuzzi L, Slakter J, Sorenson J, et al. Digital indocyanine green videoangiography and choroidal neovascularization. Retina 1992;12:199.
31. Flower RW, Hochheimer BF. Clinical infrared absorption angiography of the choroid. Am J Ophthalmol 1972;73(3):458–459.
32. Miller K. Protocols for the efficacious use of indocyanine green/sodium fluorescein angiography. J Ophthal Photog 1993;15:63.
33. Nyberg W. Re-injection technique for establishing landmarks in late phase ICG angiography. J Ophthal Photog 1993;15:66.
34. Hope-Ross M, Yanuzzi L, Gragoudas E, et al. Adverse reactions due to indocyanine green. Ophthalmology 1994;101:530–531.
35. Cohen SY, Quentel G, Coscas G, et al. Safety of a dye without iodine for indocyanine green angiography. Invest Ophthalmol Vis Sci 1995;36:S248.
36. McQuaid K, Saine PJ. Intra-arterial injection of indocyanine green dye. J Ophthal Photog 1997;19:66.
37. Fineman MS, Maguire JI, Fineman SW, Benson WE. Safety of indocyanine green angiography during pregnancy: a survey of the retina, macula, and vitreous societies. Arch Ophthalmol 2001;119:353.
38. Young DS. Effects of Drugs on Clinical Lab Tests. Philadelphia: American Association for Clinical Chemistry Press, 1990.

Chapter 5

Ocular Angiography: Instrumentation and Technique

Patrick J. Saine

Introduction

The view is challenging through the dark blue exciter filter. You appreciate little contrast between the blood vessels and the fundus as you squint through the tiny viewfinder in the darkened room. The injection site is being prepared for the administration of fluorescein dye. On your signal, a syringe filled with a bright red fluid is emptied into your patient's antecubital vein. Quickly, you start the timer and insert the barrier filter—completely obscuring your view of the retina. Then suddenly, magically, your patient's retinal blood vessels fill with glowing sodium fluorescein, and you are witnessing bright yellow-green fireworks! Your urge is to stop taking pictures and stare at the show. You are transfixed by the natural beauty of a unique event to which only you and the camera are witnesses. You are performing your first fluorescein angiogram.

Ocular angiography describes the diagnostic tests that document the dynamic flow of dye in the blood vessels of the eye. After sodium fluo-

A   B   C

FIGURE 5-1
Although the same fundus camera is used to capture fundus photography **(A)**, retinal angiography **(B)**, and choroidal angiography **(C)** images, each of these tests reveals very different visual information.

rescein or indocyanine green (ICG) has been injected into the patient's veins, a rapid sequence of photographs records the dye as it flows through both the choroidal and retinal blood vessels. Fluorescein or ICG acts as a marker, detailing precise areas of vascular leakage, or conversely, the absence of dye. The ophthalmologist uses these photographs both for diagnosis and as a guide to patient treatment.

This chapter begins with a description of the instrumentation and procedure used to perform film fluorescein angiography (FA), including practical advice about common problems and advanced techniques. Information on ICG angiography follows. This chapter concentrates on the angiography procedure itself; for digital imaging issues, please refer to Chapter 7.

The following essential topics are discussed elsewhere in this book:

- Fundus photography technique (Chapter 2)
- Injection preparation (Chapter 4)
- Normal side effects and potential complications associated with the injection of sodium fluorescein and ICG (Chapter 4)

Fundus photography and ocular angiography are both similar and, at the same time, quite different procedures (Figure 5-1). Both use a fundus camera and its requisite alignment and focusing techniques. Ocular angiography adds the requirements of an exciter/barrier filter set and specific timing.

Time is an important aspect of both procedures, but for different reasons. Fundus photography documents the retina at a specific moment in time. Retinal changes are followed over days, weeks, months, or years. Angiography records, usually in still pictures, the dynamic process of dye flowing through and leaking from ocular blood vessels. Significant changes can occur over fractions of seconds. During angiography, the pace of photography is faster, and the timing of the photographs is more critical.

Successful ocular angiography is contingent on your mastery of fundus photography. If you are comfortable taking color photographs of the retina, then ocular angiography will be simple to learn. One way to think of ocular angiography is as rapid-sequence fundus photography using colored filters.

What Is a Filter?

A filter is a device used to separate items. An everyday example is the filter in your furnace. Dirty air is drawn into your furnace through a filter. The filter separates the clean air from the dirt particles by trapping the dust in the fibers of the filter. Clean air then exits the furnace through the vents. Optical filters separate light into different wavelengths in much the same way. White light strikes a blue filter, and blue light exits: The blue light is separated from the white light. Actually, one of two very different mechanisms is at work.

Optical filters can be divided into two categories: absorption filters and interference filters. Most standard photographic filters are absorption filters. They absorb the unwanted wavelengths of light in the same way that the furnace filter traps the dirt from the circulating air. Available in glass (sturdy but not optically neutral) or gelatin (easily scratched but more optically neutral) and in a wide variety of colors, absorption filters are relatively inexpensive to manufacture. Absorption filters are both less efficient and less precise than interference filters (Figure 5-2). The Kodak publication *Filters for Scientific Uses* is a useful guide to absorption filters.[2]

Interference filters reflect rather than absorb unwanted wavelengths of light, allowing sharper wavelength cut-off and greater efficiency. Although they are more expensive to manufacture, their performance is closer to the ideal.

Novotny and Alvis used commercially available absorption filters (KW47 for excitation and KW58 coated with copper for the barrier) in their early fluorescein work.[3] Haining and Lancaster suggested narrow-band interference filters in 1968. Delori et al. described an improved set in 1976.[4,5] Standard fluorescein filter sets are now almost exclusively interference filters.

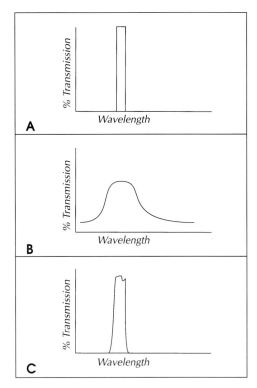

FIGURE 5-2
The transmission curve of an ideal filter is represented with a steep, vertical slope that represents the sharp separation of wavelengths **(A)**. Its efficiency is evidenced by the 100% transmission of the desired wavelengths. The transmission curve of an absorption filter **(B)** has a gradually sloping curve and a lower level of transmission. Monochromatic interference filters **(C)** exhibit the best real-world separation of wavelengths and efficient transmission levels.

Instrumentation

Almost any type of mydriatic fundus camera may be adapted for fluorescein angiography: narrow-angle, wide-angle, hand-held, film-based, or digital. Most modern fundus cameras are supplied as ready for angiography by the manufacturer, although a few are not.

If you are performing film angiography, use separate 35-mm camera bodies for color and black and white to reduce both film waste and barrier filter mishandling. This arrangement also adds a measure of security to the fundus photography system: A spare film back should always be available in the event of a breakdown. The camera bodies should be motorized and capable of triggering an electronic flash sequentially for at least 30 seconds at a minimum rate of one frame per second.

Fluorescein angiography requires a fluorescein filter set, consisting of an exciter and a barrier filter (see the sidebar What Is a Filter?).[1] Sodium fluorescein molecules absorb blue light between 485 and 500 nm, become excited, and consequently emit green light between 520 and 530 nm (Figure 5-3).[6] In a fluorescein angiogram, the filters optimize the illuminating wavelengths and discriminate between the illuminating wavelengths and the emitted wavelengths.

The exciter filter is blue in color, having a peak transmission of 490 nm. It is placed in the optical pathway in front of the light source for fluorescein angiography. This ensures that the retinal illumination is only within the wavelength range that maximally excites the circulating sodium fluorescein.

When this blue light is projected into a normal patient's eye after a sodium fluorescein injection, it is either (1) absorbed by the circulating

FIGURE 5-3
The absorption and emission spectra of in vitro sodium fluorescein.

sodium fluorescein or (2) reflected by surfaces that contain no dye. If the blue light is absorbed by the circulating sodium fluorescein, then the fluorescein molecules become excited and emit a green light. If the blue light is reflected by areas containing no dye, then the blue light reflects unaltered toward the film. After being illuminated by blue light, returning wavelengths of both green and blue light exit the pupil and continue toward the film.

The fluorescent green light contains important diagnostic information; it tells us where in the retina the sodium fluorescein has traveled. The blue light does not contain important diagnostic information; its task of exciting the sodium fluorescein is complete. We discriminate between the two wavelengths of light by placing a barrier filter in the optical pathway between the subject and the film plane. This filter (peak transmission: 525 nm) allows only the green light to continue on toward the film (Figure 5-4).

Exciter filters are routinely placed in the optical pathway after the flashtube and viewing light (Figure 5-5). The barrier filter can be situated either in front of the eyepiece and film or just before the film plane. If it is placed in front of the eyepiece and film, you will view directly through this filter during fluorescein angiography. This makes camera positioning more difficult during the initial phases of the angiogram because you see virtually nothing through the viewfinder (note: you can check your alignment by quickly sliding one of the two filters in and out). On the other hand, this placement allows a clearer view of the circulating sodium fluorescein once the dye has reached the retina.

If the filter is placed directly in front of the film plane, you will view the circulating fluorescein without the benefit of the barrier filter. It may be more difficult to detect the presence of fluorescein in the eye; however, you will have the advantage of more easily appreciating the standard

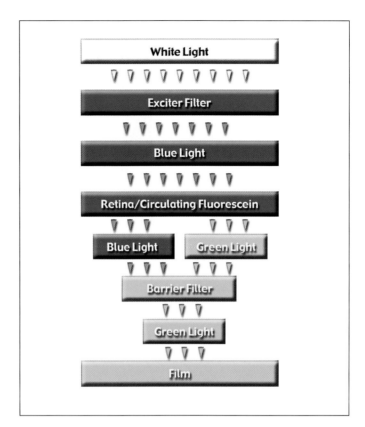

FIGURE 5-4
The exciter and barrier filter. White light enters the exciter filter, which transmits only the blue portion of the light. The blue light enters the eye, where it is either absorbed by the fluorescein or reflected by the retina. The light absorbed by the fluorescein is emitted as green light. The green excited light and the reflected blue light leave the eye. The blue light is rejected by the barrier filter, whereas the green light passes through the barrier filter and is recorded on film or digital chip.

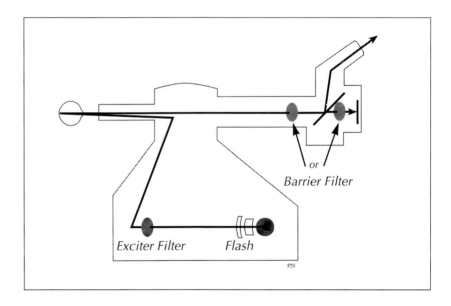

FIGURE 5-5
Filter location. The exciter filter is located after the light source but before the light enters the patient's eye. The barrier filter can be placed in one of two positions: either in front of or behind the single lens reflex mirror. The photographer views through the barrier filter during angiography if the filter is placed in front of the mirror and does not if it is placed behind the mirror.

crescent and haze positioning artifacts during angiography. Check your manual to ascertain the precise location of the filters in your particular fundus camera.

The perfect position for a barrier filter has often been debated among veteran ophthalmic photographers. The topic has cooled with the introduction of solenoid-activated barrier filters, which pop in and out of position when activated by a manual switch or the shutter release. This mechanism allows you to choose your view, with or without the barrier filter in place. The manual option is important because the exciter filter may also be used for nerve fiber layer photography.

FIGURE 5-6
Note the discoloration of these barrier filters. When was the last time your filters were inspected?

Table 5-1. Fluorescein Angiography: Step by Step

Prepare and position	Prepare the room
	Plan the procedure
Patient contact time ⟶	Perform color fundus photography
	Switch cameras and filter
	Photograph name tag and green filter
	Expose a control photograph
	Re-educate your patient
	Double-check everything
	Solicit injection
Expose	Signal injector
	Begin series—shoot earlies
	Pictures at 1, 3, 5, and 10 minutes
	Close the session
Follow-up	Process and edit the images
	Deliver finished product
	Review your work

Note: Review these steps before or during the procedure to help establish your routine. Post a copy of these steps near your fundus camera for reference.

Like all colored objects, fluorescein filters eventually degrade (Figure 5-6). Age, exposure to light, and high humidity are some of the factors that contribute to filter failure. Increased pseudofluorescence (see the section Pseudofluorescence and Autofluorescence) is a sign of worn-out filters.

Fluorescein filters should always be replaced as a matched pair to ensure efficiency. In busy offices in warm, humid climates, filters may need to be replaced each year. Smaller practices in cooler climates may need to change their filters every 3 years. When were your fluorescein filters last changed?

Procedure

This section describes a step-by-step procedure for performing fluorescein angiography (Table 5-1). The nomenclature used in this chapter primarily describes fluorescein angiography using film. The procedure is similar when capturing images electronically, with the proviso that you are interacting with a computer and monitor as opposed to film cassettes

Table 5-2. Fluorescein Angiography Supply Check List

Filled syringe	10-cc syringe with 5-cc 10% sodium fluorescein
	5-cc syringe with 2.5-cc 25% sodium fluorescein
Needle	20-gauge straight needle
	23-gauge butterfly, 12-in. tube, $^3/_4$-in. needle
	23-gauge catheter
Wound cover	Adhesive bandage
	Gauze or cotton ball with tape
Tourniquet	$^3/_4$-in. tubing
Cleansing aid	Alcohol pads
Personal protection	Gloves, mask, and safety clothing as needed
	Syringe disposal unit
Miscellaneous	Emergency supplies
	Emesis basin

Note: Prepare the injections and gather all supplies before the patient enters the room. Choose specific supplies to maximize convenience and value.

Table 5-3. Disease-Specific Fluorescein Angiograms

Disease	Primary Views (Earlies)	Angle of View (Degrees)	Recirculation Phase (Lates)
Macular diseases (e.g., ARMD, CME, CSR, POHS)	Macula	30	Macula (CME: 15-minute)
Occlusive diseases (e.g., CRVO, BRVO, CRAO, BRAO)	Macula	30 or 45	Macula and periphery as needed
Systemic diseases (e.g., diabetic retinopathy)	Macula	30 or 45	Macula and seven standard fields
Site-specific diseases (e.g., tumor, macroaneurysm)	Area of lesion	30 or 45	Area of lesion, include borders

ARMD = age-related macular degeneration; BRAO = branch retinal artery occlusion; BRVO = branch retinal vein occlusion; CME = cystoid macular edema; CSR = central serous retinopathy; CRAO = central retinal artery occlusion; CRVO = central retinal vein occlusion; POHS = presumed ocular histoplasmosis syndrome.
Note: Fluorescein angiography records the dynamic process of fluorescein dye flowing through the blood vessels of the eye. In an abnormal eye, the dye can leak or be blocked from view at different times during this process. Determine the patient's working diagnosis and then use the simple table above to plan your angiogram. Experienced workers should refer to Table 8-6 for extended recommendations. It is usually better to take too many photographs than too few.

and a darkroom. Learning fluorescein angiography is like driving a car: Once you become comfortable with the process, you can drive any car using your accelerating, braking, and steering skills. In the same way, different brands of cameras or different recording media (film versus electronic) pose few difficulties for the experienced angiographer.

Prepare and Position

1. *Prepare the room.* Tidy the room. Complete all billing and paperwork. Adjust the stool height and the fundus camera's mechanical controls to their approximate midpoints. Load both camera backs with film—one with color slide film and one with fast black and white negative film—or enter the patient's name in the digital angiography database. Confirm that the illumination and flash settings, the filter wheel, and the diopter compensation control are in their standard positions. Set your eyepiece reticle. Prepare the sodium fluorescein injection and injection supplies (Table 5-2).
2. *Plan the procedure.* Have a photographic plan in mind before you escort the patient into the room. Review the photograph request form and examine any previous photographs. Note the patient's visual acuity and working diagnosis. Determine the fields to photograph. Select your camera and angle of view, the areas of the patient's retina you intend to document (Table 5-3), and the timing of your photographs (Figure 5-7). If multiple angles of view are required, be certain that each variation is shot both in color and as

FIGURE 5-7
Timing fluorescein frames. Examples of common strategies used in timing fluorescein angiograms are shown. A contact-printed, 36-exposure film of mono-fluorescein exposures is represented at the left. The slots in the fifth row of images may also be dedicated to stereo. A stereo angiogram composed of original negatives mounted as 35-mm slides is shown below. Adopting a standard angiogram pattern streamlines routine angiography. The experienced photographer departs from the standard when interesting patients require more photographs or when difficult patients limit the amount of photography. (Inj. = injection; OD = right eye; OS = left eye.)

A

B

FIGURE 5-8
Standard color fundus photographs exposed after a fluorescein injection convey an adulterated coloration of the retina. When performing fluorescein angiography, expose colors before the injection **(A)** rather than after **(B)**.

an angiographic frame. Ask pertinent questions: On which retinal level should you focus? Should the periphery be scanned during the recirculation phase? Should the iris be documented for signs of rubeosis?

3. *Perform color fundus photography.* The physician compares color fundus photographs with the fluorescein angiogram frames when reading an angiogram. Take color images (slides or digital) at the same session as the fluorescein dye test and before the dye is injected (Figure 5-8).[7]

4. *Switch from the color camera body to the black and white camera body.* Exchange the camera bodies, making sure to flip the camera selection switch if necessary. Check the diopter setting if the camera backs include the eyepiece. If you use a single camera body, load the appropriate film and check that the barrier filter is in place.

5. *Photograph a name tag.* Using the green filter and a low flash setting, photograph a name tag. This identifies the patient's images throughout processing, editing, and filing. You will probably need to increase the viewing light's intensity to focus clearly while the colored filters are in place.

6. *Photograph the fundus using a green filter.* Select the angle of view and the focus you will be using during the fluorescein angiogram. Insert a green filter and select a low flash setting to photograph first the nonaffected eye, and then the affected eye. Imaging the affected eye last correctly positions the camera for the early photographs. (Note: The barrier filter located at the film plane will not affect these photographs.)

This is a good time to practice stereo shifts and to determine the best camera placement in eyes with a compromised view. Focus carefully, because this focus will remain unchanged throughout the angiogram (at least until you are more experienced).

7. *Expose a control photograph.* Set the flash for the fluorescein setting (see sidebar How to Determine the Proper Exposure), remove the green filter, and insert both the exciter and the barrier filter. Take a photograph. This will be your control photograph. The section Pseudofluorescence and Autofluorescence explains how examining

How to Determine the Proper Exposure

Begin with the manufacturer's exposure recommendations found in the owner's manual. Tweak this setting by performing a sequence of exposures during the recirculation phase (between 1 and 3 minutes) of a fluorescein angiogram in which you are most interested in the late photographs (for minimal impact on patient care). If no recommendations are available, then use the green filter and take one picture at each flash setting. Choose the best exposure and increase it by two or three exposure steps for your initial fluorescein exposure.

Judge your exposure from original negatives, not from contact sheets. Look for a full range of densities from clear film to dense blacks. The negative image of the control photograph (assuming efficient filters and a young, clear-eyed patient) should be completely clear. The "earlies" should progress from clear to grays to rich blacks. "Lates" will be gray.

A good negative yields a fine print, given proper darkroom technique. Of course, the instant feedback of electronic imaging shortens this testing process.

Remember that your exposure is a balance between actual film speed (film sensitivity plus exposure plus development) and patient comfort. Fine-grain photographs with full tonality are useless if the required flash setting is too much for the patient to tolerate.

Indications for increased exposure during fundus photography may or may not suggest exposure compensation during angiography. If fundus photography exposure was increased to compensate for a smaller pupil, it is wise to increase the angiography flash setting. On the other hand, if the flash increase in fundus photography is due to darker patient pigmentation, do not increase the angiography flash setting. In general, fundus photography is exposed for the pigment in the retinal pigment epithelium, and fluorescein angiography is exposed for circulating dye in the blood vessels (which do not contain pigment).

Exposure for digital angiography follows the same principles, but corrections can be made immediately.

---

this frame can help you determine the integrity of your filters. Reset your timer to zero.

8. *Re-educate the patient.* Remind the patient about the common side effects of the dye injection and prepare him or her for the upcoming test. The patient should have been adequately informed by the physician (who also obtains a signed consent form that details potential complications), so a lengthy discussion is probably not needed. Here's what we tell patients: "What I am going to do now is to go get Dr. _____, who will make a dye injection into your arm. Then I'm going to take a lot of blue pictures of the dye as it flows through the blood vessels in the back of your eyes. Two things you'll notice from the dye are that your skin will be a little yellow for the next 8 hours, and your urine will be a bright yellow-orange for the next day and a half. Don't worry about either of these things; it's just the dye leaving your body. Do you have any questions?" Make eye contact during the explanation with both the patient and any companions. Use a reassuring tone of voice. A light touch on the patient's hand is optional. Some photographers spend considerable time discussing potential reactions just before the test. In other offices, the physician or nurse thoroughly discusses complications with the patient before the patient visits the photographer.

If you are photographing a light-sensitive or otherwise difficult patient, you may want to insert a "pep talk" here, hoping that it will help the patient cooperate during the early, rapid-sequence photographs. Try this: "I'll be taking a lot of blue pictures right after Dr. _____ makes the injection. These are some of the most important pictures that we'll take today. I'm going to need your help in holding extra still during these pictures. They won't be as bright as the first pictures we took, but there will be a lot of them. Let's try and get some good photographs for Dr. _____, OK?"

If the patient is a less than optimal candidate for intravenous injections (as some large, diabetic, or frail patients are), have the patient hang his or her arms down and suggest that he or she clench and release a fist while you summon the health care worker who will perform the injection.

Before leaving the room:

9. *Double-check everything.* Develop the habit of reviewing major variables just before the test. Make sure that film is loaded in the camera and check the flash setting. Make sure your computer settings (timer, sensitivity, filter) are correct for digital capture. Check that the fluorescein injection and supplies are readily available. Confirm your angiographic plan. Have a stopwatch ready to help you keep track of time.

10. *Solicit help for the injection.* Depending on your specific office procedures and your state's laws, ask the attending physician or a registered nurse to perform the injection.[8,9] Better-quality angiograms result when someone other than the photographer performs the injection, especially when the photographer is inexperienced. As the photographer, you should concentrate on just one task—obtaining the best retinal photographs. In addition to performing the injection, the other person should monitor the patient for potential reactions, hold lids as needed, and be trained in emergency health care.

In 1998, the Ophthalmic Photographers' Society, Inc., issued the following policy statement on performing venipuncture and intravenous injections:

The OPS wishes to make its members aware that OPS has no legal authority to determine who may perform venipuncture or intravenous injections. The current position of OPS, taken through its Board of Directors, is that OPS neither advocates nor opposes venipuncture or the administration of intravenous injections, such as dyes, by photographers. The OPS also wishes to inform its members that: OPS is unaware of any federal laws which address who may perform venipuncture or intravenous injections; and the scope of practice of medical professionals has been established traditionally on the state level, meaning that the states determine the activities each medical specialty is allowed to perform under their state license. Accordingly, OPS recommends that each individual photographer check with the appropriate agency or agencies in the state in which they practice to determine whether the performance of venipuncture or the administration of intravenous injections falls within their scope of practice.[10]

Expose

11. *Begin the test.* While the injection site is being prepared, realign the patient, viewing first with the green filter (checking your focus) and then switching to the blue exciter filter. Confirm your alignment by monitoring saturation and crescent artifacts. If you are shooting stereo, perform some practice shifts. Recall your angiographic plan. Take a (quiet) deep breath and feel confident!

    When you are ready for the injection to begin, signal the injector with an "OK" or a thumbs-up sign (you risk losing important early photographs if they begin injecting before you let them know you are ready). In turn, they should signal you with an "OK" or "injection started" as soon as the injection begins. For a good bolus of dye, the injection should last 3–5 seconds. Simultaneously start the camera timer or stopwatch, or both, and insert the barrier filter into the optical pathway. Take a photograph when the injection is completed to record the injection duration.

    If the barrier filter is placed at the film plane, your view of the blue retina remains the same. If you view through the barrier filter during angiography, your view becomes black as soon as the barrier filter is inserted. Do not panic. Until this point, you had been viewing the fundus with the blue exciter filter. With the barrier filter now in place and no fluorescein dye yet in the retina, there is no light reaching the eyepiece. Your view of the retina will return as fluorescein dye fills the blood vessels.

12. *Begin taking pictures almost immediately.* Count to five and begin taking photographs at a rate of one image every 2 seconds—even if you do not see anything in the viewfinder. It is important to record the progress of the dye as it fills the choroid. This happens before you can clearly perceive the dye through the viewfinder. Your first few pictures may be blank, but you can edit these out later. This timing technique assures you of excellent early-phase photographs—photographs that are critical in diagnoses such as macular degeneration. If you are photographing the angiogram in stereo, remember to shift the camera side to side for each picture.

13. *Increase your picture-taking rate.* Begin taking pictures at a rate of one image per second as soon as you see dye in the blood vessels or approximately 10 seconds after the injection (whichever comes first). These initial photographs (the transit phase or "earlies") document the rapid initial dynamics of the fluorescein dye in the choroid and retina. The dye first flows into the choroidal vessels, fills the retinal

arteries, and then empties through the retinal veins. It may be difficult to appreciate these changes through the viewfinder, but they will be easy to see in your photographs. The earlies will be among your brightest and sharpest fluorescein frames.

14. *Pause picture taking at approximately 30 seconds.* This flurry of photographs can continue only so long. Stop taking pictures when 30 seconds are up, when you run out of film or computer space, or when you can no longer appreciate any changes in the dye. With more experience, you will better appreciate the flow of the dye and develop your own unique shooting rhythms.

    Allow patients to take a short break by asking them to close their eyes but keep their head in the headrest. Reassure them that the test is going well. We let them know that "the hard part is over with—there are no more injections, just some more pictures." This is also a good time to evaluate the need to reload film or edit digital images.

    If the patient is going to have a reaction to fluorescein, it will most likely occur between 30 seconds and 2 minutes after the injection. Practical suggestions for managing patient reactions are offered later in this chapter.

    The person injecting should check the injection site and apply a bandage. (We use bright adhesive bandage strips decorated with popular animated characters. Patients always smile when they discover their—or their grandchild's—favorite cartoon character at the injection site.)

15. *Take recirculation and late photographs.* Photographs taken after the injection at regular time intervals will reveal the extent to which the sodium fluorescein did or did not leak. There is no specific standard for the timing of these photographs; intervals vary both by office and by disease. The minimum acceptable timing of "lates" is 3- and 5- to 7-minute pictures. A complete series would contain 1-, 3-, 5-, 10-, or 15-minute—and perhaps even 30-minute—photographs. We routinely expose stereo pairs of both eyes at 1, 3, 5, and 10 minutes after the injection, taking later pictures as requested by the physician and in cases of suspected cystoid macular edema or optic nerve head drusen.

    Complete requested peripheral photographs, or scan the periphery per Tables 5-3 or 8-5. Advanced fundus photography techniques, such as scleral depression and auxiliary lenses, may also be pursued.

16. *Close the session.* Let the patient know that he or she did well (even if it's not true) and that you obtained the needed photographs (which you should have). Remind the patient that the colors they are seeing are from the bright flashes. Reassure them that these spots will go away soon. Release patients with a smile, making sure that they feel fine and know where their next clinic stop is. Complete all paperwork, including signing the chart. An uncharted procedure is an incomplete procedure. Finish completely with one patient before beginning another.

Follow-Up

17. *Process the film or save the digital images.* Follow the instructions for developing film found in Chapter 6 or save your digital images as described in your owner's manual. Edit your raw images before presenting them to the physician. Only show the images that are clinically significant and represent your best work. A complete

stereo film fluorescein angiogram contains the following stereo pairs both properly exposed and well composed:

- Monochromatic green stereo fundus photographs of both eyes
- A preinjection control photograph documenting any pseudo- or autofluorescence
- At least one blank frame taken immediately before the fluorescein dye is present in the choroid
- Choroidal filling of the affected eye in stereo at a rate of one frame per second
- Arterial and venous filling phases in stereo of the affected eye at a rate of one frame per second
- Recirculation (arteriovenous) phase stereo photographs of both eyes (including stereo photographs of the periphery as needed)
- Mid- and late stereo photographs of both eyes (at 3, 5, and 10 minutes)

Of course, not every single fluorescein procedure will contain the complete set of photographs described. Patients may not cooperate, you may begin taking pictures too late, or your office may have a different routine for late photographs. Electronic fluoresceins routinely contain fewer images to minimize electronic storage space. On the other hand, if you appreciate the structure of a complete test, you can make informed decisions about routine fluorescein angiography at your office.

Always take some time during the editing process to review your work with an eye toward quality control. Ask yourself how this particular angiogram could have been made better.

18. *Deliver the finished product.* Deliver the patient's photographs and chart to the referring physician in a timely manner. In a busy retina practice, angiograms may be requested "stat," or immediately. Many of these stat patients are scheduled for laser treatment the same day. It is up to you to provide the results quickly without compromising quality. Film images usually take 25 minutes to 1 hour to cycle through a complete development process. Electronic images can be made available to the physician in a matter of minutes.

19. *Review your work.* You should endeavor to not only understand pertinent photographic principles but also to appreciate the various disease processes and their effects on the eye. Learn to look at fluorescein studies from the physician's point of view. Schedule regular conferences or ask impromptu questions, but routinely review your fluorescein angiograms with your physician.

Troubleshooting

What a wonderful world it would be if all of our angiograms were perfect! However, filters may not work properly, our timing can be off, and patients can be light sensitive or uncooperative. This section suggests practical solutions for common angiographic problems. The technical problems of filters and timing are followed by a discussion of managing patients and reactions.

Pseudofluorescence and Autofluorescence

Pseudofluorescence indicates an inefficient fluorescein filter system. Autofluorescence describes the "glowing" phenomena of certain entities

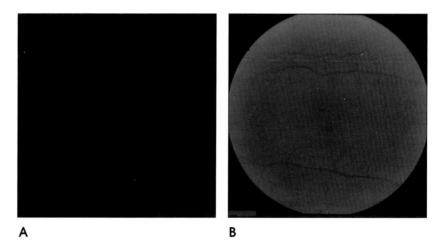

A   B

FIGURE 5-9
When an efficient set of fluorescein filters is in place, the control photograph will be devoid of retinal details **(A)**. If the control photograph reveals retinal details **(B)**, then the filter set is either poorly matched or faded.

——— New Filter Set
■ Pseudofluorescence
········· Faded Filter Set
▨ Pseudofluorescence

FIGURE 5-10
Pseudofluorescence. New fluorescein filter sets (*solid line*) exhibit a minor amount of filter overlap or pseudofluorescence (*black triangle*). As filters age, they transmit greater amounts of light (*dotted line*), creating more pseudofluorescence (*gray triangle*).

found within the eye. The status of both of these phenomena can be determined by examining a control photograph.

The control photograph (see Expose a Control Photograph) is part of every complete fluorescein angiogram. It is exposed with both the barrier and the exciter filters in place and before sodium fluorescein is injected. In a normal patient photographed with efficient, well-matched filters, the control photograph is completely blank (Figure 5-9). This indicates that the barrier filter is properly excluding blue illuminating light and that there is no sodium fluorescein (or anything else) emitting fluorescent light.

Both barrier and excited filter transmission curves overlap slightly (Figure 5-10). If ideal filters—those with extremely sharp transmission curves—were used, then this overlap would not exist. In the real world, however, even new filters exhibit some crossover. Furthermore, as filters age, their transmission characteristics become less discriminatory. Factors that degrade filters include age, high humidity, and exposure to light. As each filter in the pair deteriorates, it begins to pass more wavelengths that overlap with the other. As this supplementary light increases, it crosses the exposure threshold and is recorded on film. This additional light is called *pseudofluorescence*—literally, false fluorescence. Pseudofluorescence contributes to the overall exposure. It masks fine retinal details by overexposing highlights (the fluorescent areas) and decreasing overall contrast (Figure 5-11). Remember that correct angiography exposure is a balance between filtered light intensity, film exposure, and development. If you are experiencing pseudofluorescence, closely examine your exposure and development techniques.

FIGURE 5-11
Pseudofluorescence masks fine details by effectively overexposing the highlights. An efficient fluorescein filter set **(A)** is compared with a mismatched set **(B)**. Note the better overall definition in **(A)**, and the decreased sharpness and brighter highlights of **(B)**.

FIGURE 5-12
Optic nerve head drusen **(A)** are photographed using both a barrier and exciter filter **(B)**—but no sodium fluorescein—to illustrate autofluorescence. Astrocytic hamartoma also displays this phenomena. You would expect no retinal details in a normal patient's control photograph with a well-matched set of filters.

Autofluorescence also causes identifiable retinal details in a control photograph. This happens when structures in the eye act like sodium fluorescein: They absorb blue light and emit green light. Autofluorescent properties have been documented in the cataractous lens, optic nerve head drusen, and astrocytic hamartoma (Figure 5-12). In the second two instances, the autofluorescent images can help the physician determine the appropriate diagnosis.

Fluorescein Timing

A crucial difference between fundus photography and fluorescein angiography is the rate at which the pictures are exposed. It is easy to get to know the patient during fundus photography. The changes you are documenting usually occur between visits, allowing images to be exposed at a more leisurely pace. Alternately, the "earlies" are a very important phase of fluorescein angiography that come and go within 30 seconds. Timing is clearly of the essence.

Begin shooting before you see any dye within the blood vessels. Once the dye fully fills the retinal blood vessels, sodium fluorescein's rate of visual change is measured in minutes rather than seconds. Inexperienced photographers may get caught up in the moment and continue to shoot rapidly after the dye has progressed through its initial changes. Remember that the most important images occur as the dye is filling the blood vessels. If you have missed these pictures for some reason (perhaps the patient moved or you forgot to insert the barrier filter), taking a rapid sequence of photos after the dye has filled the blood vessels is of little consequence.

Use consistent timing during the late phases of your angiography. Presenting consistent results will help the interpreting physician gauge the normalcy of dye distribution. Similar timing of late photographs in

A   B

FIGURE 5-13
Asteroid hyalosis. A green filter **(A)** shows the extent of these vitreal calcium-lipid deposits, which disappear on angiography **(B)**. (Courtesy of Peter Hay, Retina Vitreous Surgeons on CNY, Syracuse, New York.)

two fluorescein tests from different dates allows better comparison of the relative activity of a lesion.

When You Can't See the Dye

Particularly unsettling to the inexperienced angiographer are the instances when no fluorescein dye can be seen in the blood vessels after a seemingly successful dye injection. Keep your head and remember that this can be the result of a number of circumstances. Check first with the person injecting: Was there infiltration, extravasation, or an arterial injection?

The patient may have circulation problems. If you don't see dye by 20 seconds after the injection, continue to shoot—but shoot more slowly (1 frame every 2–3 seconds). Admittedly unusual, angiogram earlies may begin as late as 90–120 seconds after the injection. Arm position can affect dye flow: Exorotation and abduction of the upper arm and antecubital vein should be minimal.[11]

It is often difficult to distinguish dye flowing through the retinal blood vessels of high myopes with clear media and in many patients with small pupils and hazy media. If the injection was successful and you are confident of your alignment and filter selection, the final images almost always will look better than your view through the finder. If your view is compromised, pay special attention to crescent and haze artifacts for alignment, flip to your green filter for viewing, and use standardized timing. More often than not, you will be rewarded by a readable angiogram.

Dense asteroid hyalosis is a good example of a condition that offers a poor view but results in an adequate angiogram. Because these vitreous deposits are not stained with circulating sodium fluorescein, they are rendered invisible using the exciter/barrier filter system (Figure 5-13).[12]

Be aware of potential exposure problems, monitoring your exposure on the screen if you have a digital angiography system. A poor view through a small pupil in a clear eye may yield a better angiogram with an increased flash setting. Brunescent cataracts can act as an additional filter. Their reddish-brown color blocks the blue exciting light and transmits little of the fluorescent green. Turn up the flash power to compensate.

Attitude and flexibility are two important angiographic tools. Before each dye test, consciously decide to produce enough images for a full series of clear, sharp pictures throughout the color, early, mid, and late phases of your stereo angiogram. Each patient deserves your best efforts and undivided attention. At the same time, recognize that a perfect angiogram may be all but impossible in some patients. Although not the norm, in some instances as few as two different images taken at different times of the same eye may show enough change to be considered a useful angiogram.

Reactions to Sodium Fluorescein

Fluorescein angiography's relatively low adverse reaction rate is balanced by the very real possibility of severe adverse events.[13] Review the contraindications, the type and frequency of reactions, and the standard emergency kit as described in Chapter 4. This section deals with the practical aspects of managing these situations.

All angiography locations should have a written emergency plan. Specific responsibilities, a list of emergency supplies (see Table 4-4) and their locations, and multiple scenarios—from mild reactions (nausea) to moderate reactions (urticaria) and severe reactions (vasovagal reactions)—should be addressed. Involve all photographers, the individuals responsible for injections, the physician, and the risk manager in the process of writing the emergency plan. Review the plan regularly with all staff involved in day-to-day angiography and make it required reading for new employees.

Nausea and vomiting are the most common adverse reactions to injected sodium fluorescein; these usually occur within the first minute after the injection. Clinical experience indicates that this reaction occurs more often in agitated or nervous patients (and when the photographer is agitated or nervous!), in younger patients, and when the room is warm.

If a patient becomes nauseated, remain calm, ask him or her to sit back and take slow deep breaths through the mouth with eyes open. A reassuring attitude is important. We suggest to the patient that "the nausea usually passes as quickly as it comes" in even, calming tones. Try humor ("Not many people react to this dye—you are one of the lucky 2%") or distraction ("The pictures are timed—do you think we can take some more now?"). Nausea does not always lead to vomiting. If it does, offer your patient an appropriate container. A plastic lined wastebasket is more useful than the often too small emesis basin.

Most minor reactions do not need medical intervention. If you think that the reaction may be more severe, stay with the patient and dispatch another person for a physician or registered nurse (a reminder: the person injecting should remain in the room for at least 1 minute after the injection). Signs of a more severe reaction include lightheadedness, difficulty breathing, fainting, and tightness in the chest.

Moderate adverse reactions to sodium fluorescein include urticaria (hives), which may occur 3–10 minutes after the injection. Urticaria is the result of an allergic reaction that releases histamine. The physician may prescribe an injectable or oral antihistamine to abate the problem. The patient should be monitored until all itching has stopped.

Both vasovagal and more severe reactions require decisive action. Obtain trained medical help immediately. Do not leave the room; rather, make the patient comfortable, perhaps helping him or her to lie on a stretcher or the floor and loosening any clothing around the neck. Locate the emergency supplies and assist emergency personnel. Help with transporting the patient or performing cardiopulmonary resuscitation as needed.

Keep in mind that your patients may be sick or fragile. The population that is likely to have fluorescein angiography includes the elderly as well as patients with diabetes. Learn about the special health and communication needs of these patients.

Advanced Angiography Techniques

Oral Fluorescein Angiography

Intravenous injection of sodium fluorescein is the administration method of choice. In patients who are unable to receive an injection, it may be advantageous to administer the sodium fluorescein orally.[14,15] Photographing the injected dye reveals a full range of phases: choroidal, arterial, arteriovenous, and "lates." Oral fluorescein photographs disclose only the late phase of angiography. Oral administration is useful for determining the status of late leaking retinal conditions such as clinically significant macular edema or cystoid macular edema.

Double the intravenous dosage of sodium fluorescein and dissolve it in cold tomato or vegetable juice, or milk for children. Tomato juice masks some of the taste and most of the color. Staining of the patient's teeth can be reduced by using a straw. Powdered sodium fluorescein in capsules is available in Great Britain and Japan but not currently in the United States. Performing oral fluorescein on a patient with an empty stomach will avoid unwanted dye absorption, resulting in brighter images. Normal side effects, including staining of the skin and urine, are present. Expose a control photograph and record the dye at 5, 10, 15–20, and 30–40 minutes postingestion. This timing allows comparison of any leakage sites at multiple time intervals.

Angiography in Children

As with any medical procedure designed for adults, special considerations must be made for children. The dose of sodium fluorescein should be adjusted specifically for the child's weight using the manufacturer's recommendations in the package insert. For example, if a package insert for a 500-mg (5-ml) ampule of 10% fluorescein sodium lists the children's dose as 3.5 mg/lb, then a 50-lb child should receive 1.75 ml. The following two equations, showing labeled units, demonstrate the mathematics:

$$50 \text{ lb} \times 3.5 \text{ mg/lb} = 175 \text{ mg}$$
$$175 \text{ mg} \times 5 \text{ ml}/500 \text{ mg} = 1.75 \text{ ml}$$

How many milliliters would the same child receive if a 750-mg (3-ml) ampule of 25% sodium fluorescein (recommended dose: 5 mg/lb) were used? (The answer is found at the end of this section.)

This reduced dose also holds true for smaller adults. We use the "100-lb rule"; if the patient weighs less than 100 lb, we calculate a lesser dose. Larger than normal patients generally do not need their dose increased, because their greater bulk rarely reflects a larger vascular volume.

Another method of calculating a reduced dose of sodium fluorescein is to refer to Table 5-4. This table can be used for children (example: the dose for a 42 $^3/_4$ lb child would be 1.4 [40 lb] + 0.07 [2 lb] + 0.026 [12 oz] = 1.496 ml) or small animals (example: the dose for a 1 lb 4 oz rodent would be 0.035 [1 lb] + 0.009 [4 oz] = 0.44 ml).

Excellent patient management skills are essential when working with children. Explain the procedure fully (using appropriate vocabulary) to both the child and the parents. Reassure them of the safety of the procedure and the importance of taking multiple photographs. Talk the patient and parents through the procedure, encouraging them and keeping their attention focused. Expose a minimal number of fundus photographs, keeping the patient fresh for the fluorescein series. A flawless injection technique is crucial. Consider using an intravenous team member or anesthesiologist who may first numb the injection site topically. Shoot for quality, not quantity.

We have successfully performed office fluorescein angiography on patients as young as 3 years. For younger children, consider performing the test during an examination under anesthesia (Figure 5-14).

Table 5-4. Weight-Specific 10% Fluorescein Doses

Weight (oz)	Dose (ml)	Weight (lb)	Dose (ml)	Weight (lb)	Dose (ml)	Weight (kg)	Dose (ml)	Weight (kg)	Dose (ml)
1	0.002	1	0.035	20	0.7	0.1	.008	1	0.077
2	0.004	2	0.07	30	1.1	0.2	0.015	2	0.154
3	0.007	3	0.105	40	1.4	0.3	0.023	3	0.232
4	0.009	4	0.14	50	1.8	0.4	0.031	4	0.309
5	0.011	5	0.175	60	2.1	0.5	0.039	5	0.386
6	0.013	6	0.21	70	2.5	0.6	0.046	6	0.463
7	0.015	7	0.245	80	2.8	0.7	0.054	7	0.54
8	0.017	8	0.28	90	3.2	0.8	0.062	8	0.617
9	0.02	9	0.315	100	3.5	0.9	0.069	9	0.695
10	0.022	10	0.35	110	3.9	1.0	0.077	10	0.772
11	0.024			120	4.2			20	1.543
12	0.026			130	4.6			30	2.315
13	0.028			140	4.9			40	3.087
14	0.031			143+	5.0			50	3.859
15	0.033							60	4.63
16	0.035							64.9+	5.0

Courtesy of Mark Croswell, Henry Ford Health Systems, Detroit, Michigan.

A

B

FIGURE 5-14
Angiography during examination under anesthesia (EUA). Fluorescein angiography may be performed in the operating room EUA. Use a hand-held fundus camera capable of angiography. Alternately, lay the patient on his or her side and use a standard fundus camera **(A)**. Rotate the photographs 90 degrees for proper viewing **(B)**.

(The answer to the dose question: 50 lb × 5 mg/lb = 250 mg; 250 mg × 3 ml/750 mg = 1 ml.)

Anterior Segment Angiography

Abnormal blood vessels in the conjunctiva, cornea, or iris may be the subject of fluorescein angiography (Figure 5-15).[16,17] Multiple strategies for recording anterior segment angiography have evolved: A 35-mm

A

B

FIGURE 5-15
Anterior segment angiography. Angiograms of the cornea or iris may reveal important vascularization information. These early **(A)** and late **(B)** iris angiograms were photographed by Dennis Cain, Baltimore, Maryland.

Table 5-5. Anterior Segment Angiography

Camera	Illumination System
Fundus camera	Standard
Photo slit-lamp	"Coffee can" attachment
35-mm single lens reflex mounted to fundus camera lens barrel	Fundus camera

Note: Some strategies for illuminating the anterior segment during angiography are listed.

camera equipped with a macro lens has been mounted along the barrel of a standard fundus camera, a rapid recycling flash (affectionately dubbed the "coffee can attachment") for the Zeiss photo slit-lamp has been marketed, and a 25-mm microscope lens has been mounted in front of a 30-degree fundus camera objective (Table 5-5).[18]

Whichever imaging system you use, choose your plane of focus carefully. The focal plane and the specific instrumentation are the major departures from the standard angiography procedure. The flash exposure for anterior segment fluorescein angiography is usually at least two steps higher and should be based on empirical exposure tests for your particular instrumentation. As a dark iris may block fluorescence, the most successful iris fluorescein angiograms are of patients with light irises.

Color Fluorescein Angiography

High-speed color film may be substituted for black and white film during fluorescein angiography; however, the result is little different than what is seen through the viewfinder. A technique to record retinal fluorescence on a normally colored fundus photograph was developed by Matsui in the late 1960s (Figure 5-16).[19,20] A magenta excitation filter (Wratten number 31 or 34) and a yellow (Wratten number 12) barrier filter were used with a medium-speed color film.[21] The resulting photographs document the circulating fluorescein with the fundus in natural color. Alternate methods include exposing color film using just the exciter or barrier filter. Although suitable for the occasional teaching

FIGURE 5-16
Color fluorescein angiography highlights fluorescence while representing the fundus in close-to-realistic color. (Reprinted with permission from S Shikano, K Shimizu. Atlas of Fluorescence Fundus Angiography. Philadelphia: Saunders, 1968.)

slide, color fluorescein angiography has not gained wide acceptance as a clinically useful technique.

International Perspectives

The natural viewpoint of this textbook's authors is to describe procedures and technical information as is currently practiced in the United States and European community. Taken for granted is relatively easy access to film supplies and digital equipment, the latest modern fundus cameras, easy access to manufacturer service departments, and a ready supply of retinal specialists to interpret our work. It seems painfully obvious to state that such is not the case worldwide. In a number of countries, resources for fluorescein angiography are minimal. Some local strategies that have evolved are noted here because they may help guide angiographers who find themselves in similar situations.

In Mexico City, high-speed negative color film is substituted for the standard black and white film used in the United States. The color film is push processed at the local 1-hour film processing laboratory; the resulting snapshot-type prints are then viewed by the ophthalmologist (Figure 5-17). Flash settings are higher, vessel resolution is lower, and prints display a green cast. A color fundus photograph is also available immediately.

As an island, Cuba has always been in an import situation. Film and other manufactured items are currently especially dear there, so when fluorescein angiography is performed, three patients are fit on a single 36-exposure roll of film. Much tighter shooting is involved: With just 12 frames per angiogram, stereo is sacrificed and earlies are kept to six frames. All that is required is good timing and the discipline to shoot for quality rather than quantity. The standard stereo angiogram can seem downright wasteful when compared to this barebones approach.

Fluorescein Angiography in Fiction

Although I have yet to read a novel where a retinal angiographer is the primary protagonist, the test we so frequently perform has made a num-

FIGURE 5-17
Color fluorescein images exposed on color negative film from Mexico. (Courtesy of Alejandro Dalma, MD, Mexico City, Mexico.)

ber of appearances in recent fiction.[22–24] This subject is mentioned here for two reasons: These fictionalized accounts may be a first exposure our patients have to a fluorescein angiogram, and, especially in the case of the monologist and humorist Spaulding Gray, they provide feedback on how our patients actually perceive this test.

In Kathryn Harrison's 1992 novel *Exposure*, Ann, a photographer who also has diabetic retinopathy, visits her ophthalmologist's office and is diagnosed as having a macroaneurysm. "We'll take an FA today," the physician says. Continuing, he explains that a "fluorescein angiogram is a picture of the inside of your eye." He "injects one of the prominent veins in Ann's arm with an orange dye that travels to her eyes and illuminates their minute blood vessels with a blue light at which the doctor grunts and mumbles. She feels a wave of nausea as the dye enters her bloodstream. . . . The angiogram machine produces a picture of what it sees: on its screen the vessels of her left eye are lit up like some freakish tree hit by lightning, the burning bush. . . ." Ann goes on to have successful laser surgery.

The ophthalmologist Dr. James Harte is a character in Jodi Picoult's 1998 book *The Pact*. He performs an angiogram on his patient Mrs. Neely who is afflicted with macular degeneration:

He directed Mrs. Neely to a big camera and seated her in front of it. Then he took the hypodermic of fluorescein and injected it into Mrs. Neely's arm. "You might feel a burning sensation in your arm. It is the dye we are looking for," he said. "It will travel from your vein to your heart, then around your body, eventually getting up to your eye. The dye stays in the normal blood vessels, but will ooze out of the abnormal hemorrhaging ones that caused your macular degeneration. We'll figure out where they are, exactly, and treat them." It took twelve seconds, James knew, for the dye to travel from the arm to the heart to the eye. The light, in the back of the eye, illuminated the fluorescent dye. Like the tributaries of a river, the normal blood vessels of Mrs. Neely's retina branched out in fine, tentative lines. The abnormal blood vessels were sunbursts, minuscule fireworks, which softened into puddles of white dye.

Early in the 1994 book *Gray's Anatomy*, Spaulding Gray discovers that he has a macular pucker. The rest of the book is devoted to his personal experiences with this condition, including his exploration of various healing methods that are not aligned with the teachings of modern medical science. His description of his fluorescein angiogram is as accurate as any light-sensitive patient's could be:

> *He put me in an exam chair, got out a huge syringe, and told me he was going to shoot me up with colored dye. Well, I thought, why not, he's the doctor. I had to get him to explain everything to me. Why the dye? Well, it turns out that he wanted to take some photographs of my eye, and in order to photograph the vessels you have to have some dye in them.*
>
> *He shoots me up. My vessels get filled with colored dye very quickly. He and the nurse tilt me forward and put me in some kind of brace. I'm looking through two holes, into what I didn't know at the time was the camera, and they begin to take photos, and the camera turns out to be a flash camera, and the flashbulbs are going off right in front of my eyes. It's like torture. I feel like I'm being blinded and I try to pull my head back but the nurse keeps pushing my head forward–flash, flash, flash! It's like a* Clockwork Orange *situation. It's really like torture. I come out reeling; all I can see is spots.*

Every light-sensitive angiographer who has been on the other side of the fundus camera will appreciate Gray's insight.

Indocyanine Green Angiography

Ocular angiography with dyes other than fluorescein sodium has been explored. The most clinically promising angiography technique for the posterior segment has been ICG angiography.

ICG has been used in medical imaging since 1956[17] and was first photographed in the eye by Kogure and Choromokos in 1969.[25] Flower and Hochheimer continued developing the procedure throughout the 1970s, with Destro and Puliofito updating it in the late 1980s.[26,27] It was not until 1992, however, that Yannuzzi et al. first described a practical method for achieving clinically significant ICG angiographic images.[28] Yannuzzi's work has led to ICG angiography becoming an important adjunctive technique to fluorescein angiography.[29]

This section describes the principles of ICG angiography and provides a step-by-step procedure for performing it. It assumes that you are familiar with the physical and physiologic properties of ICG as discussed in Chapter 4 and with electronic fluorescein angiography.

Choroidal Angiography versus Retinal Angiography

The principles of fluorescein angiography provide a framework for understanding ICG angiography. Both tests use a fundus camera to document ocular blood vessels after a colored dye has been injected intravenously. Fluorescein angiography documents the dynamic flow of fluorescein sodium primarily in the retinal vasculature (Figure 5-18); ICG angiography documents the staining characteristics of ICG in the choroid.

These complementary dyes have differing physical characteristics. Fluorescein sodium is a red, water-soluble dye that is excited by blue (465–490 nm) light and emits yellow (520–530 nm) light. ICG is a green, water-soluble, tricarbocyanine dye that becomes excited in the near infrared range: maximal excitation, 805 nm; maximal emission, 835 nm (Figure 5-19).

FIGURE 5-18
This 4-up demonstrates a red-free image, bright transit phase, isofluorescent mid phase, and late inversion phase of indocyanine green angiography.

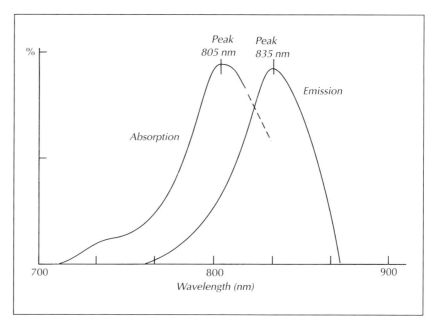

FIGURE 5-19
The excitation and emission spectra of indocyanine green dye.

The image sequence of fluorescein and ICG angiography is similar. Fluorescein angiography is usually referred to as *retinal angiography*, and ICG angiography as *choroidal angiography*; however, both sets of blood vessels are visible in the normal phases of each test. In a normal fluorescein angiogram, dye is captured in the early transit phases (patchy choroidal filling, arterial filling, and laminar flow as veins fill in the arteriovenous phase) and the 5- and 10-minute late phases. In a normal ICG angiogram, the dye is captured in the early choroidal transit phases (medium-sized choroidal arteries fill, then large choroidal veins—with a possible watershed effect).[30] At the same time, the ICG fills the retinal blood vessels in the familiar way: arterial filling then laminar flow as veins fill in the arteriovenous phase. The ICG angiogram continues through the isofluorescent mid pictures of 8–12 minutes and the late inversion phase photographs of 20–30 minutes.

There are practical differences between these two dye tests. Fluorescein sodium is provided in solution, whereas ICG must be dissolved shortly before use. Circulating fluorescein sodium can be recorded using either film or electronic media, whereas ICG angiography can only be practically recorded using electronic imaging. Different exciter and barrier filter pairs maximize the appropriate wavelengths for each test. As we shall see, the plane of best focus and timing is unique to each test. Dye changes during fluorescein angiography are visible in the optical viewfinder, whereas those during ICG angiography are not. Fewer complications and a less fatiguing flash intensity make patients more comfortable during ICG angiography.[31]

However, the duration of ICG angiography (up to an hour versus 15–30 minutes for a complete fluorescein angiogram) balances the patient comfort scales. Procedures for obtaining optimal exposure vary between the two tests. Fluorescein angiography has a relatively constant dynamic range, which is easily captured within the recording range of either film or electronic imaging systems. ICG angiography has a much larger luminescence range, which falls within the infrared portion of the spectrum. Both the flash and the electronic camera sensitivity must be manipulated throughout the procedure to obtain consistent tonal qualities throughout the study. One reason for the large range of fluorescence may be the difference in the percentage of each dye that is bound by proteins in the blood.[32,33] Only one-half of the circulating fluorescein sodium is protein-bound; the rest remains independent to circulate freely through the blood. On the other hand, the more than 90% of the ICG that binds to protein begins by circulating freely, making the early post-injection photographs very bright. Within the first minute after the injection, however, most of the ICG becomes protein-bound and thus unavailable for exposure. As the test continues, less and less ICG is available for fluorescence, creating a need for increased flash and camera sensitivity.

Performing Indocyanine Green Angiography

Two different instruments are currently being used to perform choroidal angiography: the traditional fundus camera and the scanning laser ophthalmoscope (SLO). Not every fundus camera can be used for choroidal angiography because of issues with the efficiency of infrared radiation illumination. Advantages of using SLO technology include the ability to perform simultaneous FA/ICG angiography and full-motion video studies.[34,35] SLO technology and angiography is discussed in Chapter 7. If you are making a choice between these two types of instruments, you should know that with each instrument there are instances in which the identical ICG-filled eye may look very different.[36]

ICG angiography with the fundus camera uses the same basic ophthalmic photography techniques as fluorescein angiography. This section delineates a step-by-step procedure for ICG angiography using a fundus camera, based on the "prepare, position, expose, and follow-up" format. The experienced angiographer who is proficient in the electronic imaging of fluorescein angiography can quickly become successful in ICG angiography.

Conduct a step-by-step review before or during the procedure to help establish your routine. Post a copy of the steps near your fundus camera for easy reference.

A   **B**

FIGURE 5-20
Red filter photograph **(A)** and indocyanine green frame **(B)** showing nevus and resulting hypofluorescence.

Focusing with Infrared Light

The range of electromagnetic radiation extends from gamma rays and x-rays through ultraviolet, visible, and infrared radiation to radiowaves and microwaves. Our eyes, our optical instruments, and our recording media are all optimized for that small band of the electromagnetic radiation that we call light.

We record infrared radiation (IR) during ICG angiography. Although its longer wavelength allows visualization through some pigments and thin hemorrhages, IR does not focus in the same plane as visible light. An additional 0.25% of the focal length added to the lens-film distance is a standard correction.[37] The red index mark on 35-mm interchangeable camera lenses simplifies this process. After the lens is focused, the indicated distance is shifted to the red index mark. Both the standard calculation and the index mark options for correction are impractical for fundus photography.

Two different strategies have been used to ensure the sharp focus of IR wavelengths in ICG angiography. Real-time IR-sensitive video viewing (with or without a barrier filter) is available on some systems. An IR-sensitive video camera replaces the viewfinder and displays real-time images on a medium-resolution monitor. Advantages include feedback from real-time focusing. Capital expense and lower viewing resolution are obvious disadvantages.

A technologically simpler strategy is to bias the focusing system manually by adding two positive diopters to your reticule setting. In this instance, you will see a blurry reticule when looking through the viewfinder. Focus on the choroid while keeping the blurred reticule as blurry as it looked when you first viewed it. The instant feedback of electronic imaging makes this method practical. Inexperienced angiographers may have some initial problems, but the experienced ophthalmic photographer will readily adapt. Although this solution is admirably inexpensive, it introduces the potential for photographer error.

Whichever focusing system is used, target the focus to the choroid by visually dissecting the retina as described in Chapter 2. Focus past the retinal blood vessels and the pigment in the retinal pigment epithelium to the larger choroidal vessels. Remember that even with the best possible focus, the spongy choroid will always seem less sharp than the retinal blood vessels you are accustomed to imaging.

PREPARE AND POSITION

1. *Perform color fundus photography.* Expose stereo photographs that document the status of the retina, including any hemorrhage and edema. After obtaining these photographs, switch from film to electronic image acquisition.

2. *Expose monochromatic images.* Capture green and red monochromatic images. The green images are establishing shots that provide landmarks for overlay and indicate the status of retinal blood vessels and hemorrhages. Use a low flash setting and normal camera sensitivity for the green photographs.

   The red monochromatic photographs provide a correctly focused view of the choroid without ICG dye (Figure 5-20) and document potential hypofluorescent areas (e.g., nevus, dense hemorrhage, or dense pigmentation). Exposure with a red filter can be problematic: You may need to abandon the flash and carry out the exposure using only the viewing light and perhaps some gain in camera sensitivity. Empirical testing will lead to a correct exposure.

3. *Prepare the camera.* After these monochromatic photographs are obtained, prepare the fundus camera and electronic imaging unit for ICG angiography. Double-check the exposure (we suggest a high flash intensity: 300 w/s), camera sensitivity (low), infrared exciter and barrier filter position (in), aperture setting (fully open), and focus (see the sidebar Focusing with Infrared Light). Remember that the exposure values are suggestions only: Empirical experimentation will yield the proper starting point for your particular instrument.

   Ascertain that the injection (25- or 50-mg ICG powder diluted in 3 ml of sterile aqueous solvent) and all necessary supplies are ready. Solicit an injection from the appropriate health care professional.

EXPOSE

4. *Photograph the "earlies."* As with your fluorescein technique, expose a control photograph and time the actual injection using photographs. Stereo imaging during ICG angiography adds important visual information (Figure 5-21). Using established injection techniques, have the health care professional inject the patient with ICG. If you are viewing the retina through the ocular, there will be no visual indication of the dye. You will see instant feedback after the choroidal arterial phase on the computer image monitor. If your system is equipped with an infrared camera viewfinder with monitor, and you are viewing with a barrier in place, you may see the

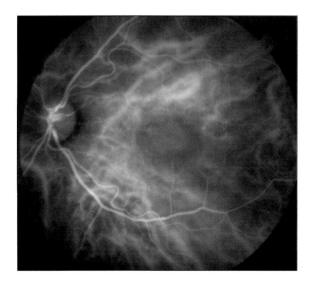

FIGURE 5-21
This red-cyan stereo indocyanine image clearly demonstrates an elevated, well-defined area of choroidal neovascularization beneath the retinal pigment epithelial detachment in a patient with choroidal neovascularization secondary to age-related macular degeneration. (Courtesy of Dennis Orlock, Ophthalmic Consultants of New York.)

dye on the monitor. As with fluorescein angiography, begin capturing early images before your eyes can detect the dye.

Constantly monitor the exposure during ICG angiography. ICG earlies will begin at approximately the same time as standard fluorescein earlies. Fluorescence peaks quickly (approximately 10–20 seconds) and then steadily decreases.

Keep a hand on the exposure control. Your earliest choroidal images will be correctly exposed at 300 w/s. The ICG images will quickly become overexposed unless you rapidly decrease the flash setting. Try decreasing the flash setting in full f-stop or greater increments. Continue to ride this wave of exposure, adjusting the flash setting all the way down to 18–25 w/s, if needed. The correct exposure will be a moving target: With experience, you will begin to anticipate the changes.

There is some controversy over whether the earliest photographs are clinically significant, but because these pictures are the sharpest choroidal images and show the retinal blood vessels, we suggest that you include them (Figure 5-22). There will be few significant changes throughout the early images: Edit this phase liberally, saving only the sharpest and best exposures.

5. *Expose the "lates."* Continuously monitoring the instant feedback of electronic imaging, and increasing the flash setting and camera sensitivity as needed, continue to photograph the ICG at 2, 5, 10, 20, 40, and, perhaps, 60 minutes. The ICG dye will be quite bright during the first 1–5 minutes after the injection. Then, at 8–12 minutes post-injection, the images will become isofluorescent (ICG equally distributed between the choroidal vessels and the surround). We suggest terminating the test when the "inversion phase" phase has been clearly identified (usually approximately 20 minutes). In the inversion phase, the choroidal vessels have emptied of ICG, making them appear dark against a brighter background of ICG in the interstitial space.[38]

The exact timing of the lates is open to interpretation. Some offices routinely expose 1-hour late images; some use a logarithmic timing series (2, 4, 8, 16, 30 minutes); others ignore the early photographs altogether.

Although the usefulness of early choroidal images is being debated, current clinical practice suggests recording the early

A

B

FIGURE 5-22
Early indocyanine green angiography reveals filling of the medium-sized choroidal arteries **(A)** followed by filling of the large choroidal veins **(B)**.

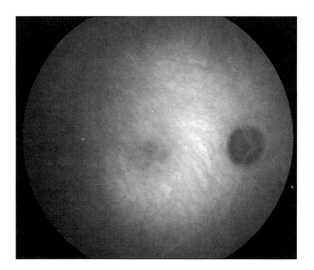

FIGURE 5-23
Late image of indocyanine green (ICG) shows a dark optic nerve, in contrast to the late hyperfluorescent optic nerve in a fluorescein angiogram. Notice that the tonality of the choroidal blood vessels inverted when compared to an early ICG frame.

choroidal and retinal phases until it is proved that they are not clinically useful. Thirty minutes may be the minimal time for the lates. The actual timing of your latest photograph is limited only by the tenacity of your imaging system.

The amount of illumination from ICG decreases dramatically as time from injection increases. It is not unusual to have to maximize both the intensity of the flash and the sensitivity of the electronic imaging camera to provide adequate exposure for late photographs. Increasing the viewing light to maximum output may help increase the illumination in the late phase.

Normal late ICG photographs show a darkened disc where retinal blood vessels cannot be distinguished (Figure 5-23).

6. *Close the session*. Reassure patients that all went well. Release them with a smile, making sure that they feel fine and know where their next clinic stop is. Complete all paperwork, remembering to sign the chart.

7. *Complete the process*. Edit, save, and print a hard copy of the completed electronic angiogram. Take the time to evaluate your work for quality and to discuss the results with the physician. ICG angiography is still an emerging technology. Professional ophthalmic photographers keep informed of the cutting edge of ophthalmic imaging.

Practical Indocyanine Injection Issues

Multiple modified injection techniques have been suggested, including simultaneous fluorescein/ICG injection, pulse ICG angiography, and landmark injection.[39–41]

Most FA/ICG combined angiography is performed using sequential injections. Stopcocks and intravenous sites can be used to advantage if only a single needlestick is desired. The inexperienced worker may prefer keeping the angiography separate: first performing fundus photography, then requesting the familiar fluorescein injection, followed by the ICG injection after the 10-minute fluorescein lates have been completed. The experienced angiographer may start with the color images, then request the ICG injection, photograph the ICG earlies to approximately 7–8 minutes, switch the camera to the fluorescein settings, have the fluorescein injected and photograph it to the 5 minutes, switch back to ICG for 15-minute lates, then to the fluorescein 10-minute lates, and finally to the ICG 20- to 30-minute lates. If these two angiographies are embedded together in this way, be very careful to follow through on all exposure, filter, and focus settings. This second method saves a significant amount of time when compared to sequential angiography.

Sodium fluorescein and diluted ICG can be mixed in the same syringe. Injecting this mixture for a simultaneous FA/ICG has two possible outcomes. If a standard fundus camera is being used, one usually concentrates on the earlies of the fluorescein angiography, not beginning to expose ICG frames until 5 or 10 minutes after the injection. This saves a few minutes of time and requires only a single patient injection. The fluorescein angiogram is usually chosen for transit phase. In fundus camera ICG angiography, this technique saves time at the expense of one of the two early phases. Newer SLO models are capable of performing simultaneous angiography. The sacrifice here is that only one fundus level (choroidal versus retina) can be in sharp focus at a single time.

Recording the wide swings of ICG intensity during the early and late phases of fundus camera-based digital ICG choroidal angiography is problematic. Standard retinal angiography technique requires a bolus injection of fluorescein dye. When the same bolus injection technique is used for choroidal angiography, the relatively high initial post-injection concentration of circulating ICG often causes portions of the transit phase to become overexposed. To compensate, the photographer adjusts the fundus camera flash intensity or the digital gain control, modifying the exposure in direct response to the angiographic screen image. As the test progresses, the amount of circulating dye decreases dramatically, requiring the ophthalmic photographer to maximize both the flash intensity and camera sensitivity.[42]

Because the ophthalmic photographer manipulates the exposure and sensitivity scales during the choroidal angiogram to create a successful image, the tonalities within each of the images are based on different light intensity and camera sensitivity values. Consequently, in choroidal angiography, the intensity of early phase and the intensity of late-phase hyperfluorescence are not specifically comparable, as they are during fluorescein angiography.

Using a pulse injection technique increases the clinical information available in ICG angiograms. Divide the usual ICG dye dose into thirds, inject the first third, wait 30 seconds, inject the second third, wait 30 seconds, and then inject the final third. The transit images will be more evenly exposed, the late-phase ICG photographs will be easier to image, and areas of late hyperfluorescence will be visualized earlier. The pulse method increases transit phase choroidal vascular detail by decreasing the circulating ICG dye early in the angiogram. It increases the amount of ICG dye available for imaging during the late recirculation phase, resulting in lower camera sensitivity requirements for the late photographs. When these mechanisms are combined, less photographer manipulation of exposure variables is required.

Another technique for exposing late ICG photographs that includes retinal blood vessels as landmarks has been reported by Nyberg.[40] He suggests that the small amount of the ICG that remains in the original bottle be diluted and the patient reinjected slowly. Photographs are exposed until the intensity of the retinal blood vessels matches the intensity of the choroidal blood vessels. Unwanted frames are deleted. The additional ICG in the various retinal blood vessels acts as anatomic landmarks. The landmark injection creates useable late images by reintroducing fresh dye, in essence creating a new transit phase.

ICG angiography has a very low rate of adverse reactions. However, because ICG incorporates iodine in the dye preparation process, patients should be screened for iodine allergy. The personnel, procedures, and supplies for systemic reactions to fluorescein angiography should be readily available. Although the dye does not pass through the placenta, fetal toxicity tests have not been performed, and thus this test should not be performed in a pregnant patient.

As with any exciter/barrier filter system, aging filters can result in pseudofluorescence. Autofluorescence has not been reported. Successful anterior segment angiography is being evaluated in research settings.[43]

References

1. Wolfe DR. Fluorescein angiography basic science and engineering. Ophthalmology 1986;93:1617.
2. Eastman Kodak Company. Kodak Filter for Scientific and Technical Uses. Rochester, NY: Eastman Kodak, 1981.
3. Novotny HR, Alvis DL. A method of photographing fluorescence in circulating blood in the human retina. Circulation 1961;24:82.
4. Haining WM, Lancaster RC. Advanced techniques for fluorescein angiography. Arch Ophthalmol 1968;79:10.
5. Delori F, Ben-Sira I, Trempe C. Fluorescein angiography with an optimized filter combination. Am J Ophthalmol 1976;82:559.
6. Emmart EW. Observations on the absorption spectra of fluorescein, fluorescein derivatives, and conjugates. Arch Biochem Biophys 1958;73:1.
7. Saine PJ, Bovino JA, Marcus DF, Nelson PT. Timing of color fundus photographs and intravenous fluorescein angiography. Am J Ophthalmol 1984;97:783.
8. Szirth BC, Wong GD, Bate R, Bartlett DA. Legal ramifications of administration of sodium fluorescein. J Ophthal Photog 1989;11:66.
9. Scott JR. Dye injection by ophthalmic photographers (letter). J Ophthal Photog 1999;21:7.
10. Ophthalmic Photographers' Society. OPS position on performing venipuncture and intravenous injections. OPS Newsletter 28:6, November 1998.
11. Norel J, Biesen PR, Groen GJ, Norren D. Hold up of dye in the arm during fluorescein angiography. Am J Ophthalmol 2000;129:551.
12. Hampton GR, Nelsen PT, Hay PB. Viewing through the asteroids. Ophthalmology 1981;88:669.
13. Yannuzzi LA, Rohrer KT, Tindel LJ, et al. Fluorescein angiography complication survey. Ophthalmology 1986;93:611.
14. Kelley JS, Kincaid M. Retinal fluorography using oral fluorescein. Arch Ophthalmol 1979;97:2331.

15. Garcia CR, Rivero ME, Bartsch DU, et al. Oral fluorescein angiography with the confocal scanning laser ophthalmoscope. Ophthalmology 1999;106(6):1114–1118.
16. Fetkenhour CL, Choromokos E. Anterior segment fluorescein angiography with a retinal fundus camera. Arch Ophthalmol 1978;96:711.
17. Brancato R, Bandello F, Lattanzio R. Atlas Iris Fluorescein Angiography. Milan, Italy: Kugler & Ghendini, 1995;1.
18. D'Anna SA, Hocheimer BF, Joondeph HC. Fluorescein angiography of the heavily pigmented iris and new dyes for iris angiography. Arch Ophthalmol 1983;101:289.
19. Schatz H, George T, Liu J, et al. Color fluorescein angiography: its clinical role. Trans Am Acad Ophthalmol Otolaryngol 1973;77:254.
20. Matsui K, Oka Y, Matsui T. Fluorescein fundus angiography in color. Acta Soc Ophthalmol Jap 1969;73:653.
21. Shikano S, Shimizu K. Atlas of Fluorescence Fundus Angiography. Philadelphia: Saunders, 1968;9.
22. Harrison K. Exposure. New York: Random House, 1993;78.
23. Picoult J. The Pact: A Love Story. New York: William Morrow and Company, 1998;79.
24. Gray S. Gray's Anatomy. New York: Vintage Books, 1994;7.
25. Kogure K, Choromokos EA. Infrared absorption angiography. J Appl Physiol 1969;27:154.
26. Bischoff PM, Flower RW. Ten years experience with choroidal angiography using indocyanine green dye: a new routine examination or an epilogue? Doc Ophthalmol Proc Ser 1976;138:3.
27. Destro M, Puliofito CA. Indocyanine green video angiography of choroidal neovascularization. Ophthalmology 1989;96:846.
28. Yannuzzi LA, Slakter JS, Sorenson JA, et al. Digital indocyanine green videoangiography and choroidal neovascularization. Retina 1992;12:191.
29. Guyer DR, Yannuzzi LA, Slakter JS, et al. Digital indocyanine-green videoangiography of occult choroidal neovascularization. Ophthalmology 1994;101:1727.
30. Hope-Ross M, Yannuzzi LA, Gragoudas ES, et al. Adverse reactions due to indocyanine green. Ophthalmology 1994;101:529.
31. Stevens RA, Saine PJ, Tyler ME. Stereo Atlas of Fluorescein and Indocyanine Green Angiography. Boston: Butterworth–Heinemann, 1999;24.
32. Baker KJ. Binding of sulfobromophthalein (BSP) sodium and indocyanine green (ICG) by plasma alpha-1 lipoproteins. Proc Soc Exp Biol Med 1966;122:957.
33. Desmettre T, Devoisselle JM, Mordon S. Fluorescence properties and metabolic features of indocyanine green as related to angiography. Surv Ophthalmol 2000;45:15.
34. Bischoff PM, Niederberger HJ, Torok B, Speiser P. Simultaneous indocyanine green and fluorescein angiography. Retina 1995;15(2):91–99.
35. Flower RW. Experimental studies of indocyanine green dye-enhanced photocoagulation of choroidal neovascularization feeder vessels. Am J Ophthalmol 2000;129:501.
36. Flower RW, Csaky KG, Murphy RP. Disparity between fundus camera and scanning laser ophthalmoscope indocyanine green imaging of retinal pigment epithelium detachments. Retina 1998;18:260.
37. Sansone SJ. Modern Photography for Police and Firemen. Cincinnati: WH Anderson, 1971;312.
38. Soubrane G, Seres A, Coscas G, Flower RW. Suggested terminology for different phases of indocyanine green angiogram. Retina 2000;20:319–320.
39. Miller K. Protocols for efficacious use of indocyanine green/sodium fluorescein angiography. J Ophthal Photog 1993;15:63.
40. Nyberg WC. Re-injection technique for establishing landmarks in late phase ICG angiography. J Ophthal Photog 1993;15:65.
41. Saine PJ, Stevens RA, Cavender JC. A new technique for administering ICG during choroidal angiography. J Ophthal Photog 1999;21:44.
42. Yannuzzi LA, Flower RW, Slakter JS. Indocyanine Green Angiography. St. Louis: Mosby, 1997.
43. Chan TK, Rosenbaum AL, Rao R, et al. Indocyanine green angiography of the anterior segment in patients undergoing strabismus surgery. Br J Ophthalmol 2001;85:214.

Chapter 6

The Ophthalmic Darkroom: Processing and Printing Fluorescein Angiograms

Lawrence M. Merin

Introduction

In one of his famous paintings, the surrealist artist Magritte painted an image of a pipe with the caption, "Ceci n'est pas une pipe" (This is not a pipe). Similarly, a fluorescein angiogram is obviously not dye in the retina and choroid, but rather a two-dimensional monochromatic representation of that reality. In this case, the painter and the ophthalmic photographer have the same challenges and opportunities: to ensure that their images communicate effectively.

Ophthalmic photographs use commonly accepted characteristics to convey information. Line, form, and especially tonal gradation are all essential components of the image and represent the physical attributes of the subject. Photographers must carefully choose their materials and master the processes that will reveal these qualities and thus imbue their photographs with veracity and eloquence.

For many, the craft of black and white film processing and printing is an enormously satisfying pursuit. In a world where more and more tasks may be accomplished by the computer and results appear through a sequence of button pushing, exposing film and processing it yourself is an intensely personal and human experience. There is also a magical quality to this activity. I confess that I often still feel a thrill as an image gradually appears on a plain sheet of paper in the developing tray, just as I did when I made my first print in my uncle's basement darkroom three decades ago.

That amazement is certainly in keeping with the almost miraculous detail provided in fluorescein angiography. If you pause to linger over a properly exposed and processed fluorescein angiogram, you may find yourself enchanted by the magnificent detail and delicacy in the image.

The materials and processes of black and white photography have distinct capabilities for the reproduction of shades of gray, black, and white. In conventional fluorescein angiography, these attributes are of paramount importance, as film and paper materials are the only way to share the clinical information that the photographer witnesses privately through the camera eyepiece.

This chapter introduces you to the ophthalmic darkroom. The chapter offers a little of the theory and quite a bit about the practice of film development and touches on the methods of viewing and storing the angiographic negatives. Positive printouts in transparency and print formats are often generated from these negatives, and specific recommendations for fine-tuning this process are provided. Printing for exhibition or publication requires the highest level of technical skill, and I offer several suggestions to maximize the aesthetic as well as the informational qualities of the fine photographic print.

Each photographic procedure presents the photographer with choices. The first choice to be made is which camera and film to use to photograph the patient. The proper flash setting is then chosen to produce the correct exposure. Next, you must select a film developer, along with the time and temperature needed to produce proper negative contrast. If a positive version of the original negative is required, you must again choose the positive film or paper and its dedicated processing parameters. The place where the processing occurs, the ophthalmic darkroom, contains hardware and supplies chosen to facilitate the production of informative clinical images.

A note of caution: Just reading this chapter will not be enough to master film processing and printing. If you want to become proficient, you must work with and refine the techniques yourself. This chapter provides enough theory to help you understand why things happen and suggests practical measures to help you understand the capabilities and limitations of photographic materials and processes. By reading and experimenting, you should learn how to make photographic choices confidently and enhance your skills as a capable scientific communicator.

The Darkroom

Designing the Ophthalmic Darkroom

The darkroom has been typecast as a gloomy and claustrophobic place where mechanical, boring, or otherwise distasteful tasks occur. By adopting modern design features, however, your darkroom can be a cheerful venue that is conducive to the creation of high-quality ophthalmic images.

As with other design projects, the first step in designing an efficient new ophthalmic darkroom (or renovating an older one) is to assess your specific needs. You should consider such things as the present and potential volume of the photographic service, the number of employees who may need to work in the darkroom simultaneously, whether the facility will process black and white materials exclusively or whether color film and prints will also be processed, and the degree of automation you may desire. The answers to these service-related questions will logically suggest hardware and physical plant decisions and, in turn, will help determine the budget for the project.

Chromogenic Film

The image that is formed on conventional black and white negative film is composed of metallic silver. There are many different processes available for processing such materials, and that variety means that there is no "universal" method to achieve standardized results. Professional photographers test extensively and use their own custom processing parameters to achieve the results they desire.

Ilford's XP-2 film initially captures the image using silver halides but, during processing, replaces the silver with semitransparent color dye clouds to form a "black and white" photograph. This film is designed to be processed in color negative processing solutions (process C-41), commonly found in automated mini-lab facilities associated with amateur film photoprocessing. Portraiture is the most common subject matter for amateur photographers, and flesh tones in these snapshots can be printed accurately only through tight processing control. For this reason, C-41 chemistry is designed to be used within very narrow limits of time and temperature. Conveniently, this also provides a consistent processing standard for fluorescein angiograms.

XP-2 has a film sensitivity of ISO 400 and thus is similar to conventional films used for fluorescein angiography. It is panchromatic and responds accurately to the specific wavelengths of light used during the study. Its image structure and resolution compare favorably with its silver counterparts, and the film's granularity is actually much finer than that of conventional black and white 400-speed emulsions. The image seen in XP-2 negatives has a magenta cast rather than the gray typically seen in conventional film media but is nonetheless eminently readable.

Most mini-labs routinely produce 3.5-in. × 5-in. or 4-in. × 6-in. prints, and XP-2 angiograms can be machine printed the same way. These angiographic prints may appear to have a sepia cast, but this will not obscure diagnostic information. The total turnaround time for negatives and prints from such a facility is approximately 1 hour. If specialized printouts are required, such as contact sheets or exhibition prints, XP-2 negatives can be used the same way as conventional black and white negatives. Because of these attributes, XP-2 can be a useful alternative to setting up a dedicated darkroom for small-volume practices.

Table 6-1. Comparison of Three Types of Ophthalmic Darkrooms

Minimal	Standard	Advanced
Negative processing	Negative processing Contact prints	Negative processing Contact prints Enlargements

Obviously, the first question is whether a darkroom is a necessary feature of a particular photographic service. For many practices, concerns about quality control, cost-effectiveness, and immediate availability of processing can best be addressed when the darkroom is located within the office or institution. To maximize quality, you can alter film processing at will to adjust for unusual pathology or physical characteristics of the subject. Consistent quality results from careful attention to detail, and this comes from having all the processing parameters under your control.

Probably the most important aspect of providing your own processing service comes from rapid availability of the photograph. No outside processor can provide angiographic results as quickly as in-house film processing, a crucial benefit for patients requiring urgent treatment for vision-threatening disorders.

The direct costs of in-house processing are typically less than those paid to send the film out. Consumables, such as the cost of processing chemicals, usually come to less than $1 per roll. If you factor in indirect costs (space, equipment, labor, and benefits) you may still save money, particularly if you process several angiograms simultaneously.

For an extremely low-volume practice or one in which there is no space for a darkroom, using a professional extramural service for conventional film processing may be a logical choice. Alternately, such a practice might consider using a chromogenic film (see the sidebar Chromogenic Film) for expedient processing in the same locality. Of course, practices that acquire digital angiographic equipment may not require a conventional darkroom at all. However, the theories of tonal reproduction included in this chapter are equally applicable to electronic imaging, even though electronic, rather than chemical, means are used to obtain and process the angiographic information.

Color slide processing for fundus photography and the printing of such slides are outside the scope of this chapter. However, only the busiest ophthalmic practices have the volume that would make color film processing cost-effective, considering supply and labor costs.

Black and white processing, on the other hand, can be either simple or complex, depending on the sophistication required of the service. Three levels of technology are typically encountered in ophthalmic darkrooms: minimal (film only), standard (film and contact sheets), and advanced (film, contact sheets, and paper enlargements). Each category has specific requirements for space, hardware, and supplies (Table 6-1).

What is a darkroom? First, it is a dedicated space designed to control ambient illumination when processing light-sensitive materials. Such a place should incorporate three different lighting situations: (1) white light, typically provided by fluorescent or tungsten light fixtures and used for chemical mixing, setting up hardware for processing tasks, and general maintenance; (2) total darkness, for loading film into processing tanks; and (3) "safelight" illumination of a specific color (typically amber or red) for paper and sheet film processing. Although other parameters (such as plumbing, ventilation, access, and total area) are all important, the defining character of the darkroom is light control.

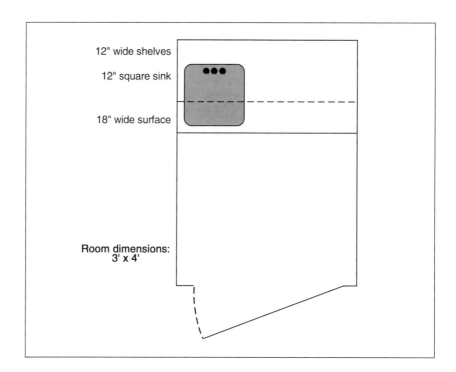

12" wide shelves

12" square sink

18" wide surface

Room dimensions:
3' x 4'

FIGURE 6-1
Plan and elevation of the minimal darkroom. In a space of only 12 square feet, angiographic negatives can be developed, washed, and dried.

Regardless of size and space, a major consideration in designing a darkroom is the division between wet and dry work areas. Because sensitive materials (i.e., unprocessed film and paper) are particularly susceptible to contamination from water, processing solution splashes, and chemical dust, they must be protected from such accidents. Design the darkroom work space so that a physical barrier separates the processing sink and chemical storage area (wet side) from the film-loading area, paper storage areas, and the enlarger (dry side). That barrier might be either an aisle or a partition, depending on the configuration of the room. If floor space does not permit such a division, then the dry "side" may simply be a secure cabinet above the sink.

When planning space for the darkroom, you must anticipate the required square footage for the specific processes you will perform there. For film processing only, a spartan facility as small as 12 square feet is sufficient (Figure 6-1). For a facility to process film and a tray line for contact sheet and print production, a minimum of 36 square feet allows adequate space (Figure 6-2). An even larger space permits other nonclinical photographic tasks (i.e., copy work) to be performed (Figure 6-3).

Because film used for angiography is extremely sensitive to light, the darkroom must be totally light-proof so no stray illumination can strike the film while it is being loaded onto the processing reels. The most common sources for stray light include the gap between the door and its frame, spaces between tiles in acoustical or "drop" ceilings, and holes through which plumbing fixtures enter the darkroom. Apply flexible rubber weather-stripping material (available at hardware or home improvement stores) to the edges of doors to prevent light leakage. Rubber flanges designed to prevent air drafts are also useful to seal the bottoms of doors from errant light. Drop ceilings should incorporate tight-fitting tiles to prevent stray light from distant fixtures or adjacent rooms from entering the darkroom.

The best way to detect problems with light leakage is to simply stand in the darkroom for 15–20 minutes after all lights have been turned off inside the room, but with all lights illuminated in adjacent rooms and

FIGURE 6-2
Plan of standard ophthalmic darkroom. If you have a 36-square foot space, both negative processing and positive printout production may be handled.

FIGURE 6-3
Diagram of an advanced darkroom. This plan of the Jones Eye Institute darkroom indicates the space allocation for enlarging, processing, drying, and ancillary production activities required to support an academic department of ophthalmology.

hallways. This allows you to adapt to the dark and permits even small points of light to be seen. Using opaque black photographic tape, block any tiny lights observed in the ceiling, and apply additional pieces of foam rubber to the door frame if any similar leaks are detected there.

Because proper light-proofing also restricts air flow, arrange for forced air ventilation in the darkroom.[1] Light-proof louvers and fans, sold through professional photographic suppliers, permit fresh air to replace contaminated air freely while they simultaneously prevent light from

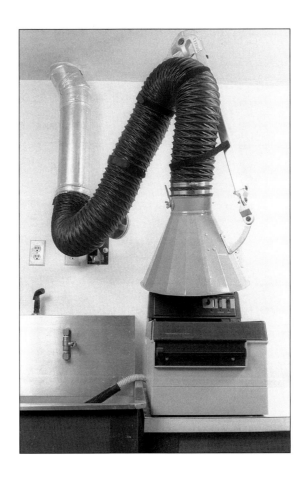

FIGURE 6-4
Vent hood. To satisfy Occupational Safety and
Health Administration requirements and to make the
darkroom safer and more pleasant, this vent hood
helps rid the darkroom of noxious fumes.

entering the room. Because many processing solutions emit noxious
odors and even toxic fumes, assisted ventilation is highly recommended
for health and safety reasons and may be mandated by law in your state
(Figure 6-4). To be certain that the air quality will be sufficient, considering the number of workers in the darkroom and the nature of the
processes used, consult with an industrial hygienist or a ventilation engineer when planning any new facility.

Equip the darkroom with its own thermostat for heating and cooling.
If the air temperature is kept at the same setting as the required temperature for processing (typically 68–72°F), then you can use stored chemical
solutions immediately without requiring water baths to heat or cool them.

For most standard and advanced darkrooms, standard line voltage
should be sufficient to operate timers, safelights, and enlargers. In North
America, this means a 110-volt, 20-ampere circuit. Because the darkroom
is a damp environment, use ground fault interrupter outlets to prevent
electrical shocks. Make sure that outlets are placed behind the sink to
provide electrical power for processing timers, adjacent to the enlarger
for its own power requirement, and proximal to the film or print dryer.
To compensate for warm, ambient water temperature in warm climates,
water chillers may be necessary and require a 240-volt circuit. The
enlarger should be on a separate circuit to avoid voltage fluctuations.
Safelights should have their own switch-controlled outlets. White-light
switches are often mounted a foot or so above the safelight switches to
avoid confusion. Many photographers arrange for a single master power
switch next to the door so all circuits may be shut off when processing
and printing have been completed.

Exposed film is at its most vulnerable state when being transferred
from its cassette to the processing reel and daylight tank. The film will be

FIGURE 6-5
Drum door. These allow entry into the darkroom without permitting outside lighting to change the illumination chosen for work within the area.

FIGURE 6-6
Thermostatic mixing valve. Photographic-quality valves allow the water temperature to be easily selected and maintained. This valve includes a water filter to ensure a clean water supply.

ruined if someone inadvertently opens the darkroom door at that moment. The most elegant way of avoiding such a catastrophe while providing easy access to the facility is the rotating drum door. These devices allow easy entry and exit without affecting existing darkroom lighting conditions (Figure 6-5). A less expensive alternative is to equip the door with a sliding lock operable only from the inside, although some means of alternate entry from outside may be useful in an emergency. Illuminated "in use" signs may alert others to darkroom activities if they are mounted conspicuously outside the darkroom.

Although the design of the minimal darkroom does not absolutely require its own water supply (as you can use another room in the clinic to mix processing solutions and wash film), professional installations need both hot and cold running water. Depending on the cleanliness of the water supply, an inline water filter may prevent suspended grit or organic matter from adhering to the film. Typical black and white processing requires a flow rate of at least 3 gallons per minute and a temperature of 65–75°F; if your practice is in a warm climate, you may need to install a small refrigeration unit or "chiller" to cool the water in the summer. A photographic-quality thermostatic mixing valve is highly recommended (Figure 6-6) for convenient temperature control. These valves incorporate a gauge that allows the temperature of the water to be precisely set and easily maintained.

Standard and advanced darkrooms require a processing sink. These fixtures are designed to be set into a cabinetry base or may be supported by their own leg and shelf assembly and are used to provide a work surface to process film and printout media. The typical darkroom sink is approximately 4–6 in. deep. Determine its area by counting the number and size of processing trays to be used simultaneously, plus the area of the print washer. The ophthalmic darkroom should be able to process 8-in. × 10-in. material, as that is the minimum size for an angiographic contact print. Thus, a 2-ft × 4-ft sink is the minimum size for four 8 × 10 trays, though a larger sink will allow the trays to be manipulated with less congestion. On occasion, exhibition printing up to 11 in. × 14 in. may be called for. Rarely will the next larger size, 16 in. × 20 in., be requested.

Typical darkroom sinks are constructed of either fiberglass or stainless steel. Fiberglass sinks are lighter and less costly than steel but are also easier to scratch. They must be cleaned with special care using only nonabrasive cleaners. Stainless steel sinks are impervious to chemicals and last for many years with no sign of wear or breakdown of their surface. When either type of sink is installed, use shims under the sink or its legs to ensure that sufficient gradient is provided for proper water drainage. Without the slope, water will tend to pool in the sink instead of flowing out through the drain.

The last construction detail to consider is the finish for the walls, cabinetry, and floor. For a pleasant workplace that is easy to clean, paint the walls with washable high-gloss white enamel. White allows the room to be maximally bright under safelight illumination but will not contribute to fogging of sensitive materials.[2] Finish the walls directly behind or adjoining the enlarger with flat black paint to absorb stray reflected light when printing. Consider white plastic laminates for all work surfaces, table tops, and cabinet faces, as this material allows chemical spills to be easily cleaned. If color materials are processed and evaluated for color balance, then white or neutral gray sinks, cabinets and walls are essential. The floor must be waterproof, of course, and a central floor drain is good insurance against accidental water damage to adjacent offices if the sink leaks or a hose becomes disconnected. Either vinyl tile or sheet flooring material is a good choice. Install cushioned flooring material (i.e., Ace Koralite) on top of the standard floor to help prevent leg pain if darkroom workers must stand for prolonged periods.

Equipping the Darkroom

Because the array of hardware required for black and white processing is task-specific, the minimal darkroom requires only a few items. Standard and advanced darkrooms need a greater array of tools. These specialized materials are best found at professional photographic suppliers.

The following basic equipment is required for manual film processing:

1. Thermometer. An accurate thermometer is required because processing is a chemical reaction influenced by the temperature of the solutions. Fluid-filled glass thermometers are extremely accurate but quite fragile and difficult to read. Metal thermometers with dial faces are more durable and may be read even under safelight illumination. For the ultimate in accuracy, digital units are available. When first purchased, thermometers should be calibrated against a laboratory-quality instrument to verify their accuracy.
2. Timer. Timing the duration of the processing steps requires a timer that shows both minutes and seconds. Although one could use a

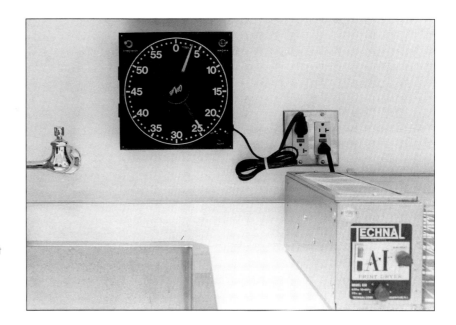

FIGURE 6-7
Laboratory timer. This unit features luminous hands that count down to zero, and a loud buzzer (that may be turned off) that announces the conclusion of each processing step. The timer is plugged into a ground fault interrupter receptacle that provides an extra measure of electrical safety in this wet environment.

standard clock with a sweep second hand, a far superior choice is a laboratory timer that counts down from the total required time to zero (Figure 6-7). Such timers typically have large luminous numbers and hands and also have an audible alarm buzzer that may be set to sound at the end of the time interval.

3. Tanks and reels. Film-processing reels and tanks are available in either plastic or stainless steel. The two materials have significant differences. To load steel reels requires greater manual dexterity, and thus practice is needed before loading can be confidently accomplished.[3] However, steel is impervious to chemical contamination and is an excellent thermal conductor (important when adjusting solution temperatures in a water bath). To load a steel reel, attach the end of the film to the center of the reel (with a spring clip, slot, or pair of prongs, depending on the model and brand) and then slowly turn the reel while the slightly bowed film is fed into it. Stainless steel reels may be loaded successfully when damp. However, if a steel reel falls to the floor, it may be permanently bent (although this is less of a problem if high-quality, heavy-gauge reels are purchased).

Plastic reels use a ratchet mechanism that semiautomatically pulls the film onto the spiral reel. Their construction style and material make thorough cleaning difficult. Even minimal moisture in the film track can prevent proper loading. The plastic tank is a poor thermal conductor, and thus its contents cannot be cooled or heated easily in a water bath. On the positive side, however, many novices find the semiautomatic loading feature much easier to master than loading a steel reel. If your darkroom uses an automatic film processing machine that uses plastic or stainless steel reels, then you have no choice in the type of reel to use.

Once loaded, the processing reels are placed in "daylight" tanks, containers that have two-piece tops that allow the processing solutions to be poured in and emptied, rapidly, in bright room illumination (Figure 6-8). Tanks to accommodate one, two, four, and eight 35-mm reels can be acquired. I have found it useful to equip my own darkroom with three tanks (one each of one-, two-, and four-reel sizes). With this selection, I can always process films efficiently.

FIGURE 6-8
"Daylight" style tanks incorporate a two-part top that permits solutions to be poured in and drained without allowing the film to be struck with light.

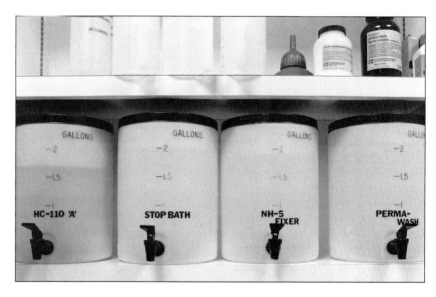

FIGURE 6-9
Two-gallon storage tanks with spigots. These allow solutions to be easily poured into measuring containers by simply opening the valve. The labels are created with self-stick black vinyl lettering. Be sure to follow Occupational Safety and Health Administration labeling guidelines for hazardous substances.

4. Solution storage tanks. Mixed processing solutions must be stored in containers that limit evaporation and oxidation. Plastic or glass bottles with tight-fitting tops may be equally effective for small batches of solutions. However, if space permits, the use of storage containers with built-in spigots permits the easy transfer of solutions (Figure 6-9). These containers are available in 1-, 2-, and 5-gallon sizes and come with floating lids to limit oxidation caused by the large area of fluid surface in contact with the air. If the standard solutions are premixed to working strength and stored in these containers, then it is simple and quick to decant the required quantity.

Another alternative storage method is to use multiple small bottles to store chemistry. If 1 gallon of liquid is prepared, it may be stored in four quart-size bottles, each filled to the top, to limit oxidation.

Because many photographic processing solutions are colorless, be sure to label each storage container with its contents. Once the containers are labeled, you can avoid future contamination by only refilling the container with its labeled contents. If you use a label-making machine to identify these containers, avoid red labeling tape, since it cannot be read under safelight illumination.

5. Graduates, beakers, funnels. Assorted measuring devices are required when processing film. Although photographic supply houses offer a variety of these items, try discount stores that sell them inexpensively as houseware items. Before use, verify their accuracy by comparing their marked volumes with a laboratory-grade graduate. Plastic is preferred over glass because of its durability and break-resistance. Translucent plastic allows the fluid level to be readily ascertained. (Although measuring utensils are also available in stainless steel, they are costly and are more difficult to read, as you cannot determine the exact location of the fluid meniscus for accurate measurements.) A set of three each of 1-pint and 1-quart graduates, and a 1-gallon plastic bucket will be needed for solution mixing and film processing needs.

6. Film washer. After processing the film, it must be washed. You can wash film simply by setting the tank underneath a running faucet, but much more thorough washing can be accomplished (with less water!) by using a dedicated film washer. Such devices typically use a length of plastic tubing to connect to the faucet. The wash water is sent into the unit where residual processing chemistry is washed out of the film. Some washers introduce the water at the bottom of the unit, and it then exits by overflowing from the top (Figure 6-10). Others bring the water into the top and the waste water exits from the bottom. Still others use siphon action to completely fill and empty the washer in cycles. Each style of washer has its adherents, and each can be effective provided sufficient time is spent washing the film.

7. Film dryer. After washing has been completed, the film must be dried. For many years, film manufacturers recommended that the film be "hung to dry in a dust-free place." Although that suggestion is still applicable, film dryers speed the process and allow the angiogram to be safely examined in a fraction of the time air-drying requires. Film dryers incorporate a heater and a fan mounted in an enclosure, allowing the films to be suspended in a stream of warm air. Filters are used to ensure that the air is dust-free. The fastest dryers use a high-speed fan and allow the film to be dried on the processing reel; some will dry a single roll of film in as little as 2 minutes (Figure 6-11). If you use a machine that dries film while still on its reels, be sure to scrub the reels in hot soapy water thoroughly after removing the dried film. Otherwise, residues from dried wetting agent will accumulate on the reels and contaminate the development process for subsequent rolls of film.

The items described allow standard processing of black and white camera film. The preferred method of angiographic analysis consists of directly viewing the processed negative. However, if positive copies are required (i.e., to send a copy of the study to the referring physician), a contact sheet may be produced. Either sheet film or paper may be used for this purpose, and either medium requires the following additional equipment for processing:

1. Contact printer. Contact prints are produced by placing the emulsion side of the negative onto the emulsion side of the paper or sheet

FIGURE 6-10
Film washer. These devices allow flowing fresh water to cleanse the film of residual fixer and washing aid chemistry.

FIGURE 6-11
Forced-air film dryer. This unit is one of the fastest dryers available and is capable of drying a roll of film quickly while still attached to the processing reel.

film, pressing the two materials into firm contact, and then exposing the print medium through the negative to a timed light source (Figure 6-12). Specially designed contact printers may be used. These machines consist of a series of individually controlled lights, a fully adjustable timer, and a pneumatic pressure plate that maintains firm contact between the negative and the printout material (Figure 6-13). Such contact printers are perfect for ophthalmic use because you can customize their light pattern to produce multiple prints with precisely matched characteristics, but they are expensive.

A low-tech, low-cost alternative consists of a standard photographic contact frame, comprised of a sponge rubber or felt pad

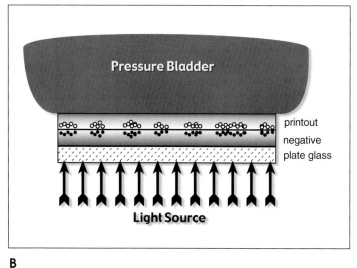

A

B

FIGURE 6-12
Professional contact printer **(A)**. Ideal for producing high-quality single printouts or multiple matching prints, this Arkay (Regal/Arkay, Milwaukee, WI) contact printer features a pneumatic pressure device to create maximum contact pressure **(B)**.

FIGURE 6-13
Orientation of negative and printout material. In contact printing, the negative's emulsion layer must be in firm contact with the positive printout material's emulsion layer to create a perfectly sharp copy.

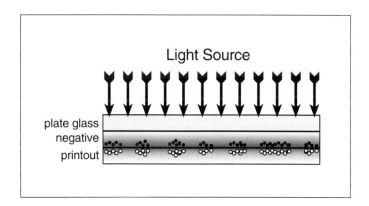

with a hinged plate-glass cover. With this device, the negative-printout sandwich is placed into the unit, the glass cover is closed, and the regulated light source is provided by either a low-wattage bulb suspended over the work or an enlarger with a timer to regulate exposure duration. For the ultimate in simplicity, some photographers use a single piece of plate glass and simply lay the glass on top of the negative-printout sandwich beneath the enlarger when contact printing. For either simple method, make sure that firm pressure is applied to the sandwich to counteract the natural curve of the film. If the negative and the printout medium are not in tight contact, the positive will not be sharp.

One problem associated with the use of high-contrast sheet film as the printout material is the inadvertent production of dust spots on the printout. These tiny white spots are caused by dust particles that are caught in the beam of light and produce tiny unexposed shadows that appear white. Most of these artifacts can be prevented by changing the illumination from a point source to a broad, diffused one. This can be simply accomplished by fastening a thin sheet of frosted plastic (i.e., milky Plexiglas like that used on the front of x-ray viewboxes) or opal glass to the glass top of the printing frame. When the enlarger's illumination strikes this diffusion material, the

FIGURE 6-14
Sodium vapor safelight. This Thomas Duplex safelight produces enormous quantities of safe illumination from its sodium vapor bulb. Suspended from the ceiling, its light shines on the ceiling and walls, creating indirect illumination.

Testing Safelight Illumination

In spite of their name, safelights are not completely "safe." If the orthochromatic photographic material remains under safelight illumination that is too bright or for too long, some fogging may occur. Under certain conditions, virtually all safelights may cause fogging.

To test your safelight, in total darkness place a sheet of printout material you usually use (paper or sheet film) in the same location as the tray line would normally be and place several coins or other opaque objects on the sheet. Turn on the safelight and allow it to illuminate the sheet for two or three times the duration of the longest processing time. Next, turn off the safelight and, in total darkness, develop, stop, and fix the sheet. Turn on the room lights and inspect the printout. If you can see where the coins were placed, this indicates that the safelight fogged the adjacent areas. Either move the safelight farther away, replace its bulb with one of lower wattage, or shorten the exposure time for the next test until you have determined the maximum "safe" time or brightness, or both.

---

frosted medium in turn becomes a broad, diffuse light source that virtually eliminates pinholes without changing the sharpness of the contact sheet. The diffusion sheet must be homogeneous to produce suitable diffusion, so avoid rippled or textured materials.

2. Safelight. The film used in the camera for angiography is panchromatic (sensitive to the full spectrum of visible light). Before processing, this material must be handled in total darkness. Photographic paper and contact sheet film are usually orthochromatic (relatively insensitive to red or amber light). Safelights are designed to produce illumination that will usually not expose these orthochromatic materials (see sidebar Testing Safelight Illumination).

   Most safelights incorporate a low-wattage tungsten bulb in a fixture with a glass filter that limits the emitted wavelengths to either amber or red. The most efficient safelights use a sodium vapor lamp and adjustable louvers for maximal "safe" illumination (Figure 6-14). These lamps produce amazing quantities of light and thus enhance the working environment.

   The color of the safelight illumination must be matched to the printout material. Many photographic papers require the use of an "OC" filter that produces a yellowish-orange illumination, whereas certain sheet films specify that a "1A" filter be used, producing a fairly dim red light. If your filter does not match the spectral requirements of the printout, fogging may result!

3. Photo trays and tongs. After exposure, the printout material (sheet film or paper) must be processed. For manual laboratories, processing occurs in print trays. Sized for 5-in. × 7-in., 8-in. × 10-in., 11-in. × 14-in., and 16-in. × 20-in. print material, these are usually made of plastic. To minimize eye fatigue when working under safelight illumination, all-white trays are preferred to those made of red,

FIGURE 6-15
Plexiglas print washer. Properly designed print washers continually bathe both surfaces of prints with fresh water to remove processing chemistry.

black, or other colors. The bottoms of the best trays feature either raised ribs or buttons; these facilitate removal of the print when processing is completed. To prevent cross-contamination of chemistry, label each tray and tong (i.e., developer, stop-bath, and fixer).

Use a set of stainless steel or plastic tongs to transfer the paper from tray to tray. Some developing agents, such as metol, have the potential to cause an allergic skin reaction, so use tongs instead of bare fingers to decrease your chances of developing metol poisoning or contact dermatitis.

Of the tongs currently available, stainless steel ones are the most durable, although plastic tongs work well if they are handled carefully. Avoid those made of bamboo with rubber tips, as they retain chemistry and cannot be cleaned adequately to avoid future contamination of print materials.

4. Paper safe. A paper safe is a light-tight box with a hinged door that permits individual sheets of film or paper to be easily removed under safelight illumination. The safe uses baffles to prevent its contents from being accidentally exposed to white light. Even though the original packing container for paper or film may be used for its storage, the use of a paper safe streamlines printmaking.

5. Print washer. After processing the contact sheet, residual chemistry needs to be washed out of its emulsion. The simplest, least expensive washers permit you to use a standard processing tray to wash prints; these use a siphon that attaches to the tray to constantly circulate fresh water and drain contaminated water. More sophisticated units are made of Plexiglas and use water jets to continually bathe each print with clean water (Figure 6-15). Because fixer-laden water is heavier than clean water, one might assume that washers that drain from the bottom would be superior, although the turbulence caused by entering clean water keeps the fixer well circulated. Thus, either style of washer may be effective, provided that the prints are allowed to move around in the water stream and that sufficient time is permitted for maximal chemistry removal.

6. Squeegees and print dryers. After the wash has been completed, the print needs to be dried. If rapid turnaround times are not important, you may squeegee them to remove excess water and then clip the prints to a thin overhead wire or string (akin to a clothesline)

Machine Processing Options for Film and Positive Printouts

Within the last decade, automation has made steady advances in the ophthalmic darkroom. If your practice produces a high volume of angiograms, some degree of machine-processing technology may prove beneficial, as it may free the photographer from the darkroom and allow more time for patient contact. Of the various methods of processing automation, the two types most commonly used in ophthalmology are the rotary tube processor and the roller transport method.

Both technologies automate the series of processing steps, and thus you only need to load the film and retrieve it from the machine when the steps have been completed. With manual processing, you must take care of each step yourself; machine processing permits you to leave the darkroom for the largest portion of the processing time.

In rotary tube processing, the film is threaded onto a processing reel, just as with manual "daylight tank" processing. The loaded reels are placed into the processing chamber. In some machines, this looks similar to the manual tanks, whereas others use a covered trough-like chamber. When the process begins, a motor starts rotating and sometimes oscillates the reels. Developer is automatically introduced into the processing container or trough. When the required development time has concluded, a valve opens automatically, permitting the used developer to exit the chamber. A brief water rinse typically ensues, followed by draining. Fixer is then admitted and the agitation cycle commences, followed by a water wash cycle. The film is manually removed from the machine for conventional drying.

In the health care field, roller transport machines were first used in radiology and dental departments. They consist of separate chambers that hold developer, fixer, and wash water. The rollers are made of rubber and consist of paired units that are motor-driven; they gently squeeze the film and pull it sequentially through the processing solutions. To begin processing, the film is removed from its cassette and taped to a leader card. This stiff piece of plastic sheet is then inserted into the first pair of rollers, and the angiographic film follows the card through the different chambers.[4] Several rolls of film can often be processed simultaneously, and once the film is inside the processor (or enclosed in a light-proof loading chamber), room lights may be turned on. Roller transport processors often incorporate a forced-air dryer, so the completely processed film emerges from the machine dry and ready to view. In addition to roll film, roller transport processors can also process sheet film and paper prints, often with the same processing chemistry.

Provided that regular and thorough maintenance is performed on the machines, films processed automatically are indistinguishable from those processed manually. In fact, the motorized agitation and the timer-regulated fluid transfer enable machine processing to potentially achieve a higher degree of uniformity and absolutely consistent results. These benefits are in addition to the fact that automatic processing frees valuable photographer time.

Although this technology is not inexpensive, a careful assessment of labor costs, personnel utilization, and patient volume may reveal a clear application for processing automation in your department.

FIGURE 6-16
Printout drying. One of the simplest methods for drying sheet film or resin-coated paper prints is to hang them up to dry. This darkroom has been equipped with a sturdy metal wire line above the darkroom sink. Regular wooden spring clothespins are drilled and threaded onto the line and securely grasp each print for air drying. Note the tray line set up in the sink.

and allow them to air dry (Figure 6-16). Some dryers use a heated forced air system to dry prints quickly, whereas others use an infrared drying element. Stationary units that direct the air flow onto the prints may be used for either paper or sheet film materials. Roller transport dryers that move the materials through the hot-air chamber can usually be used only for paper materials.

One of the best methods of drying fiber-based paper prints consists of placing the squeegeed prints onto clean fiberglass screens. This technique allows the prints to dry slowly in room air. Avoid the use of blotters or drum dryers for paper prints; both are prone to contamination and cannot be cleaned easily.

The Advanced Darkroom

The advanced ophthalmic darkroom has the capability of producing enlargements on paper. The following items are required for this assignment (see sidebar Machine Processing Options for Film and Positive Printouts).

1. Enlarger. The enlarger projects the image of the negative onto photographic paper to produce a positive print. Component parts of this device include a light source, negative carrier, lens board with an enlarging lens, support column, and baseboard. Condenser enlargers collimate the light and direct it evenly over the negative, although after-market light sources are available to change the illumination quality.

   Some ophthalmic photographers prefer point-source enlargers that produce extremely sharp prints but are prone to image dust, dirt, and scratches with equal precision. Others prefer "cold light" enlarging and use a fluorescent lamp light source. These enlargers minimize dust spots on the print. Like many other aspects of ophthalmic photography, the choice becomes one of personal preference, provided your enlarger produces the print quality you and your clients demand.

   When properly adjusted, the enlarger's baseboard, lens board, and negative carrier are all perfectly parallel with each other and are held in rigid alignment. A well-designed enlarger column per-

FIGURE 6-17
Photographic enlarger. Although 35-mm enlargers can produce acceptable work, those designed to accommodate larger negatives, such as this Beseler 23C enlarger (Linden, NJ), produce a wider field of even illumination.

mits this to occur and allows the enlarger head to be raised off the baseboard for selected magnifications while maintaining structural rigidity.

For most applications, the best enlarger for any format is one capable of accommodating the next larger negative size. If 35-mm work is to be done, an enlarger capable of handling 6-cm × 6-cm negatives would therefore be chosen (Figure 6-17). This ensures that the negative is kept well centered within the illumination of the instrument and that no fall-off of density caused by diminished light intensity will appear at the edges of the resulting prints.

Most enlarger manufacturers offer negative carriers in a variety of sizes. Carriers are usually made of metal. Avoid those that incorporate glass windows that contact the negative, as the glass surfaces attract dirt. Many carriers have an aperture that is too small to permit the entire frame to be projected. If you cannot see clear film surrounding the entire image when it is projected onto the easel, you may wish to use a fine metal file to slightly enlarge the aperture. Following this operation, carefully apply flat black paint to the shiny metal edges.

2. Enlarging lens. The focal length of the enlarging lens is designed to provide a reasonable degree of enlargement at the baseboard and is different for each film size. A 50-mm enlarging lens is typically used to enlarge 35-mm camera negatives, although a longer lens (i.e., 80-mm) produces a slight improvement in the evenness of illumination. Unlike camera lenses, enlarging lenses are optically corrected for the limited range of magnifications typically needed to produce prints. Their maximum aperture is seldom faster than f2.8, and lenses with wide-open settings of f4 or f5.6 are common. Because

FIGURE 6-18
Enlarging timer. The Zone VI (Calumet, Bensonville, IL) enlarging timer shown here **(A)** uses a photocell that reads the actual light intensity from its matching cold light enlarging head **(B)**, providing accurate exposure control for lengthy printing sessions.

A   **B**

FIGURE 6-19
Paper easel. This simple paper easel is designed exclusively for 5-in. × 7-in. paper and permits rapid production of paper enlargements.

print sharpness and resolution are a direct result of lens quality, it is logical to pay more for a high-quality optic, rather than to accept compromised quality for the sake of saving a few dollars.

If a condenser illuminating system is used, it must be adjusted to match the lens, not just the film size. Maximal sharpness and contrast can only be achieved with a precise match between the enlarging lens and the condenser.

3. Enlarging timer. When printing, minor differences in the duration of the enlarging exposure can show up as significant changes in print density. To do a proper job of enlarging, the enlarger must be controlled by a dedicated timer that turns its lamp on and off with precision. The simplest enlarging timer is the standard laboratory timer mentioned above; this unit allows the duration of each exposure to be set directly. More sophisticated timers incorporate an automatic reset feature that can be useful for local exposure control. The ultimate timer is a digital unit that incorporates a photocell in the lamphouse so the timer monitors the actual light output of the lamp in addition to the time (Figure 6-18); this feature is important with cold light enlargers, as the light output from fluorescent tubes is known to vary considerably.

4. Paper easels. Enlarging paper must be held flat on the baseboard and must be positioned to include the selected portions of the negative. A paper easel is designed to accomplish both of these tasks. Most easels allow for a narrow (approximately $1/4$-in.) border to remain unexposed around the paper's perimeter. Adjustable units can accommodate paper of varying sizes and have either two or four blades that may be independently set for the desired image size. Those designed for fixed sizes of paper (Figure 6-19) permit speedy operation.

A **B**

FIGURE 6-20
Grain focuser. To assist in obtaining optimal print sharpness, a grain focuser **(A)** is used to examine the projected image while the enlarger is being focused **(B)**.

5. Grain focusers. The image must be critically focused when it is projected onto the easel. Because many modern films have fine grain, it is difficult to do this without optical assistance. A grain focuser is a low-powered microscope that uses a mirror to project the negative image to its eyepiece (Figure 6-20). While observing carefully through the focusing device, adjust the enlarger's focusing knob until a distinct grain pattern, representing the image itself, is observed clearly. Because grain focusers ensure critically sharp results, choose a high-quality instrument. The best grain focusers use precision glass optics and a reticle eyepiece. Avoid those that project the image onto a ground-glass surface, as the actual grain pattern cannot be detected.

6. Variable-contrast filter set. There are two basic types of photographic paper. One style is "graded" paper and is available in fixed levels of contrast. The levels may be assigned numbers or words; grade 1 ("soft") has low contrast, whereas grade 5 ("ultra hard") has high contrast. The grade of paper is chosen based on the contrast of the negative; if the negative is "contrasty," a low-contrast paper would be used. Obviously, to handle a variety of assignments, one should maintain a supply of each contrast grade, which can be expensive.

   The other type of paper is known as *variable-contrast paper* (Polycontrast, Multicontrast, and Multigrade are trade names for this type). Variable-contrast papers incorporate two emulsion layers of different contrasts, each designed to respond to light of different colors. The low-contrast emulsion is sensitive to yellow-green wavelengths exclusively, whereas the high-contrast layer responds to magenta light. A set of variable-contrast filters can thus be used to make the one paper act like four or five different contrast grades (as well as half grades between each full grade), depending on the relative amounts of each color of light the filter transmits. The most common set of filters are designed to be mounted below the lens (Figure 6-21), although some filters can be placed above the negative carrier. For the ultimate in sophistication (and cost), a dichroic color enlarger head, primarily designed for producing color prints,

FIGURE 6-21
Below-lens variable-contrast filter holder. Variable-contrast papers require the use of filters to modify the projected light from the enlarger. Filters in plastic holders are designed to be placed under the enlarging lens.

may be used to print on variable-contrast black and white paper by simply dialing in the required color of light.

Processing the Negative

To process black and white materials, four separate basic steps are required: development, stop-bath, fixation, and washing. Each of these is responsible for another stage toward the completion of the final product: a permanent record of the pattern of fluorescent light that entered the camera from the patient's retina.

Film Processing: Concepts

Why is it important to understand the underlying concepts of film processing, when so many aspects of photography have become automated? If you are to be a professional, with the attendant self-esteem and respect from your peers and colleagues, then you should have a strong understanding of the reasons your photographic product looks the way it does. Professional photographers continually search for ways to improve their images, and this quest will help improve the quality of your diagnostic photographs. By understanding how each component of the various chemical baths influences the final image, you will be able to manipulate the process to solve difficult imaging problems, as well as to troubleshoot if something goes awry.

FILM

Of course, before decisions about development, the first choice to be made concerns the type of film to be used. In fluorescein angiography, the typical camera film is a black and white negative stock with a sensitivity rating of ISO 400. Black and white films are typically comprised of several layers, including the base with an antihalation backing, emulsion, and overcoat. The base provides a stable support for the film and is typically made of a transparent plastic material. The antihalation backing absorbs any light that passes through the emulsion from ricocheting off the back surface of the film and degrading image sharpness. The overcoat is a transparent coating applied to the front surface of the film to make it more resistant to scratches.

The actual light-sensitive layer is the emulsion, which is made up of silver halide crystals suspended in a gelatin layer. The thickness of this layer and the physical shape of the silver halide crystals both play a large role in determining the characteristics of the final image. Historically, the emulsion layer was rather thick. At the instant of exposure, incoming light (image-forming rays) traveled through this layer, striking crystals

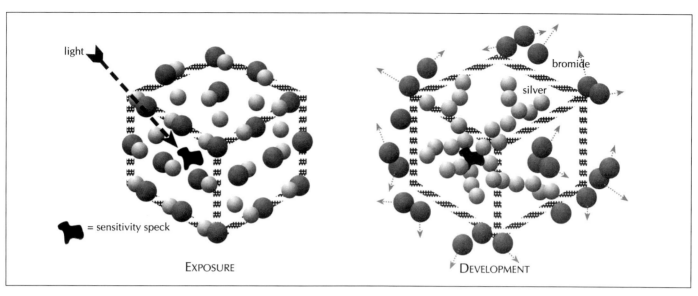

FIGURE 6-22
Photographic development. When film or paper is processed, developing agents convert the exposed silver halide crystal to metallic silver and then spin out filament-like strands of metallic silver to create a visible silver grain.

haphazardly and spreading out as it traversed the emulsion. The resulting image was not critically sharp. Today's films incorporate thinner emulsion layers with flattened silver halide crystals that are more efficient at capturing the image-forming rays. Thus, the resulting image is significantly sharper.[5]

Another important aspect of film design is the manner in which the normally blue-sensitive silver halide crystals are made sensitive to a much wider visible light spectrum with sensitizing dyes. For fluorescein angiography, panchromatic (sensitive to the complete visible spectrum) film is used. In addition to broadening the color response, these dyes also increase the film's sensitivity, measured as ISO speed. The film's speed rating or sensitivity indicates that there is a specific quantity of light required to render it developable. If there is too little light, then the film remains unexposed and no image-forming density will be evident, even with prolonged development.

When the silver halide crystal is struck by a photon of light, a very subtle change occurs within the crystal. The light changes the makeup of the crystal at a point in its structure known as a *sensitivity speck*. This change primes the crystal to be developed.

FILM DEVELOPMENT
During the process of development, the developing agent adds negatively charged particles (electrons) to those crystals that have been struck by light. The result of this reaction is the formation of a black, metallic silver image and the release of by-products into the developer (Figure 6-22). Chemists recognize this as an oxidation-reduction type of process, as silver is reduced to its metallic form while the developer is oxidized. Development is extraordinarily efficient at amplifying the effects of light on film. By making the sensitivity speck visible, development increases its size by well over a million times.

When developing film in daylight tanks, development requires periods of agitation followed by intervals when the tank is allowed to stand undisturbed. The agitation cycles introduce fresh quantities of processing solutions to the emulsion and remove waste products from it—the chemical action involves every part of the image during agitation. The quiet cycles allow the development of the highlights to slow down, as the relatively large areas of reduction liberate a commensurate quantity of waste products that prevent further highlight development from occurring. The regions of the film that have less exposure release fewer waste products and are thus permitted to continue development during the still interval.

As with any other chemical reaction, time and temperature play crucial roles. The reaction occurs more quickly at higher temperatures, and as the time increases, so do the number of silver halide crystals that are developed.

As development continues, contrast rises. Contrast denotes the separation between tones. The dark tones in a high-contrast image are extremely dark, the light tones are very bright, and the visual separation among the intermediate tones is likewise expanded. This fact is essential to the nature of black and white film materials; just as exposure creates density, development influences contrast. Excessive times or temperatures are harmful, however, as unexposed crystals may be converted to silver as well as those that were struck by light. This results in a "fogged" image of inferior quality. The physical size of the metallic silver grains also increases with prolonged development, and the resulting image appears "grainy"—almost sand-like in appearance.

Developers may be chosen depending on the type of negative desired. They are formulated with a variety of ingredients that work together to create an image with unique characteristics. Typically, these ingredients include developing agents, preservatives, restrainers, and activators. Angiographic negatives must be "readable"—that is, the information they record must be easy to ascertain through visual inspection. Areas of fluorescence, rendered as dark regions of the negative, must not be so dark that tonal variations cannot be differentiated. There should be only a few areas of maximum, deep black surrounded by regions of very dark gray, depending on the exact pathology recorded.

The developer's most important ingredient is the developing agent. Traditionally, two agents are combined: metol and hydroquinone. Developers, such as Kodak's D-76, D-19, and D-11 (Rochester, NY), feature these two chemicals in varying proportions. Ilford's Ilfotec (Paramus, NJ), Kodak's HC-110, and other modern developers have used phenidone and other agents to replace the problematic metol, which can cause contact dermatitis. A preservative is added to reduce premature oxidation. Sodium sulfite is commonly used and allows the mixed solution to be stored for several weeks in a closed container without any deterioration.

The restrainer is used to help prevent fogging or unintended development of unexposed silver halide crystals. Restrainers also are capable of increasing negative contrast. Potassium bromide is often used for this purpose.

The activator provides an alkaline environment that facilitates the action of the developing agents. Sodium carbonate and sodium hydroxide are two such activators. The latter is used in high-energy formulas, whereas sodium carbonate is a milder chemical that allows a slower rate of development.

Some developers are sold as liquid concentrates, whereas others are purchased as powders. Of the two choices, liquid allows fast mixing at temperatures at or near those used to process film. Thus, there need not be any delay between mixing the solution and using it. To mix powdered developers, a time-consuming regimen of alternately adding powder and stirring must be followed. Even after mixing, precipitates can form at the bottom of the storage container. If hot water is used to mix the powder, the solution must be cooled before use. Furthermore, mixing powdered chemistry liberates fine dust that may be harmful if inhaled. A properly designed ventilation system can reduce chemical contamination in the darkroom. If you choose a powdered developer, be sure to use a mask and eyeshield when mixing.

Current practice in the United States for angiogram development sees a variety of developers in use. There are two families of developers used in angiographic processing: high-contrast and pictorial. High-contrast developers, such as Kodak D-11 and, to a lesser degree, D-19, are carryovers from the early days of fluorescein angiography when wideband filters were used and the resulting exposure allowed a significant amount of nonfluorescent light to strike the film. High-contrast development was required to expand the tonal values so a positive print could be made with adequate dye representation. These developers are chemically vigorous and disproportionately favor areas of hyperfluorescence. The darker areas of the angiogram are thus rendered too dark whereas the brighter areas may become excessively bright. Prints from 35-mm negatives processed in these solutions have moderately high granularity.

Developers, such as Kodak's D-76, HC-110, and T-Max developer, on the other hand, are designed primarily for pictorial photography in which an extended range of gray tones and fine grain are desired attributes. The gray tones associated with fluorescein angiography are at least as important as specific areas of total hyperfluorescence or hypofluorescence. Angiograms processed in these pictorial developers exhibit a broad array of tones throughout the image.

Regardless of the particular developer chosen, it should be used only once and then discarded. Some developers offer a system of replenishment in which the chemical activity is maintained by adding more components to the solution, but this can be complicated and time consuming while offering little in actual cost-saving. Black and white processing solutions are quite inexpensive, and the only way to ensure consistency is to use fresh chemistry for each batch of film.

FILM AFTER-PROCESSES

Once development has reached the desired level of completion, the chemical activity of the developing agents must be halted. The solution known as *stop-bath* accomplishes that goal. Because the developer is usually alkaline, a weak acid effectively neutralizes it. A solution of acetic acid is used, either with or without a chemical indicator that turns purple when the acidity drops below a certain point.

Some laboratories use a brief water wash after development instead of an acid stop-bath. Although water can slow the activity of the developer, it does not halt it completely. If any developer is carried over into the fixing bath, a subtle staining of the emulsion (dichroic fog) may result. To avoid this, and to obtain the most accurate timing (and thus consistency in processing), use an acidic stop-bath.[6]

After treatment in stop-bath, the film consists of a metallic silver image surrounded by areas of unexposed (and therefore nonreduced) silver halides. The developing solution has now been neutralized, but the silver halides remaining in the emulsion are still susceptible to darkening through exposure to light. To remove these crystals from the emulsion, you must use a fixing bath. Conventional photographic fixers mixed from powders use sodium thiosulfate as the active ingredient and typically require 5–10 minutes for adequate fixation to occur. When processing fluorescein angiograms, a rapid fixer is preferred to shorten the processing time. Fixing baths that are based on ammonium thiosulfate, available as liquid concentrates, typically require less than half the time of conventional fixation. Just as with development, fixation requires periodic agitation to allow fresh solutions to be brought to the emulsion surface.

At the end of the fixation process, the film is comprised of the metallic silver image surrounded by clear areas where the unexposed crystals have been removed. The entire emulsion layer is now impregnated with fixer. However, fixer acts as a bleach over time. Thus, the film must be washed free of this chemical contaminant so the image will remain stable throughout its required life span. Washing aids facilitate this procedure.

After fixation, rinse the film with water to remove the majority of fixer from the emulsion surface. Next, bathe the film for 1 minute in washing aid solution (sold by Kodak as Hypo Clearing Agent and by Heico as Perma Wash [Delaware Water Gap, PA]; other manufacturers have their own proprietary formulations). Without the washing aid treatment, at least 30 minutes in running water is needed to ensure an adequate wash. The washing aid converts the remaining fixer into readily soluble compounds and thus shortens the final washing step. Washing aids are recommended because they not only facilitate archival processing but also are ecologically sound—ethical darkroom work is "earth friendly." Biodegradable compounds should be used and resources conserved whenever possible.

After the washing aid treatment, the final wash removes the remainder of chemicals from the emulsion. Washers should create some turbulence in the water flow to break bubbles free from the film surface and allow fresh water to flow continuously through the processing reels. Fixer diffuses out of the emulsion layers, so at least five full changes of water or 5 minutes in a well-designed film washer are required.

When the wash cycle is completed, bathe the film in a wetting agent (such as Kodak's Photo Flo 200) to lower the surface tension of the water and promote even drying. Without such treatment, water spots are likely to form. These may be impossible to remove and can be seen in the final print.

Finally, the film must be dried. Air drying is effective but slow. Special care must be exercised to avoid a dirty or drafty place for air drying, as dirt and dust that come into contact with the wet emulsion are virtually impossible to remove, even with rewashing. To speed the diagnostic information to the physician, most ophthalmic darkrooms use a heated forced-air dryer.

Film Processing: In Practice

Manual processing of film in a small tank may seem daunting to a novice darkroom worker, but the task can be thought of as a series of simple steps: preparation, loading, processing, and finishing (Table 6-2).

If this is your first time doing film processing, do a practice run before attempting to process patient photographs. You might want to photograph some nonophthalmic subjects at home on a roll of black and white film, using a regular 35-mm camera, to provide the test roll for this first attempt. Alternatively, an evening class on basic black and white processing at a local college may provide you with enough experience to approach this task confidently.

PREPARE

To prepare for film processing, organize your work space and prepare your materials. Once the lights are turned off, it will be nearly impossible to locate any materials or supplies that are not first placed in a convenient location. Your sense of touch will be the only way to identify these items in total darkness.

Selecting a Film Developer and Its Proper Processing Parameters

Experienced ophthalmic photographers use developers and associated times and temperatures based on a long process of testing, analysis, and revision. Newcomers to the field must rely on previously published data to get started.

Manufacturers often include suggested exposure and development information in the film package. However, that information is not applicable to the special requirements of angiographic imaging.

In 1995, several combinations of fundus cameras, films, and development parameters for fluorescein angiograms were in common use. Sample data are published in Table 6-3. Published data, no matter what the source, should always include a cautionary statement (i.e., "these data suggest starting points for individualized testing") because there are always local variables that influence the results. Although power supplies of fundus cameras are marked similarly, the output of the individual flash tubes may vary, and the light that actually reaches the film may have marked intensity differences between similar instruments. In spite of these differences, however, the data published above should provide usable negatives for direct viewing and interpretation.

When assessing the quality of an angiographic negative, you should make sure that the film leader and the angiographic timing data appear to be black on the negative and that the "clear" area surrounding the angiographic image is quite transparent and lacks obvious fog. For a more detailed account of the testing procedures for negative development, see Tyler's article on unusual film and developer combinations.[7]

Emergency Processing to Salvage a Study

Even though the majority of angiograms are executed properly, on rare occasions technical difficulties arise during the photographic session. One such event that can create a terribly thin negative is the accidental extravasation of dye during the injection. In such an occurrence, only a small amount may be injected into the vein. The photographer may not visualize any fluorescence or a pronounced decrease in intensity through the eyepiece. To attempt to salvage useful information, you will need to overdevelop the film.[8]

Normally, processing times are selected to achieve a good balance between angiographic information and minimal granularity and fog. In an emergency, however, doubling the development time increases the density of fluorescent areas and may allow even faintly fluorescing structures to become visible on the negative. The range of tones will be skewed, much detail in relatively hypofluorescent areas will be missing with such vigorous underexposure coupled with overdevelopment, and the background will exhibit moderate fog. However, such radical processing may provide sufficient diagnostic information so that a repeat injection at a later date will not be required.

Table 6-2. Manual Film Processing Steps

Prepare	Set out film, reels, scissors, opener, tanks
	Fill graduates with correct quantity of temperature of developer, stop-bath, fixer, and washing aid
	Turn lights out
Load **Total darkness** →	Open film canister
	Cut film end
	Load film onto reel
	Place reel in tank and cover securely with lid
	Turn lights on
Process	Set timer for development time
	Pour developer in rapidly, start timer, begin agitation
	Agitate
	Pour developer out, pour stop-bath in, agitate
	Agitate
	Pour stop-bath out, pour fixer in, restart timer
	Agitate
	Pour fixer out, pour washing aid in, restart timer
	Agitate
	Pour washing aid out, place film in washer, restart timer
	Bathe in wetting agent
	Dry

Fill three beakers or other graduated containers with the proper quantity of developer, stop-bath, and fixer (see sidebar Selecting a Film Developer and Its Proper Processing Parameters). If you use stainless steel tanks and reels, use these amounts: 1 reel = 10 oz; 2 reels = 16 oz; and 4 reels = 32 oz. The amount of chemistry is based on the size of the tank, not the number of rolls of film. All solutions should be at the same preselected temperature.

If your darkroom's air temperature is kept steady at the setting you select for processing, then it is a simple matter to pour the solutions from their storage containers and use them immediately. If the ambient storage temperature is too hot or cold, fill the sink with water at the correct temperature and then immerse the storage containers until their contents assume the temperature of the water (see sidebar Emergency Processing to Salvage a Study).

Next, lay the daylight tank, top, lid, and reels on the countertop. The reels should be oriented so that their loading slots all face the same direction. Place the film cassettes together on the counter and, next to these, a pair of scissors and a standard bottle opener. Remember precisely where these items are placed, because when the lights are extinguished, you will use them to complete the loading process.

LOADING

When all is ready, turn out the lights. (Caution: If your darkroom has fluorescent worklights, wait a minute or two before commencing, as fluorescent fixtures may have a residual "afterglow." Also make certain that any equipment indicator lights, or even telephone pushbuttons, are extinguished or covered before proceeding!) The darkroom must remain completely dark until the film has been loaded onto a reel, placed in the tank, and the tank lid is in place.

Select a film cassette and hold it so the protruding end of the spool is facing downward. Use the bottle opener to remove the opposite, flat end cap of the cassette. Remove the spool and film and cut off the leader with the scissors—you will need to do these operations by touch; the leader is narrower than the rest of the film. Next, feed the end of the film into the

Table 6-3. Angiographic Film Processing Parameters

Camera	Flash Setting	Film	Developer	Time, Temperature
Zeiss FF4	240 w/s	TMax 400	D76 straight	12 mins, 72°F
Zeiss FF4	240 w/s	Neopan 400	HC110 dil. B	6 mins, 72°F
Zeiss FF4	240 w/s	Tri-X	D-19 (1:1)	6.5 mins, 68°F
Zeiss FK30	300 w/s	Tri-X	HC110 dil. B	9 mins, 70°F
Canon	Angio setting	TMax 400	D-11 (1:1)	7 mins, 75°F
CF60UV	Angio setting	Tri-X	D-11 straight	6 mins, 72°F
Canon 60S	3	TMax 400	D-11 straight	8 mins, 70°F
Topcon 50VT	75 w/s	Tri-X	D-11 straight	5.5 mins, 72°F

processing reel emulsion side inward. If you use stainless steel reels, insert the end of the film under the spring clip located at the reel's center or into the central opening if there is no clip. Curl the film slightly by compressing it between the thumb and index finger while the other hand rotates the reel. The film is thus fed into the reel from the inside toward the outside of the spirals (Figure 6-23). In the beginning you made need to lightly touch the film (base side only) to monitor the progress as the loading proceeds. It should smoothly fit into the spiral reels without bending. If the film starts to feel crooked, unwind it, and begin again.

If you use a plastic reel, hold the film so it is parallel to the spirals of the reel. Slip the film end into the spiral groove at the outside edge of the reel; typically, there are small plastic bumps adjacent to the loading spot to facilitate locating it in the dark. Then simply ratchet the film onto the spool by rotating the top and bottom flanges of the reel in alternate directions. The film will automatically feed into the reel.

To gain confidence and accuracy in loading film, repeatedly practice with a scrap roll of film until you can load the reel successfully (with your eyes closed!), allowing your fingers to provide you with all the information you need. Treat the film gently; avoid bending or crimping the film while loading it, as these acute pressures to the film's surface will result in small curved lines in the image itself, known as *cinch marks*.

When the entire roll is loaded, cut off the cassette spool and place the loaded reel into the tank. If you do not have enough rolls of film to fill the processing tank, add empty reels to avoid overdevelopment of the film. Press the top securely onto the tank, turn the room lights on, and complete the remaining processing steps in standard room lighting.

PROCESSING

Set the timer for the required development time. Start the timer and immediately pour the developer rapidly into the top of the tank. To speed this process, tilt the tank slightly to allow air to escape while filling the tank. During the pour, do not slow down or stop for any reason, as uniformity of development will be compromised. It is better to accidentally spill a few drops of developer while rapidly filling the tank! As soon as the tank is full, place the cap on it and bang the tank strongly on the sink or countertop. This dislodges air bubbles from the film that would otherwise cause undeveloped spots ("air bells") on the negative. After rapping the tank, begin agitation. Agitation techniques typically require a cycle of quickly inverting and righting the tank for a set period. This removes waste products from the film and allows fresh developer to act on the emulsion.

A typical agitation pattern consists of 5 seconds of agitation (one inversion per second) for each 30 seconds of development. Be sure to rap the tank on the counter after each agitation cycle. To promote uniform development across the entire surface of the film, a random movement should

A

B

C

D

E

FIGURE 6-23
Film loading, using stainless steel reels. First, assemble the tank, film, reels, opener, and scissors on the countertop **(A)**. Next, open the flat end of the cassette **(B)**. Cut off the leader **(C)**, and insert the cut end into the center of the reel **(D)**. Gently squeeze the film's width into a convex curve as you roll the film onto the reel, and be sure to lightly feel the film to ensure proper tracking **(E)**. Finally, cut off the film spool, place the reel into the tank, and cover with the top.

be used during agitation. To simply achieve this, rotate the tank approximately one-third of a turn when you complete each agitation cycle. After each agitation period, the tank is allowed to sit undisturbed.

Developing is a highly individualized task. If several veteran photographers are asked to explain their technique, each may provide a different explanation. Like all other scientific disciplines, an extremely important aspect of photographic darkroom work is consistency. By working in a precise and repeatable fashion, you can more easily identify and remedy any problems that arise. Timing and agitation patterns are crucial to film devel-

Silver Recovery

Used fixer contains dissolved silver that is toxic to the environment and is not biodegradable. Many municipalities have strict laws that prohibit the discharge of heavy metals (including silver-laden used fixer) into local sewer systems. Furthermore, silver is a nonrenewable resource that is essential to the photographic process. For these reasons, you should reclaim the silver from used fixer and make the solution safe for discharge into the sewer system.

Silver recovery machines are available in various sizes, and you should choose the model that is appropriate for the number of gallons of used fixer your facility produces. One of the least expensive units is the Silver Magnet (USI International, Inc., West Bend, WI). This device consists of a low-voltage power supply connected to a small, perforated plastic tray containing an anode and a cathode. This is placed in a storage container of used fixer, and the electric current slowly precipitates metallic silver out of the solution and into the tray. When the tray is full, it may be sent to a smelter for reclamation. The smelter then sends a check to you for the current market value of the reclaimed silver. Once the silver has been removed, the remaining solution may be safely poured down the drain, as it no longer represents an environmental hazard.

If your laboratory is located within a hospital, an alternative to purchasing a silver recovery unit may be available. Some hospital-based radiology departments may allow you to add your used fixer to the x-ray machine's discharge for commercial silver reclamation. You may not receive any compensation for the reclaimed silver, but at least you will no longer be contaminating the local water supply.

opment, so be sure to time the process and agitate the tank in exactly the same way for all standard angiographic film processing.

Fifteen seconds before the allotted time is up, begin emptying the tank. Time this so that the solution is completely drained as the timer reaches zero.

Quickly pour stop-bath into the tank. After a rap of the tank on a hard work surface, at least 30 seconds of continuous agitation in the stop-bath should provide for total cessation of development. This solution is then poured out.

Now reset the timer and pour the fixer into the tank. Three minutes is required for rapid fixer. Agitation cycles are required for fixation, just as with development, to ensure that the unprocessed silver halide is completely dissolved. As the timer nears zero, pour the used fixer into a temporary storage container. Rather than pouring used fixer down the drain, it should be saved for subsequent reuse and silver recovery (see sidebar Silver Recovery).

After fixation, the film is processed and can be exposed to light without changing the image (see sidebar "Stat" Film Processing).

After fixation, wash the film. Fill the tank with water at the same temperature as the other solutions, agitate for approximately 1 minute, and then drain. This step removes much of the surface fixer. Next, fill the tank with a washing aid (i.e., Perma Wash) and set the timer for 1 minute. Agitate to ensure complete chemical conversion of the remaining fixing solution. When the timer reaches zero, drain the tank.

FINISHING

Remove the reels from the tank, and place them in the film washer. Set the water flow to a moderate rate (two to four changes per minute) and allow the film to wash for at least 5 minutes. If small bubbles seem to stick to the film, manually raise and lower the reels and tap the washer to liberate them and enable fresh water to cleanse the film. When the time is completed, turn off the water, assuming this will allow the water in the washer to remain in place.

Finally, according to its dilution directions, place some concentrated wetting agent into the water. Allow the film to rest in this solution for 1 minute, and then drain and dry in either a forced-air dryer or by evaporation. Although some photographers wipe the film with sponges, this practice may permanently mark or deform the film. When wet, the film's surface is very soft and fragile, so allowing it to dry in air provides the greatest margin of safety.

NEGATIVE STORAGE AND VIEWING

Once dry, the angiographic information is contained on a strip of plastic approximately 1-in. wide by 5-ft long. This format presents a rather unwieldy method of reviewing and filing clinical information. Furthermore, unprotected film is susceptible to physical damage. Dust, dirt, and fingerprints can each leave an indelible impression, and repeated exposure to such damage lessens the amount of information clearly visible at subsequent viewings.

The importance of caring properly for the angiographic negative cannot be overstated. In the representational aspect of scientific photography, the negative remains the only evidence of the transit of dye through the choroid and retina. The events recorded during angiography live on as delicate metallic silver tracings; for present and future review and analysis, the negative must remain in pristine condition.

Archiving requirements for medical images are based on legal requirements for record storage. In many cases, records must be retrievable for a minimum of 7 years after the patient's visit. Thus, photographic materials must be stored in inert materials that will not cause noticeable deteri-

"Stat" Film Processing

Although most fluorescein angiograms can be processed efficiently in batches once or twice a day, occasionally the film will need to be processed while the patient waits. This may be due to medical necessity, as in the case of a patient with a choroidal neovascular membrane that threatens central vision and requires immediate laser photocoagulation. Rapid processing may also be requested for the sake of convenience. If the patient has traveled a great distance to the clinic, the physician may want to plan future visits or treatment strategies based on today's angiogram.

Using conventional film processing techniques, temperatures, washing aids, and efficient film dryers, it is possible to completely process a fluorescein angiogram in less than 30 minutes. The time allotted for each portion of the stat process is detailed below. Bear in mind, however, that the total elapsed time depends on the time required for each individual step (Table 6-4). The time in developer is crucial to image quality, and cannot be changed. Stop-bath acts quickly and can be effective in as little as 30 seconds. Rapid-fixing baths can achieve complete fixation in as short a time as 2 minutes. Washing aids can dramatically shorten the required final wash time. Some film dryers are much more efficient than others, although some clinicians will demand a "wet" reading and will want to examine the film as it is taken right from the washer. (Note: When wet, the film is extremely delicate and easily scratched. After the wet reading, return the film to the wash tank for wetting agent and proper drying!)

Even though rapid processing is possible, in the real world of clinical photography, ophthalmic photographers may not always be able to deliver the results with this kind of speed. You may have to exercise critical judgment, and hope for the clinician's understanding, to weigh the need for prompt results against the overall workload. At times, manual processing may be faster than automated film development, but doing the job by hand will obviously prevent you from taking care of other patients at the same time.

Table 6-4. "Stat" Angiogram Processing

Load film reels	30 secs
Developer	8 mins—adjust as required
Stop bath	30 secs
Rapid fixer	3 mins
Water rinse	1 min
Washing aid	1 min
Final wash	5 mins
Dry	3 mins
Scissor and insert	3 mins

Note: The above data assume that all chemicals are already mixed at the correct processing temperature.

oration in image quality for at least a decade. Studies have shown that a variety of acids used frequently in modern paper-making are harmful to the photographic image. File folders, envelopes, and even glassine negative holders all incorporate materials that can attack and degrade processed photographs. However, by placing the angiogram in an *archival-quality* plastic holder, the image is protected from these antagonists.

Negative filing sheets of polyethylene, polypropylene, or mylar keep dirt and chemicals from harming the image and at the same time allow the entire angiogram to be viewed directly. These transparent plastic sheets typically incorporate a series of flat, narrow pockets with openings at either end. Cut the angiogram into five or six frame strips, taking care not to separate any stereo pairs, and then insert each strip into a pocket in the sheet. Once loaded, the sheet may be placed on a lightbox for viewing with a stereoviewer or loupe and then filed in the patient's chart or in the photographic records area.

An alternative method of storage requires that the negatives be individually cut, inserted into 35-mm slide mounts, and then placed into side-loading slide folio pages. This method is required for certain multicenter clinical studies.

To use a loupe or stereoviewer, rest the base of the device directly on the storage sheet or negative (Figure 6-24). These devices may be moved along at will, and detailed analysis of individual frames or stereo pairs may be made at any point during the inspection.

Viewers that are modified from microfiche or microfilm readers are an effective way of looking at angiographic negatives, as they can project an enlarged view of selected frames onto their self-contained viewing screen. However, those that incorporate a glass pressure plate require special care to make sure they do not scratch the negative if it is removed from its protective sleeve.

Negatives can also be reviewed on a video monitor. The Fotovix (Tamron, Commack, NY) uses a small video camera and a transilluminated base to allow individual frames to be shown in this manner. Certain versions of this instrument come equipped with a polarity switch, so that the angiogram can be electronically converted from a negative image to a positive image. These devices also offer a zoom control so selected portions of the negative may be enlarged, as well as brightness and contrast controls.

The Positive Printout

Why Analysis of the Negative Is Preferred

The vast majority of published fluorescein angiograms are produced as positives (dye depicted as white). Although some resident training pro-

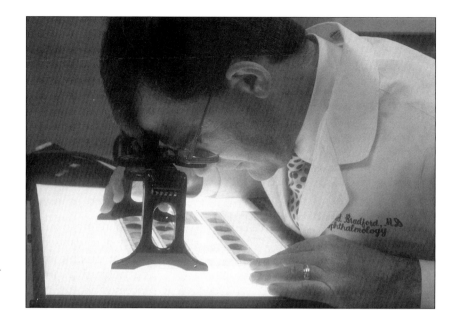

FIGURE 6-24
Viewing angiograms in stereo. When examining a fluorescein angiogram with a stereoviewer or loupe, the magnifying device is placed directly on the plastic negative sheet.

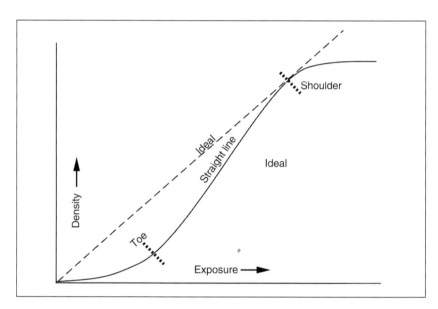

FIGURE 6-25
Characteristic curve. This line graphically shows how a film reacts to changes in exposure and development. Films cannot reproduce subject brightnesses with complete fidelity and have a tendency to compress information in the lightest and darkest parts of the image.

grams in ophthalmology use positive printouts to teach descriptive interpretation of these studies, the best way of reading and interpreting fluorescein angiograms is by direct analysis of the camera-original negatives. Issues of accuracy and timeliness support this statement.

No photographic medium reproduces the subject with complete accuracy. Every black and white film skews the reproduction of tonal values. To learn why this is true, a brief description of characteristic curves may be useful.[9]

The response of a given film and developer to changes in exposure can be graphically depicted as a characteristic curve (Figure 6-25). If a perfect film could be manufactured, it would have a constant, predictable response to changes in illumination. For every quantity of increased light exposure, the film would respond by creating density in exactly the same manner: One unit of light creates one unit of density. In reality, films do not respond well to either very low or very high levels of illumination. For low levels, seen as the "toe" portion of the curve, the film receives a fair amount of exposure before it begins to respond by creating an image.

The Angiographic Zone System

As fine-art photography experienced a renaissance in the 1930s, Ansel Adams, Minor White, and others formulated a precise methodology for equating subject brightness with the values that result in the photographic print. The key to this scheme is the zone system. By assigning shades of gray to typical pictorial subjects, the photographer is better able to expose and process negatives so that the shades of gray that were previsualized at the instant of exposure are actually seen in the final print.

Adams' zone system is comprised of a series of nine shades ranging from pure black to pure white.[10] This represents a brightness range of 256 to 1 and is closely matched to the reproduction capabilities of photographic paper. Each zone is 100% brighter than the previous zone and is 50% darker than the next higher zone. The "twice or half" relationship is the same as that between one shutter speed and another and also between one f-stop and another. Thus, after metering a subject, the photographer can, at will, make an exposure that will produce the principal tone as an exact shade of gray.

The precision associated with the pictorial zone system is made possible by the fact that natural lighting can be measured easily with a reflected light meter. Various parts of the scene can be metered independently for maximal exposure control. After determining the intensity of the light and deciding on the required exposure settings, the photographer can exercise further creative controls in the darkroom through lengthening or shortening the development time.

In fluorescein angiography, the illumination is provided by electronic flash, and even though flash meters are used in conventional photography, none have been designed to measure small changes in retinal brightness during dye perfusion. The fact that exciter and barrier filtration is necessary for angiography further complicates accurate quantification of fluorescence.

However, in spite of problems with the previsualization of lighting effects, we know anecdotally that fluorescein dye behaves predictably based on the disease process being recorded. Thus, an angiographic zone system can be formulated (Table 6-5) that helps assign values to various areas of fluorescence.[11]

Adams further believed that the values recorded in the negative were similar to the score of a symphony; the print thus became a "performance." In fluorescein angiography, the maximum angiographic information resides in the negative; the positive printout's performance must be tailored to reproduce the negative's information as faithfully as possible.

This means that the very dim portions of the subject will be disproportionately dark. A similar situation exists in the "shoulder" of the curve, representing the effects of very bright illumination. As you can see by the flattening of the line, the film reaches a point where it no longer responds to increased light. The "straight line" portion of the curve represents the film's ability to respond straightforwardly to changes in illumination. In this area, every unit of light increase results in an equivalent increase in film density.

Film can only approximate the range of brightness values that is emitted by fluorescein. The darker areas of hypofluorescence are rendered somewhat darker than they really are; maximum areas of hyperfluorescence may be inaccurately portrayed with more brightness. When using printout materials to generate positive copies of the study, this second generation further warps the portrayal of densities.

The other reason for using negatives as the prime medium for communicating the results of angiography deals with speed. Simply stated, producing a positive printout can more than double the time required in the darkroom. With conventional hand processing, an angiographic negative can be fully developed, washed, dried, and delivered in less than 25 minutes. If one must cut it into strips, contact print it, process, and finally dry the printout, these subsequent steps may add at least another 30 minutes to the wait before the diagnostic information is presented to the physician and detracts from the efficient operation of the practice.

However, in spite of these objections to using printouts as the prime method of delivering angiographic results, there are several legitimate reasons for making positive copies of angiograms. These include referral of the patient to other clinicians when the original film must be retained in the medical record, the production of teaching materials for continuing medical education, the preparation of prints to illustrate manuscripts for publication, and the production of sample prints or slides for portfolios and professional certification.

Furthermore, having the capability of standard black and white printing allows the photographic service to be more responsive, as public relations photographs, portraits, small object or surgical instrument photography, and other nonclinical assignments can be completed intramurally.

Positive printouts are produced in three basic formats: sheet film or paper contact sheets, paper print enlargements, or 35-mm positive slides. Even though there are significant differences between these media in terms of cost, ease of viewing, and brightness range, each must exhibit the proper distribution of tones (based on the characteristics of the original negative) to represent the original as faithfully as possible.

To communicate diagnostic information effectively, fluorescein angiography uses an array of blacks, whites, and shades of gray to represent the distribution of dye in the fundus. This assortment of tones can be organized into a scheme that takes into account dye concentration and the effect of overlying physical materials (such as tissue or hemorrhage). Using pictorial photography as a model, angiographic tonality can be organized into an angiographic "zone system" (see sidebar The Angiographic Zone System).

Sheet Film Contact Sheets

Sheet film contact sheets provide an expanded brightness range that allows the full range of angiographic detail to be observed. Two basic types of film are used for this printout technique: lithographic film and line film. The former is primarily designed to be processed in high-energy developers that produce black and white tones with virtually no

Table 6-5. Angiographic Zone System

Zone	Tonal/Pictorial Representation	Angiographic Representation
I	Total black	Area adjoining angiographic image
II	First visible tone above black	Retroilluminated vessels (late phase)
III	First texture in dark grays	Early choroidal fluorescence visualized through retinal pigment epithelium
IV	Normal gray value of skin in shadow	Vessels in recirculation phase
V	Middle gray (18% reflectance)	Later choroidal fluorescence
VI	Average white skin (36% reflectance)	Diffuse dye from neovascular tissue
VII	Light gray	Near-maximal dye in tissue or vessels
VIII	Lightest tone with texture	Drusen, microaneurysms, areas within neovascularization
IX	Paper base white (clear film)	Maximal dye concentration in filled vessels or in florid leakage sites (i.e., idiopathic central serous chorioretinopathy, neovascularization)

FIGURE 6-26
Dust spot artifacts. The tiny white spots that form on lithographic-type printout materials are caused by dust and dirt that is sandwiched between the negative and the printout medium. Besides their poor appearance, these may be mistaken for hyperfluorescent lesions. (Courtesy of Julie Balza, Green Bay, WI.)

intermediate steps. Dupont Cronar (Wilmington, Delaware) and Kodak Kodalith are trade names for such materials. However, processing these films in a continuous tone developer, such as diluted paper developer, can produce a range of gray tones that matches the requirements of fluorescein angiography.

In addition to accurately rendering black and white, line films can also reproduce a range of gray tones. Processing these materials (such as Kodak Fine Grain Positive film [Rochester, NY] and Angiographics Photo Supply's Angiolith film [Newton, MA]) in diluted paper developer also produces positive prints with excellent gradation.

An annoying problem associated with the use of such high-contrast media is the appearance of small white spots on the printout (Figure 6-26). These are usually caused by dust specks that become trapped between the emulsion layers of the negative and the printout and thus cause a shadow to form during exposure. The shadow represents an area with no exposure and thus appears white (clear on the printout film). Because these white spots mimic hyperfluorescence, on casual examination they could be misinterpreted as drusen bodies or microaneurysms. If your contact printer is not equipped with a frosted plastic diffusion layer, another strategy for avoiding these spots is to scrupulously clean the negatives and the contact printer before starting to print. Continuous tone or line films are less likely to produce these spots than lithographic films.

Sheet film contact sheets provide an overview of the patient's angiographic status. By reproducing the angiographic series in total, contact sheets portray, in same-size positive format, every image originally captured on the negative.

FIGURE 6-27
Placing negatives in a printer. When arranging the negatives, spend a few seconds to make sure the edges of each strip touch, and align the circular angiographic images to produce a truly professional product.

To prepare for producing sheet film contact sheets, first set up the tray line. Assuming that four 8-in. × 10-in. trays will be used, fill the first tray with at least 1 liter of diluted paper developer. Many photographers use Kodak Dektol developer, diluted 1 to 1 with water (1:1). Fill the second tray with 1 liter of indicator stop-bath, and the third tray with at least 1 liter of fixer. Follow the mixing instructions to prepare the working-solutions of the stop-bath and fixer. Finally, set up the last tray as the wash tray, or set up and fill the print washer if available. Turn on the safe-light and extinguish the room lights.

Your enlarger is a fine light source for contact printing. To use it in this manner, first turn on the lamp and adjust the height of the enlarger so that its light shines onto the baseboard in a large enough area to cover the size of the contact frame. Roughly focus the lens to produce a sharp edge of the negative carrier. You may want to mark the projected area on the baseboard with black tape to aid in positioning the contact printing frame when you are ready to expose. Once this has been checked, turn the enlarger lamp off.

If you use a simple contact frame, place a sheet of printout film (emulsion side up) onto the frame. Select a grade 3 paper for angiographic contact prints, either by using standard graded papers or by using a grade 3 filter with variable-contrast paper. Next, carefully position the angiographic negatives, keeping them in correct order (emulsion side down) onto the sheet film (Figure 6-27).

To produce a contact sheet, the negatives must be clean and already cut into strips of five or six frames (ideally, they will already be stored in negative filing sheets in this configuration). For maximal image quality, the negatives must be removed from their plastic storage sheet to be contact printed, as contact print sharpness requires intimate contact between the negative's image layer and the printout sheet's emulsion.

Lower the glass top plate onto the materials and latch if required. When assembled correctly, this "sandwich" will feature the film emulsion (right below the top glass plate) in direct contact with the sheet film's emulsion. The light from the enlarger will pass through the film first and then the printout material.

Make a test print to fine-tune the exposure time. Even though this print will be discarded later, it will still help you determine valuable exposure and processing information. To create the test print, use an 8-in. × 10-in. piece of cardboard. Set the timer to 3 seconds and cover the contact frame with the cardboard, leaving approximately 2 in. uncovered at one side. Start the timer; the enlarging lamp will expose only the uncovered strip for 3 seconds before turning off. Next, slide the cardboard laterally so that an additional 2 in. are uncovered. Repeat the exposure of 3 seconds. Repeat again and again, until the entire contact sheet has been sequentially exposed.

Next, open the frame, remove the negatives, and carry the exposed sheet of printout film to the tray line. Set the timer for 2 minutes. As you start the timer, quickly slide the print, emulsion side up, into the developer. Immediately begin agitation by lifting the end of the tray approximately half an inch and then setting it down again. Repeating this cycle rhythmically moves the solution briskly in the tray, but don't do this so vigorously that the solution spills out! Every 15–20 seconds, use the tongs to lift the film out and replace it turned over. The aim of the agitation and manipulation is to ensure that the action of the developer is uniform across the entire surface of the film. Resist the temptation to short-circuit the process because the print looks too dark; this is a typical mistake when viewing prints under safelight illumination. The printouts must all be developed for the same length of time (use 2 minutes as your initial standard).

When the timer is down to the final 15 seconds, carefully lift the film with the developer tongs by one corner and allow excess developer to drain into the tray. As the timer reaches zero, place the film immediately into the stop-bath without permitting the tongs to touch any of this solution. Make sure it is completely submerged, and agitate for at least 30 seconds in this tray.

Next, pick up the film again by a corner with the stop-bath tongs, allow excess stop-bath to drain back into the tray, and transfer the printout to the fixing bath. Set the timer for 2 minutes and again begin the agitation cycle used previously. You may turn on the room lights after 30 seconds—the remaining steps are performed in room lighting.

Drain the printout of excess fixer, and as the timer reaches zero, place it into the wash. Set the timer for 4 minutes. The print should move around in the wash water. You may want to manually move, invert, and agitate it while this process continues (you may use your bare hands for this step). When the timer reaches zero, drain excess water, place in a tray of photo-flow for 30–60 seconds, squeegee if desired, and hang it up to dry or place it in the print dryer.

Carefully inspect the test printout on a lightbox to determine the proper exposure time. Exposure primarily affects density. Examine the highlights, or areas of hyperfluorescence. The brightest regions of fluorescence should just be clear, barely lighter than very pale gray. Ideally, the strip of exposure that produced the proper highlights should be neither the first nor the last strip but instead should be located toward the middle of the strip series. Based on the exposure time for each strip, calculate the time it took to produce the correct exposure (Figure 6-28).

Next, produce another test, but this time, apply the newly determined correct exposure time to the entire contact sheet. Develop again for precisely 2 minutes, stop, fix, photo-flow, wash, and dry. Look critically at this sheet, and this time examine the darkest areas. Maximum black tones should surround the angiographic image, and there should be clearly differentiated gray tones throughout each frame. If the sheet film looks flat (without much contrast), extend the time in the developer for your next effort by another 30 seconds. If the film has too much contrast, you may wish to reduce the developing time by 30 seconds. By continually refining the processing times and exposure times, you will approach just the right combination to consistently produce good prints (Table 6-6).

Throughout this process, you should remember two fundamental concepts that influence your results:

1. Exposure creates density. The effects of exposure changes are seen primarily in the highlight areas.

FIGURE 6-28
Exposure and development testing. (For clarity, full-size images are reproduced here, rather than test strips.) Changes in exposure are shown in **A**, **B**, and **C**. **A.** An underexposed print; the hyperfluorescent areas are too light. **B.** An overexposed print; all detail is too dark. **C.** A properly exposed print, in which tonal information is seen in the highlight areas. **A**, **B**, and **C** are all exposed to the same contrast (grade 3). The development, or contrast test, will not appreciably alter the highlight tones but rather will dramatically change the darkest areas of the print, as seen in **C**, **D**, and **E**. **D.** A print made on a grade 1 paper. The detail created by the exposure found during exposure testing provides for good tonal reproduction of the highlights, but the dark values are flat and do not produce any crispness. **E.** A print produced on a grade 5 paper, resulting in good highlight detail but dark areas that are so black that no detail can be differentiated. Produced on grade 3, **C** again represents the best combination of exposure (for highlight detail) and contrast (for dark tones).

Table 6-6. Exposure and Contrast Testing

I. Make test strip for exposure. Analyze for highlight detail and select best exposure time.
II. Expose full sheet for selected time.
  A. Analyze for shadow detail.
    1. If there is adequate separation of the dark areas, adopt developer time and temperature in step I as your standard.
    2. If shadows are so black that no detail is visible:
      a. Shorten development time or
      b. Use a more dilute developer, or
      c. Use lower-contrast paper
    3. If shadows have no blacks and are just dark grays:
      a. Increase the time in the developer or
      b. Use higher-contrast paper
III. Repeat step II using new development parameters to confirm the choice.

2. Development creates contrast. Changes in development are chiefly noted in the darkest areas of the print.

Although these factors are not mutually exclusive, their effects are quite selective. Without sufficient exposure, you cannot develop to obtain a strong black. And development by itself is not sufficient to create density in the highlights—only proper exposure creates that level of tone in hyperfluorescent regions of the printout.

Of the two factors, exposure is more straightforward. By creating and analyzing test strips, correct exposure can always be determined. Correct contrast is more difficult to determine directly. If development is prolonged, you run the risk of fogging the image. If you extend the time to 4 minutes and a strong black and good tonal separation have not been achieved, you may want to use a less-diluted developer. Similarly, if the print has too much contrast (i.e., an image that seems to be made up of just black and white tones with a poor intermediate gray scale), dilute the developer further.

Another simple method for adjusting contrast is to adjust the relationships between exposure and development. To increase contrast, slightly underexpose the printout and then overdevelop. To decrease printout contrast, slightly overexpose the sheet and then underdevelop. Agitation is extremely important when underdeveloping, as positive printouts subjected to short developing times may appear mottled with patches of uneven maximum density.

Paper Contact Sheets

Paper contact sheets are the least expensive printout medium. They are relatively easy to produce and, like sheet film contact sheets, only require a printing frame and a controlled light source (i.e., an enlarger—or even a bare light bulb—connected to a timer). Although room light is sufficient to view them, paper contact sheets have some significant liabilities in terms of their ability to convey information. First, the small size of the individual frame makes magnified viewing a necessity. More seriously, the brightness range of any paper print is considerably less than transparent media (a maximum range of 50:1, compared to film's 1,000:1). However, paper prints can be used as a simple record to give an overview of the patient's angiographic status.

Most photographic papers used in routine angiographic printing are resin coated (RC). This material is comprised of a layer of paper, sensitized on one side, sandwiched between two thin layers of a plastic material. Some RC papers also incorporate a developing agent within the emulsion and lend themselves well to automated processing.

When first introduced, RC papers were considered to be inferior in quality to conventional papers, but today's RC papers are excellent for routine work. The only important processing technique to remember is the importance of accurate timing of the various processing steps. Prolonged times in fixer or in the wash may have deleterious effects on the image, as moisture can penetrate along the paper's edges, and residual chemistry is much more difficult to remove. Most RC papers require 2 minutes in fixer and a maximum of 4 minutes in the wash.

To achieve the proper exposure and development when using paper, follow the same process of test strip production and analysis described previously for sheet film contact sheets. Because photographic paper is available in a variety of contrast grades, contrast can be controlled easily by changing from one grade to another without the need to adjust developer dilution. As a starting point to determine optimal contrast, use a grade 3 paper for your printout tests.

Exposure regulation to establish proper highlight density is the same as for sheet film printouts. Remember, unless sufficient exposure is given to the printout, no amount of development will bring tone to the highlight areas.

On occasion, to maintain proper tonality within the image, the overall print contrast may need to be reduced slightly. This will result in the edges of the negatives, and the film's sprocket holes, being barely visible, rather than being processed to maximum black. However, the most important aspect of the printout is the angiographic information within, rather than outside of, the retinal image itself.

35-mm Positive Slides

Sheet film or paper contact sheets provide a single viewer with the means of viewing the entire angiogram. However, contact sheets cannot easily be used to communicate diagnostic information to a large group. The projection of individual 35-mm positive slides solves this problem. Although single frames can be cut from a sheet film contact sheet and secured into slide mounts, you must print more frames than you will use, as some frames will be discarded. Furthermore, you cannot tailor exposure and development to yield optimal quality on selected frames, because the entire contact sheet must necessarily be exposed and developed uniformly.

The alternative, producing individual frames, relies on the use of any of several styles of slide duplicators. With these, selected frames from the angiographic negative can be rephotographed onto line-type black and white negative film, processed, and placed into slide mounts. The resulting slides exhibit high sharpness and a gray scale that reproduces the tonal range of the negative. To produce these slides, use a 35-mm single lens reflex camera equipped with a slide duplicator attachment. Typically, the duplicator attaches to a macro lens capable of a 1 to 1 reproduction ratio, either via an extended helical focusing mount or by way of a bellows unit. This permits the original negative frame to be reproduced as an identically sized positive. This simple duplicator requires a separate light source.

Professional duplicating cameras incorporate a transilluminating base with tungsten or electronic flash lighting, or both, and a sturdy camera column with bellows unit onto which a 35-mm single lens reflex camera is mounted. Both duplicating systems require placing the negative into the duplicator, focusing the camera lens onto the image precisely, transilluminating the negative with tungsten or electronic flash, and finally making the exposure.

Use 35-mm line film (Kodak's Technical Pan Film is recommended for this application). If the camera's internal meter is used to regulate the exposure, an exposure index of EI 100 may provide a basis for further testing and refinement. The film may be processed in Kodak Dektol, undiluted, for 4 minutes at 72°F with regular agitation. Just as with other development data in this chapter, use this reference as an approximate starting point for additional testing. This is particularly important when testing relatively high-contrast materials, as these have much less latitude for errors in exposure and development than continuous-tone photographic media.

An especially useful modification to either a simple duplicator or a full-featured professional unit is to add the special strip film carrier from an enlarger (such as a Beseler Negatrans [Linden, NJ]) that facilitates moving from frame to frame for selected duplication.

Unlike contact sheets in which all frames received the same exposure, 35-mm positives from a slide duplicator permit the exposure to be individually tailored for each frame. With this technique, multiple slides of a single frame can be generated. This can be particularly important for teaching programs, as each resident may be given selected slides to begin their own collection of instructional materials.

Paper Enlargements

Though the brightness range of a photographic enlargement is identical to that of a paper contact print, the enlarged size allows fine angiographic detail to be more easily seen. Enlarging is a photographic skill that is useful in many clinical, research, and general photographic assignments. Good printing is an art, and mastery requires time and effort.

An important need for paper prints arises when submitting a manuscript to a medical journal. Printing for publication is challenging; high-quality work is required, and otherwise excellent manuscripts have been rejected solely because of deficient photographs. Typically, matched sets of 5-in. × 7-in. enlargements are required.

The first step in making an enlarged angiographic print is to select the image. Inspect the negative carefully with a high-quality magnifying loupe. Depending on the precise focus and the patient's tear film, there will probably be certain frames that are sharper than others within the same angiographic phase. Carefully examining the negative will help identify the best candidate for enlargement. Be sure to alert client-physicians to this fact before printing, in case a substitution is not acceptable!

To begin printing, set up the tray line with trays of paper developer (diluted 1 to 1 with water), stop-bath, fixer, and running water wash. Turn on the darkroom safelight, and if you use a cold light enlarging head, turn on its heater unit.

Clean the selected negative thoroughly before printing to minimize the need to correct dust spots on the final print. Examine the negative under strong lighting and use film-cleaning solution (either a commercial preparation or 95% ethanol) to remove any fingerprints. Next, place the negative in the negative carrier. Inspect the negative again, and use a soft brush or compressed air to remove any last specks of dust just before setting the film carrier into the enlarger.

Open the enlarging lens to its widest setting, turn on the enlarger's lamp, and adjust the height of the enlarger so the projected image is approximately the size of the required print. Place the print easel on the baseboard, roughly focus the negative onto the easel, and adjust the orientation of the negative carrier, easel, and enlarger height until the easel shows the required image projected onto its surface. Carefully inspect the edges of the easel; make sure that the projected image extends just slightly past the edges of the easel mask. Use tape to secure the easel to the baseboard, thus preventing accidental movement during the printing session. Also, lock the enlarger head height adjustment to prevent it from moving while the negative is focused. If you use variable-contrast paper, now is the time to install the filter into its holder. Begin your tests by using a grade 3 filter for an angiographic negative.

To critically focus the negative, set the grain magnifier onto a scrap piece of paper placed on the easel. The paper must be of the same thickness as the material you will use to make the final print. Look through the magnifier's eyepiece as you adjust the enlarger's focusing knob. When the image is sharp, you will see the negative's grain pattern sharply through the magnifier. Don't be surprised if you cannot recognize the image; many magnifiers use high-powered optics, so pictorial elements in the negative may not be appreciated.

Once these preliminary steps have been accomplished, turn the enlarger's light off and set a sheet of enlarging paper in the easel. Use the same process for making test strip exposures as when printing contact sheets. Incrementally expose the paper, sliding a cardboard mask across its surface so approximately an inch or two of paper is exposed for each step. Develop the print the same way you did for a paper contact print, for 2 minutes, then agitate it in stop-bath for 30 seconds. Place in the fixing tray and agitate for 2 minutes, then wash for 4 minutes. Because papers typically darken slightly when dry, assess contrast and density after the test print is dry.

Remember the all-important rule of printing: Exposure creates density, and development influences contrast. Make certain that the enlarger exposure is sufficient to render areas of hyperfluorescence that are not too bright; most vessels can be printed so they have a just perceptible hint of tone darker than the pure white of the paper base. After the highlights have been suitably printed, look at the darkest areas of the print. If they approach true black, then the contrast is probably correct. If the area surrounding the angiographic image is only gray, try switching to a higher-contrast paper or develop the grade 3 paper longer to increase the contrast. A cycle of printing, processing, assessing, and reprinting is almost always required by even the best printers.

At times, local exposure control may be required to permit the print to more closely approximate the range of values seen in the negative. "Burning in" describes the process in which a selected portion of the print is exposed longer than other areas. "Dodging" denotes lessening the exposure selectively for specific parts of the image. Both are performed manually, using either your hands or specially made tools (Figure 6-29). Both tasks require a sensitive touch; when properly done, the edges of areas that have been dodged or burned in should not be noticeable in the final print. The secret is to keep the light modifier (hands or tool) constantly moving; it must also be suspended some distance from the paper surface to cast a very soft edge to its effect.

Local exposure control has ethical implications. Photography has long been assumed to have an intrinsic honesty and objectivity—the main reason that science has adopted photography as a relatively impartial medium for recording and disseminating data. In that spirit, local exposure control should be used only to correct technical deficiencies (i.e., to overcome limitations in matching the printout medium to the negative) and not to artificially create or suppress the distribution of fluorescence.

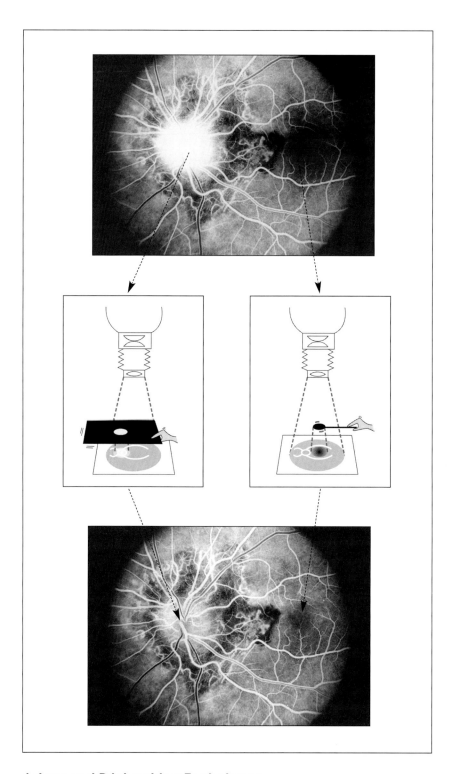

FIGURE 6-29
Presumed ocular histoplasmosis syndrome with choroidal neovascular membrane. Depending on the distribution of dye and the negative's processing, at times a straight print will show an optic nerve that is too bright and a macular region that is too dark. This can be corrected by applying extra exposure (burning) to the nerve head, while a portion of the base exposure is subtracted from the macular area (dodging) to bring the photograph into better tonal balance.

Advanced Printmaking Techniques

Even though exhibition printing usually plays a small role in ophthalmic photography, at times it may be advantageous to produce a print that reflects the highest levels of photographic quality. When producing an exhibition-quality print, the same techniques are used to determine contrast, exposure, and processing factors as discussed above. However, special photographic paper stock, exposure techniques, and processing chemistries are used to produce a print that has enhanced aesthetic qualities.

The first difference in exhibition printing concerns the choice of paper stock. Even though RC papers could be used, many experienced printers choose fiber-based paper. This stock is not coated with plastic. Instead, the image is directly incorporated in the emulsion layer bonded to the paper support material and thus appears almost tangibly closer to the viewer. The subtle texture of the paper substrate is detected within the image itself. The image appears slightly sharper, brighter, and of higher contrast than it would in an RC print. Fiber-based papers are available in either graded or variable-contrast. Most fine printers choose the "F," or glossy surface; when air-dried, this surface takes on a most pleasing luster.

A special exposure technique using the unique characteristics of variable-contrast papers also enhances the quality of your exhibition prints. This technique is called *split filter printing* and is equally applicable to RC media.

Selecting a single filter to print on variable-contrast paper always represents a compromise, as the filter works only for the average contrast value of the negative. In this case, highlight tones (i.e., hyperfluorescent areas of the angiogram) often require burning in, whereas dark areas may require dodging. Cold light heads help bring the extreme values into a closer alignment with the abilities of the paper to depict them[12] but do not solve this problem completely.

Split filter printing uses two filters: a high-contrast (magenta) filter (i.e., grade 5) and a low-contrast (yellow) filter (e.g., a grade 0 or –1). The low-contrast filter has its greatest effect on the highlights, and the high-contrast filter influences the contrast in the darkest values.

For split filter printing, first place the lower contrast filter in the enlarger. Make a test print (by sequentially exposing strips across the print), develop, fix, wash, and dry. Examine only the lightest tones; choose the final exposure to give proper density in the highlights. The low values will appear flat in this print, however. Next, make another test print giving the selected grade 0 exposure to the entire sheet and then exchange the grade 0 for the grade 5 filter and give the same sheet (already exposed to grade 0) sequential test exposures to the high-contrast filter. Process and examine the results. You will find that the grade 5 filter has little effect on the highlights, but the dark values will show much improvement. Select the grade 5 exposure strip that shows the desired contrast in these areas. To make the final print, expose first to the grade 0 filter for its proper time and then to the grade 5 filter with its distinct time requirement. Obviously, the enlarger must be locked securely and the easel taped down to prevent any movement between the two exposures. The final print will show excellent detail in the highlights, pleasing gradation throughout the middle tones, and just the right contrast in the darkest areas.

When you print on a single-contrast grade paper, you select the proper grade based on the negative's middle values. Customarily, the highlights may require burning and the shadows need dodging. With split filter printing, the highlights and shadows are each exposed through precisely matched contrast filters, and the middle values take care of themselves.[13]

Kodak Dektol or similar paper developer is used to develop fiber-based paper. A worthwhile enhancement to the developer comes from adding benzotriazole to the solution. One ounce per liter can slightly increase print contrast as well as slightly cool the print color.[14] Also, for the finest print quality, the fixer should not include hardener solution as it prevents uniform toning effects and also lengthens the required duration of the wash cycle.

Most photographic papers have a distinctive print color. Even though they are called "black and white," most papers appear to have a slightly olive-green tint once they have been processed. Many find this color to be unappealing. It can be shifted to a slightly cooler, more purplish color using a toner. After the stop-bath, fix the print for 2 minutes. Then place the print into a bath that consists of 1 liter of Hypo Clearing Agent or Perma Wash (Heico, Delaware Water Gap, PA) to which has been added 1 oz of rapid selenium toner. Caution: Selenium is toxic. Use tongs or rubber gloves when processing prints in this material! Constantly agitate the print while observing its overall color carefully (an untreated print next to the tray will provide a useful comparison). After several minutes, you will be able to detect a subtle shift in color toward a cool purplish brown.[12] When the desired color has been reached, remove the print and place it in the print washer. If the print stays too long in the toning bath, it will eventually turn noticeably brown. The intended goal of this bath should be a subtle color shift; at a glance, the finished print should still appear to be black and white.

Fiber-based papers naturally absorb more chemistry than RC materials. They must be washed much longer to ensure long-term stability. At least 1 hour in an efficient print washer is required to achieve a chemical-free condition. RC papers typically dry flat. Fiber-based papers, on the other hand, have a tendency to curl as they dry. For best results, they should be allowed to dry on fiberglass drying screens—these look like screen windows and permit air to dry both the front and the back of the print simultaneously. The emulsion surface of a wet fiber-based print is quite delicate; it is best to place these prints face-up on the screen to avoid any chance of imprinting the screen's texture on the print. Avoid the use of photographic blotters or drum dryers, as these cannot be kept perfectly clean. Drying may take anywhere from several hours to overnight, depending on the relative humidity of the environment. When completely dry, these prints may be flattened under a weight (i.e., a stack of books) for several hours.

Carefully inspect the final dried print for white specks. If they are present, they should be spotted as a last step in finishing the print. In this process, tiny white spots in the print caused by dust, scratches, or other defects on the negative can be retouched by carefully painting them with dyes. These dyes are formulated to match common print colors and are usually sold in sets of three. Use an extremely fine sable watercolor brush (i.e., size 00) to pick up a minute quantity of the selected dye. The brush must be nearly dry to avoid placing an uncontrolled drop of dye liquid onto the print surface, where it could spread and darken surrounding tones. Under strong illumination (and with the use of a magnifier), fill in the white spots by repeatedly touching the tip of the brush to the offending speck of white, periodically charging the brush with more dye as required. A light, delicate touch is needed for this work. As the pigment from the brush penetrates the paper, the spot will slowly merge into the surrounding tone. Work slowly, and periodically rotate the print's orientation to help see new spots that need correction. If the white speck is linear, it is best to first break it up into short segments and then to fill in each segment, rather than trying to paint out the line in one or two strokes. Every few seconds, sit back from the print to measure your work's progress.

ACKNOWLEDGMENT

This work was supported in part by a grant from Research to Prevent Blindness, Inc., New York.

References

1. Shaw SD, Rossol M. Overexposure: Health Hazards in Photography. New York: Allworth Press, 1991.

2. Spencer DA (ed). LP Clerc's Photography Theory and Practice. Vol. 4: Monochrome Processing. Bath, England: Focal Press, 1971.

3. Thall L. Survival of the stainless steel developing reel. Photo Electronic Imaging 1994;37:50.

4. Frohlichstein A. Automatic processing of fluorescein angiographic film with a modified MohrPro 8 print processor. J Ophthal Photography 1991;13:77.

5. Merin LM, Lewis RA. New film alternatives for high resolution fluorescein angiography. J Ophthal Photography 1988;10:36.

6. Scott ML. Understanding the Photographic Process. In JP Vetter (ed), Biomedical Photography. Stoneham, MA: Butterworth–Heinemann, 1992;14.

7. Tyler ME. Total tonal information in fluorescein angiography. J Ophthal Photography 1979;2:62.

8. Merin LM. A pragmatic approach to "technical difficulties" in ophthalmic photography. J Biol Photog 1994;62:113.

9. Hurtgen TP. Understanding photographic parameters—guides to film selection and use. In Biomedical Photography, a Kodak Seminar in Print. Rochester, NY: Eastman Kodak Company, 1976.

10. White M. Zone System Manual. Hastings-on-Hudson, NY: Morgan & Morgan, 1968;7.

11. Merin LM. Aesthetics in angiographic imagery. J Ophthal Photography 1981;4:22.

12. Picker F. Zone VI Workshop. Garden City, NJ: American Photographic Book Publishing, 1974;51–52.

13. Vestal D. The Craft of Photography. New York: Harper & Row, 1972;251.

14. Adams A. The Print. Boston: Little, Brown, 1983.

Suggested Readings

Blaker AA. Handbook for Scientific Photography. San Francisco: WH Freeman, 1977.

CBE Scientific Illustration Committee. Illustrating Science: Standards for Publication. Bethesda, MD: Council of Biology Editors, 1988.

Graves C. The Zone System for 35mm Photographers. Stoneham, MA: Focal Press, 1982.

Graves C. The Elements of Black-and-White Printing: Going Beyond Darkroom Basics. Boston: Focal Press, 2001.

Kelly J (ed). Darkroom 2. New York: Lustrum Press, 1978.

Lewis E (ed). Darkroom. New York: Lustrum Press, 1977.

Chapter 7

Electronic Imaging of the Fundus: Principles and Technique

Marshall E. Tyler

Introduction

Digital imaging provides faster results and additional diagnostic capabilities that were previously not possible with conventional photographic techniques. With advances in personal computing power and high-

Terminology Note: Photography

The term *photography* is used rather than electronic imaging or diagnostic imaging because we continue to be concerned with the properties of light and how to represent it. We would rather not dwell on the recording medium (film or silicone). It is the light that must be controlled to achieve the required images. The recording and display media in electronic imaging must be understood to be part of the total "photo-graphic" process.

resolution imaging technologies, ophthalmic digital imaging has moved from research facilities into the academic and clinical ophthalmic photography setting. Digital angiography is now the mainstream. Color digital imaging is replacing both color video and color photographic film (Figure 7-1).

We present the topic of electronic fundus imaging in its own chapter because we believe it has its own subject matter and vocabulary that is unique and separate from those of film-based fundus photography and angiography, the mainstays of ophthalmic photography.

There are several forces driving the acceptance of electronic imaging into the practice of ophthalmic photography. Electronic imaging permits the physician to receive diagnostic information in a timely manner. Computer capture of angiographic images also allow image enhancement and useful imaging tools such as image overlays. Indocyanine green (ICG) angiography, which was technically very difficult to perform with infrared (IR) photographic film, received little clinical attention until IR-sensitive electronic cameras became available. With digital, diagnostic studies can be shared with the referring physician almost instantly—via the Internet—almost anywhere in the world. Finally, the competitive marketplace demands that a patient be offered treatment in the same visit. This is particularly true if patients have traveled for hours to see the retinal specialist.

Computers and electronic imaging cameras are tools that assist in creating images (see sidebar Terminology Note: Photography). The light sources and optics of electronic imaging systems are similar to those of their film counterparts, but their "photosensitive" material is very different. These systems include video and digital cameras for color fundus, FA, and ICG angiography (ICG-A).

After an historical review, this chapter starts with a technical description of the instrumentation, followed by a description of how to use it. The differences between video and digital imaging are followed by a technical discussion of the digital components comparing film to its electronic counterparts. The components of digital systems, how they work, and how they differ from each other, as well as from comparable conventional photographic systems are discussed. Scanning laser ophthalmoscopes (SLOs) used for angiography, both fluorescein and ICG-A, are explored. Cost considerations in purchasing and using the new technology are included with equipment selection. We conclude with thoughts on the impact of digital imaging in ophthalmology.

History of Video and Digital Technology

Video Fluorescein Angiography

Amazing progress has been made throughout the history of video FA. Many manufacturers and system integrators have provided ophthalmic photographers with many new tools. As early as 1951, Ridley[1] reported television applications in ophthalmology. In 1970, Dallow[2] wrote a treatise entitled Television Ophthalmoscopy, in which he briefly discussed Image Orthicon cameras but chiefly reported on Vidicon cameras (Figure 7-2). His concepts of ophthalmic image analysis stand today as testimony to his ophthalmic and technical insight. Of particular historic interest was his advanced work on monochromatic imaging.

During the 1970s, van Heuven and Schafer used black and white video (TV) cameras to record fluorescein angiograms on videotape.[3–6] The first video cameras received images using specialized photomultiplier tubes coated with phosphors. Image intensifiers allowed FA

A

B

FIGURE 7-1
Digital fluorescein angiography system. The components include the fundus camera, optical port for digital camera, digital camera head, synchronizing "black box," computer with image grabber board, computer monitor, CD-ROM writer, and uninterruptable power supply. **A.** Escalon Imaging (Wayne, PA) and **(B)** Ophthalmic Imaging Systems (Sacramento, CA).

A

B

FIGURE 7-2
Early video fluorescein angiography. **A.** Television monitor image of selected scan lines of a monochrome image. **B.** Perspective drawing of a television ophthalmoscope. (From RL Dallow. Television Ophthalmoscopy: Instrumentation and Medical Applications. Springfield, IL: Charles C Thomas, 1970.)

images to be recorded, as conventional video camera tubes did not have adequate sensitivity. The videotaping process degrades the resolution and adds electronic and tape noise to the image. The limitations of the video camera and recorder resolution, as well as the expense, kept video fluorescein angiograms from gaining wider acceptance.

Mehu and van Heuven used a high-intensity Vidicon camera tube coupled to a three-stage image intensifier. This assembly replaced the eyepiece on a Zeiss (Dublin, CA) fundus camera. A sliding mirror was substituted for the illuminating beam splitter. This increased the intensity of the illumination at the patient's eye. They stated: "The positive public-relations aspects of this fast service are not without reward," and mentioned that recording a fluorescein angiogram as a kinetic event was of potential importance.[7]

I have always marveled at the feeling I get when seeing the true dynamic nature of a fluorescein angiogram either live on a video monitor or on a continuous medium such as videotape. Even when you take a film fluorescein angiogram, there is usually a mirror that blanks out the view of the fluorescein image each time you expose an image. The continuous visual flow of the dye is visually broken.

In the 1980s, Vidicon video camera tube(s) were replaced with silicone chips. The imaging chip technology most widely used today is a charge-coupled device (CCD).

Video Camera with Computer Digitizer

As computers became relatively less expensive, smaller, and more powerful, the next generation of imaging systems began with the introduction

FIGURE 7-3
PAR Microsystems video/digital imaging system
(Atlanta, GA).

of video frame grabbers. A computer-based video frame grabber permits an analog video signal to be digitized.

In 1980, at the University of Pittsburgh, Paul Rehkopf and Joseph Warnicki, with Stuart Brown, MD (Chairman of the Department of Ophthalmology), began developing an ophthalmic video digitizing system. In late 1982, they worked with Jim Cambier at PAR Microsystems (Atlanta, GA) to develop the first marketable ophthalmic imaging system (Figure 7-3). This system was based on a Unix-based computer running a Motorola 68000 processor on an S-100 data bus. RGB or National Television Standards Committee (NTSC) video images were digitized to a 512×512 pixel resolution with rectangular pixels using seven imaging boards. There was a capture and a memory board for each color (RGB), as well as a controller card. The color images were used for stereo glaucoma studies. The system sported an 80-megabyte (MB) HD and an optical drive for direct recording of images. The computer did not have enough hard disk space for the temporary storage of images, so all images were recorded to the optical disk. Final proof sheets could be built without any "bad" images, but they still wasted space on the non-erasable optical disk. It took approximately 1 second to record just a single memory plane for a black and white video image. The initial system was wired for the electronic interface and flash synchronization circuits of the Topcon (Paramus, NJ) fundus camera although shortly after that, supplementary interfaces were made for the Zeiss fundus camera and slit-lamp.

The program screens were in monochrome but had "windowed" control areas, and a mouse was used as a pointing device for image selection and contrast manipulation. Quite a few of the image manipulation routines seen in current systems were implemented in this system. Image sharpening took 2–3 minutes and image registration took well over 5 minutes. In a personal memorandum, Mr. Warnicki stated, "There were 24 ribbon cables with more than twelve hundred connections for just the video capture and memory boards. These connections were very touchy. We regularly had to clean them to keep the system running."

This imaging system was marketed in 1983 by PAR Microsystems as the IS-2000. The cost of the basic system was $150,000. This included an S-100–based 68000 computer with Unix operating system, two monochrome vt-100 computer terminals, two color monitors, and a 12-in. optical disk recorder, which could store 1 GB of data. The disks cost approximately $400 each. The basic system was rack mounted in a cabinet approximately 30-in. × 30-in. wide and 6-ft high.

Ophthalmic Imaging Systems, Inc. (OIS) (Sacramento, CA), founded by Dennis J. Makes and Steven Verdooner, shipped its first FA-512 system in 1986. It consisted of an Ikegami black and white video camera on a Topcon TRC-50VT fundus camera and an IBM-compatible computer using an Intel 80286 processor. Their first FA-1024 system (1989) used a Dage 1-in. Vidicon tube-type video camera, and the analog video signal was converted to a digital file in a personal computer.

In 1987, Topcon America purchased the system marketed by PAR Microsystems and released the product under the IMAGEnet name. Three models were available: fluorescein, color fundus, and stereo.

In 1988, Olendorf Research (subsequently controlled by Tomey, Inc. and now by MRP Group, Inc.) introduced its Zeiss-adapted fundus camera using a Kodak (Rochester, NY) digital camera. The camera back was mounted on a Nikon F-3 35-mm camera and used a Macintosh computer and software based on the National Institutes of Health software called Image. Later models used the Kodak DCS-100 and DCS-200 camera backs. These digital backs use the Kodak M2 and M3 chip technology, which digitizes the image at the chip level instead of remotely on the computer frame grabber circuit board.

In 1989, OIS and Topcon introduced 1024 models using the Kodak Videk camera to create the first commercially available high-resolution system with analog-to-digital conversion within the camera control unit (CCU). This was used for FA. The Intel-based computers (80386) were slow at acquiring these larger images. To speed up the process, one manufacturer skipped the recording of every other line of the image and later extrapolated it to synthesize a 1024×1024 pixel image. When computers became faster, a full-resolution system was introduced.

In 1990, Topcon, at the ICO in Singapore, integrated the Kodak Megaplus (model 1.4) into their system. This was a high-resolution video camera based on Kodak's M1 chip technology. Like the Videk, it contained a digitizing board in the CCU. The image was not digitized near the chip but several meters away.

In 1994 and 1995, OIS and Topcon America brought Microsoft Windows-based software to ophthalmic photography. This advance assisted in transferring the images onto computer networks. Systems with a single monitor showing both the menu text and the images were brought to the marketplace in the mid-1990s as a space- and cost-saving measure.

COLOR VIDEO CAMERAS

Color video cameras brought color fundus imaging to our angiography systems. First, single-chip (CCD) video color cameras, and then three-chip video cameras were used. European designed systems often used phase alternate line (PAL) standard cameras to increase the resolution of the image. The PAL systems use 625 lines with 50 fields at 25 frames per second: 576 lines are used in the image.

HIGH-RESOLUTION DIGITAL CAMERAS—COLOR

Color digital cameras with more pixels are replacing their lower resolution video counterparts. In addition to a higher resolution (greater number of pixels), the better digital cameras have increased dynamic range (bit depth). This expands the exposure latitude of the camera, increases shadow detail, and avoids the overexposure of highlight details. It is actually the well-capacity that gives the extra dynamic range of exposure to the camera (Table 7-1).

INFORMATION SHARING

In 1994 ophthalmic photographers Joseph Warnicki and Paul Montague set up the first ophthalmic photography list-server and file transfer protocol (FTP) sites on the Internet to foster communication within the ophthalmic photographic community. These capabilities permitted interested

Computers—General Operations

Computers and their software drive these digital imaging systems. Your ability to work with these tools will increase your productivity. Although the following is no substitute for a good education in how to use computers, their operating system, and applications, it may give you a few items to aid you in a successful relationship with a computer.

The hardware in a computer consists of a few major components. Their functions are:
Central processing unit (CPU): This is the brain of the computer where the processing of information happens.
Random access memory (RAM): This is the working place for data (information) to be stored temporarily. This is akin to the top of your desk.
Hard drive (HD): This is magnetic storage to keep the computer's operating system (OS), applications/programs, and data (your information). This is similar to your filing cabinet.
Input/output devices: These are the components that permit you to communicate with your computer. The main items are the keyboard, the mouse, and the display monitor. Additionally, the printer falls into this category.

When you start (power-up) your computer, it has enough information to know how to get itself started. After it checks itself out to see what components are attached, it will go to the HD and load the operating system (OS) into the RAM. After the OS is loaded, the computer knows how to display the programs (applications) that have been loaded onto the system. At this point, you may choose to run one, or more, programs. These programs may include the proprietary imaging program for your angiography system, or Photoshop (Adobe Systems, San Jose, CA), or PowerPoint (Microsoft Corp., Redmond, WA).

After you have run (used) your application (computer program), and have saved your work (data files), you may close (shut down) the application. It is important to properly exit your programs, as they open many files while they are in operation. Failing to exit properly may leave work files open on your hard drive and waste space on it. After closing all of your applications, you should then exit the OS. In Windows this is done via the "Start" button at the bottom of the monitor screen—then by selecting "Shut down" and "Shut down the computer." After executing these commands, the computer may power itself off or inform you, via a message on the monitor, that it is safe to turn off the computer.

Sometimes a computer will appear to stop functioning. When this happens on a Windows computer, you may give it a "three-fingered salute" — that is, press and hold down the CTRL-ALT keys and then press the DEL key. This will present to you the Task Manager window. You may inspect which program, if any, is failing to respond. If you can identify the offending program, you may close it down in this window. If you cannot determine the problem, repeating the three-fingered salute restarts the computer. This, or turning off the power, results in an improper shutdown of some of the programs and the OS. On restarting the computer, it may run a program called *ScanDisk* to attempt to clean up unused computer files.

Even if you do not have problems as described above, you may wish to run some diagnostic software every few weeks to ensure

(continued)

Table 7-1. Relative Resolution and Dynamic Range of Photographic Films and Various Electronic Cameras

Angiography	Tri-X film	Video B&W	MegaPlus	D-100/200
Resolution	3k × 2k	512	1024	
Bit depth	~12	8	8	8
Color	Slide film	1-chip	3-chip	MegaVision
Resolution	4k	512	512	2048
Bit depth	~10	6	512	12

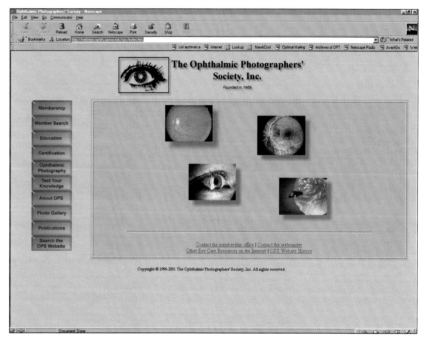

FIGURE 7-4
Web site homepage of the Ophthalmic Photographers' Society (http://www.webeye.org).

ophthalmic photographers to send messages (typically news, questions, or answers) to other ophthalmic photographers around the world. The FTP site is a depository for images to be shared with other photographers. World Wide Web (www) home pages on the Internet provide additional image sharing capabilities (Figure 7-4). For current home page addresses, contact the Ophthalmic Photographers' Society (see Appendix A) or use a Web search engine to search for "optimal," "ophthalmic photography," or "Ophthalmic Photographers' Society."

Cameras and Instrumentation: Technology Basics

For a quick course in computer basics see sidebar Computers—General Operations.

Electronic Fundus Imaging and Angiography

When film is replaced with its electronic counterpart, the digital camera, there are additional technical challenges for the photographer. The technical differences between video and digital imaging form the basis for all of the discussions that follow. Included are how the components are integrated and how to use this new technology for fluorescein and

Computers—General Operations
(continued)

that your system runs smoothly. ScanDisk is a program that looks for orphan files and pieces of files. Another is the defragmentation program—DeFrag. DeFrag brings together into one contiguous file, files that were written to your hard drive onto more than one physical part of your drive. In Windows, these programs are started via the Start/Programs/Accessories/ System Tools area.

Terminology Note: Analog Video versus Digital Cameras

Some basic vocabulary is needed to understand the remainder of this chapter. We have all heard the terms *video* and *digital*. We have even used these terms interchangeably when discussing cameras. But they have very different meanings. Two concepts are important: the nature of the signal and their typical resolutions.

Let us first think about what creates a photographic image. A photographic image represents the original scene with varying densities at locations throughout the negative or print. In a photographic negative, these potential density specks are located where the light actually falls. In the world of electronic imaging, however, there are technical limitations that define the possible locations which can represent the bright and dark "specks" that make up the image. This is either the scan lines of a tube-type camera, or the pixels of a digital camera.

A video camera is an electronic camera with a lens that focuses an image onto one to three analog electronic sensors. Currently, these sensors are usually CCDs. The signal that comes out of the camera electronics is analog. An analog signal varies in intensity and thus tracks the brightness of the original scene with a pattern of horizontal lines that are painted with an electron gun onto the phosphors that cover the inside of a television screen. These brightnesses represent the brightnesses found in the original scene. In video, a voltage of 0–1 volt represents the darkness or brightness of locations on the television screen (Figure 7-5).

Resolution is limited by the standards to which television signals must apply. Three major standards are currently in use: NTSC, PAL, and sequential color and memory (SECAM). In the United States, the standard is NTSC, which is limited to 525 vertical lines, with 485 lines being used for the image. PAL is used in countries that have ties with England, and SECAM, which was developed in France, is used there and in countries that have historical ties with France. The two versions of SECAM have resolutions of 625 and 525 lines. None of these standards is interchangeable or compatible.

In NTSC, an entire image frame is sent from the camera every $1/30$ of a second. Each television frame consists of two fields, called *odd* and *even*, that are interlaced to reduce the visual perception of a flicker. A new field is displayed on the monitor every $1/60$ of a second.

No matter how good the camera is, if the signal is displayed on an NTSC television monitor, it will be 485 horizontal scan lines. There

(continued)

FIGURE 7-5
Scan lines on a National Television System Committee television screen.

ICG-A, monochromatic imaging, and color fundus photography. There are many basic components to be discussed: fundus camera, optical interface, electronic image camera (digital camera), computer (with image digitizing board, image display board, archiving system, and network connection), software, and printer.

This section describes how the components function; the next section describes how to apply an electronic system to ophthalmic photography.

A complete explanation of the electronics of the digital camera, the computer interface, and the mathematics of image enhancement is outside the scope of this book. The information presented here describing this equipment is sufficient to allow the photographer to understand the capabilities and the limitations of digital imaging. First, however, see sidebar Terminology Note: Analog Video versus Digital Cameras.

Angiography System Components: Instrumentation Overview

Integrators of electronic fundus camera systems have combined a digital camera, computer, and software onto a film-type fundus camera to create a hybrid ophthalmic instrument. This is not a simple task. When making a photograph, you are asking the system to do the following: clear the previous image from the computer's image capture board, clear the previous image in the digital camera, and then synchronize the fundus camera's solenoid eyepiece head, electronic flash, and digital camera's image capture with the computer's image capture board. All vendors' systems use similar components to accomplish digital fundus imaging (see Figure 7-1).

SYSTEM SYNCHRONIZATION
A synchronizing device coordinates the flash, digital camera, image capture, and computer to receive the image. Each system manufacturer has its own name for this synchronizing "black box," which is one of the most important hardware components of the system. Without the synchronizer, the image capture sequence cannot be coordinated.

DIGITAL CAMERAS
Photographic film responds to light by creating image density that relates to the intensity of the light that exposed it. The resultant density is a very accurate (although not linear) representation of the degree of illumination or subject reflectance. An almost infinite number of shades of gray,

may be greater definition in these horizontal scan lines with the better cameras and monitors, but there is a practical limit of approximately 800 horizontal "lines" of resolution. Increasing resolution further is of little benefit once the horizontal resolution is more than twice the vertical resolution, as the vertical resolution limits the overall image quality.

Video is an analog signal and therefore is continuously adjustable—for example, the (audio) volume control on a radio, a tuner on an old radio, or the viewing lamp brightness adjustment (continuous type) on a fundus camera. A digital signal is expressed as a pure number or as a choice of numbers—for example, 88.5 MHz on the tuner of a digital radio, the flash power setting on a fundus camera (the number of capacitors selected is a precise number), or "0s" and "1s" in a computer.

If the signal is turned into an analog signal in the camera, then, by definition, the camera is an analog video camera. If the camera maintains the digital information all of the way from (next to) the CCD to the recording medium, then the camera and system are digital. Some cameras have a high-resolution (greater than NTSC) analog signal going to the CCU where it is digitized. An example of this technology is the Kodak Megaplus, model 1.4, which uses what Kodak calls M1 chip technology.[8] The model 1.4i has no separate CCU and has computer-adjusted controls.

The brightness of the video image is represented by a voltage level (Figure 7-6), which is changed in the computer on the digitizing board (frame grabber) into a digital signal for each relative position on the video signal (Figure 7-7). The advantages of this transformation of the video signal to a digital signal are twofold. First, the image saved in the computer is of a higher quality than the same signal recorded and played back on videotape, because the process of recording and replaying an analog videotape degrades image quality. Replication (attempts at duplication) further degrades image quality. Computers that can record continuous video signals are expensive. Duplication of a computer (digital) image is not degraded when copied, whereas in photographic or video replication, the image is modified when one attempts to duplicate it.

Second, the digitally recorded video frame may later be manipulated in the computer. Overall contrast expansion and control of brightness is similar to changing paper grade or exposure, or both, when printing in the darkroom. These brightness and contrast expansions allow the viewer to see the desired image.

A video camera can be a cost-effective input device for low-end electronic imaging systems. Do not forget that not only is the image of lower resolution, but it is not a true "digital imaging" system, because the image was once an analog signal. Thus, it should be referred to as a *digitized video imaging system*.

Resolution of a digital camera is limited only by the levels of present technology and cost. Digital cameras with image resolutions of 2k × 3k are now available.

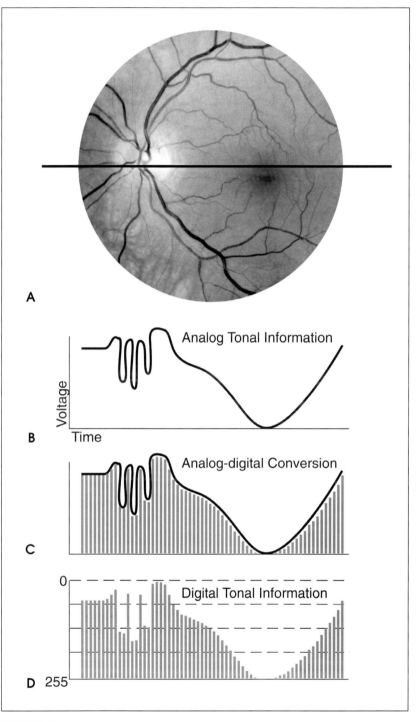

FIGURE 7-6
The fundus photograph **(A)** has a single scan line drawn through the image. Relative brightness (expressed as voltage) at approximate positions on the video screen **(B)** and its transition and conversion from analog to digital signal **(C)** are precisely recorded brightness at exact locations on the digitized image **(D)**.

with a dynamic range of 160 to 1, are created in a photographic negative. In a digital camera, electronic approximations are created to represent the illumination on the camera chip face (Figure 7-8).

The digital camera receives the image of the fundus after the fundus camera illuminates the eye with its electronic flash. A digital camera's CCD sensor contains a grid of many thousands of discrete locations, each of which is uniquely identified. These locations on the sensor are called

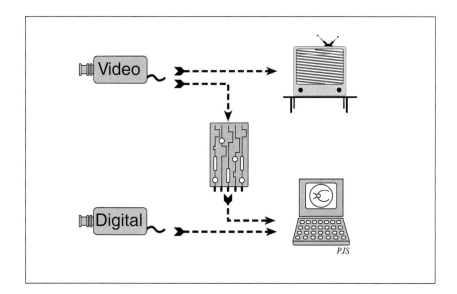

FIGURE 7-7
Integrating video or digital images. Electronic angiography systems use either a video or a digital camera. A video camera produces an analog signal, which can be recorded in analog on videotape or translated into 0s and 1s by a digitizing board in a computer. A digital camera provides a digital image directly to the computer.

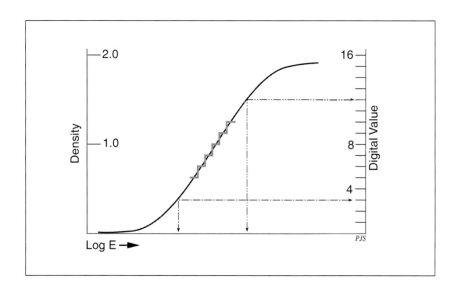

FIGURE 7-8
Analog film density versus digital camera output. The digital camera creates discrete values for each level of illumination and produces values that represent the linear nature of the imaging devices.

pixels, short for picture elements. The smaller the pixel, the finer the resolution, given the same size of active chip area.

The digital camera translates the analog world of brightness into numbers, which can be sent directly to a computer for storage. Conversely, making a photographic slide from a digital original creates an analog image from the digital file. Compared to video images, the digital camera typically has higher image resolution and a lower signal to noise ratio. When duplicating an image, the digital process does not induce image distortions (tonal shifts) or increase image noise as does replication by videotapes.

IMAGE BIT DEPTH
A digital camera receives light onto its CCD, where the light on each pixel generates a number that represents the brightness of the light. Eight-bit cameras generate a number between 0 and 255 ($2^8 = 256$); 12-bit cameras: 0 to 4,095 (2^{12}). This number, one for each pixel, approximates the amount of light that falls on that specific pixel. Some cameras use a 10- or 12-bit dynamic range for image capture but typically save the image as an 8-bit image. Although Photoshop will work with 16-bit images, all of its fea-

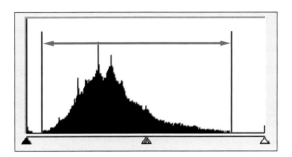

FIGURE 7-9
A 16-bit histogram showing the range of useful information that will be compressed and stored in 8 bits.

tures are not implemented. Most computer monitors use an 8-bit display system. There are also 16-bit cameras, and these store 65,536 gray-level values (2^{16}).

How the digital imaging system reduces 10 or more bits to 8 bits is important. Some systems simply reduce the entire range. Others use the first 8 bits and throw away the other information. Using the computer to look at the range of values and compress those values that have useful information may be the best system. The method and amount of compression used should be recorded for each image (Figure 7-9).

Pixels are typically numbered starting in the upper left-hand corner of the image sensor. This location is 0,0 for the row-column location. The next pixel in the first row would be number 0,1. Because the pixels are read off in order, there is little reason to note the actual location of the pixel once the total array dimension (in pixels) of the CCD is known. Just the brightness (luminance) values are noted as discrete values (e.g., 0, 127, 255). These values represent black, medium gray, and white.

PIXEL DEFECTS

Most cameras have some defective pixels. A bad pixel will return a (brightness) value of 0 (black) no matter how much light falls on it (see section on Digital Artifacts and Figure 7-23). Camera grading is based on the quality of all of the pixels and their placement. The higher the pixel defect grade, the less distracting the bad pixels will be. There is a significant cost premium for near-perfect cameras. Cameras with a few bad pixels are considered the standard grade, and cameras with multiple central defects are sold at a discount. Software can change the value of a bad pixel and give it a value similar to adjacent pixels, which visually masks the defective pixels. The location of these defects should be considered in research studies.

SENSOR SIZES AND ASPECT RATIOS

Imaging chip measurements are based on standards developed in the video industry. The first TV camera tubes, image orthicons, were referred to as *2-inch tubes*. This was the measure of the diagonal of the rectangular scan area of the image on a round tube face. Video camera chip sizes are also referenced by the diagonal measure of the active chip area. Typical diagonal measurements are $^1/_3$-in., $^1/_2$-in., and $^2/_3$-in.

Digital cameras are often referred to by the number of active pixels on the CCD and less often by the physical size of the active area of the chip. For example, 1370 × 1035 pixels and 8.98 mm × 7.04 mm (this was the Kodak Megaplus camera that was used on the OIS and IMAGEnet 1024 systems in the early 1990s). The pixel count reflects the resolution of the system, and the image area is used to calculate the magnification of the images (Table 7-2). An early series of cameras had pixel counts of 1012 × 1524 and an active image area of 14.0 mm × 9.3 mm. Later units had more

Table 7-2. Imaging Device Tube and Chip Sizes

Format	Diagonal (mm)	W × H (mm)	Pixels	Image Size (MB)	% of 35 mm
$^1/_3$-in. video	8.5	5.1 × 6.8	—	—	4
Megaplus 1.4	11.4	7 × 9	1035 × 1370	1.4	7.3
$^1/_2$-in. video	12.7	7.6 × 10.2	—	—	9
DCS-100	16.8	9.3 × 14	1012 × 1524	1.5	15
$^2/_3$-in. video	17.0	10.1 × 13.5	—	—	15.8
1-in. video	25.4	15.2 × 20.3	—	—	35.7
Nikon D1H	29	16 × 24	1312 × 2000	2.74	67
DCS-460	33.2	18.4 × 27.6	2024 × 3072	6.1	58.8
Mega-Vision S-3	43.27	24 × 36	2k × 3k	18	100
35-mm film	43.3	24 × 36	—	—	100
2-in. video	50.8	30.5 × 40.6	—	—	117

H = height; MB = megabyte; W = width.

pixels, 3072 × 2048, and a larger image area 27.6 mm × 18.4 mm. OIS and Escalon Medical Imaging offer color imaging chips in the range of 2k × 3k (k = 1024). Escalon uses a MegaVision/Phillips CCD chip, which has a sensor size of 24 mm × 36 mm—the full size of 35-mm film's image area with a full 12 bits of image bit-depth.

ASPECT RATIO

The height-to-width ratio is different for different imaging technologies: 35 mm, 2 to 3; video, 3 to 4; and round fundus images, 1 to 1. When these media are mixed, there will either be some black area added or some cropping of the images.

For comparison, a 35-mm film image size is 24 mm × 36 mm. Typically, digital chips are smaller. This means that an optical adapter is required to make the image the correct size for physically smaller electronic imaging cameras. Typically, they use an additional lens to minify the size of the image.

Optical devices (photo adapters)[9] that "relay" the image to the video or digital camera are often referred to by the diagonal size (diagonal measure) of the video image they support (e.g., $^1/_2$-in.). Calculations must be made to show the magnification of the image and therefore how the image will be displayed by a particular chip size. When selecting an imaging system, ensure that the image is filling the full area of the chip, using as much of the chip's active area as possible to create the highest resolution image. Check this by increasing the brightness control on the monitor to reveal the edges of the chip's active scan area.

COLOR FUNDUS ELECTRONIC IMAGING

Video CCD cameras continue to be integrated into electronic ophthalmic imaging devices to reduce expense. Keep in mind that the resolution of video systems (300 to 400 horizontal resolution × 525 vertical resolution) is only approximately one-third that of even the most basic digital camera (Figure 7-10).

Imaging systems sometimes use color video cameras, which provide a single color frame (image) that is "grabbed" in the computer on a special video capture card. This gives the computer imaging system color fundus recording capabilities. The quality of images from single-chip video cameras is comparable to those produced on instant film materials and perhaps, therefore, are not of adequate quality as the only documentation of the color fundus. However, these images may be used as a convenience to remind the clinician of the previously examined fundus. Three-chip color video cameras produce a clearer image than single-chip color cameras.

A

B

FIGURE 7-10
Color video fundus image. The video image **(A)** is reproduced to show the anticipated detail that would be seen on a 3-in. × 4-in. print. The enlargement **(B)** is magnified to show the detail as it would appear on a 5-in. × 7-in. print. Evaluate the image sharpness on an actual print from any system you are evaluating—does it meet your needs?

In a true digital camera, the digital signal is maintained from the sensor, the camera head, all the way to the imaging card in the computer. This card receives a digital signal directly from the digital camera. Whenever there is an analog-to-digital converter, some information is lost, whereas no information is lost with reproduction or duplication using the digital signal. The picture is then moved from the imaging card to the computer memory or, in some systems, directly to a fast HD.

Color digital cameras are as useful for color fundus photography as monochromatic digital cameras are for angiography. Color digital cameras with the resolution for both high-quality color and black and white imaging are now available. The greatest advantage achieved by replacing video with digital cameras is the freeing of the resolution of the image from the NTSC (video) standards. The first color digital cameras that were affordable in clinical ophthalmology had resolutions of 1024 × 1280 pixels. Now cameras that yield more than four times that resolution—2048 × 2048 pixels—are entering the imaging market.

At these resolutions, the digital camera matches or exceeds the resolution of the fundus camera. This statement is made particularly when including the optical interface/optical components of the subject: the human eye. Processing images of this size (~15⁺ MB) presents a significant task to the computer. Storage of these large images is also a concern.

Images may be stored in a wide variety of image file formats. Common formats for our imaging systems are TIFF, JPG, and RAW. These and other file formats have unique characteristics (Table 7-3).

COLOR IMAGES

High-resolution color imaging systems are capable of capturing the full resolution of the image created by the fundus camera. With bit depths of 12 or greater and resolution of 2k × 2k and greater, film is no longer a requirement for high-quality fundus images. Even creating a "2×" (actually 5× to the film) of an optic nerve or macular hole is extremely well documented with these new imaging systems (Figure 7-11).

Table 7-3. Computer File Formats

Format	Software Description (Manufacturer)
.TIFF	TIF Tagged Image file format (Aldus)
.JPEG	JPG compressed files (Joint Photographic Experts Group)
.PSD	Photoshop Proprietary, image compressed (non-destructive PK-Zip method), Layers, Vector text (Adobe)
.PDF	Portable Document Format (Adobe)
.EPS	Encapsulated PostScript, Sending files to PostScript printers and QuarkExpress
.GIF	Graphics Interchange Format, GIF98a supports transparent pixels
.PICT	Macintosh Picture file (Apple)
.MPEG	Motion (Joint Photographic Experts Group)
.TGA	Targa (TrueVision), interfacing with video images
.TXT	Text
.DOC	Word document (Microsoft)

FIGURE 7-11
Enlarged portion of a 2k × 3k color digital fundus image. The yellow square in the 30-degree fundus photograph shows the location of the enlargement. At this magnification (enlarged image), the full print would be 28 in. × 28 in. The subject (fundus) to print magnification is 100×.

In the future, complementary metal oxide semiconductor–active pixel sensor imaging technology may provide reduced sensor costs while providing electrical power and size advantages. In addition, there may be improved reliability through a reduced overall system component count. In 2000, Canon Electronics manufactured a consumer video camera that used a complementary metal oxide semiconductor chip.

CHARGE-COUPLED DEVICE COLOR STRIPPING

Color digital cameras generate an RGB value for each pixel location. To enable a monochrome CCD chip to create a color image, its pixels are filtered, in a prescribed pattern, with RGB filters. Because green is the color where most of the definition takes place in our visual system, half of the pixels are stripped with a green filter; 25% are red, and 25% blue. The filter pattern is green, RGB. The pattern is offset on the next row of pixels (Figure 7-12). Due to the RGB filters that have been placed in front of the pixels, color chips are usually 28–30% less sensitive to light.

COLOR CCD CHIPS USED FOR ANGIOGRAPHY

Because each pixel has a red, green, or blue filter in front of it, a value only for that color can be assigned to it. To assign a value for the other colors for that pixel, the pixel is assigned an average value for the adjacent pixels of that color. This creates an image file three times the size of the original sensor's resolution.

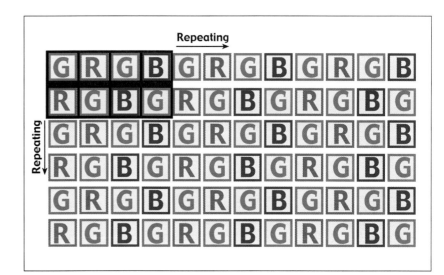

FIGURE 7-12
Color striping pattern of color digital cameras. Green
(G), red (R), and blue (B).

Using a color camera for angiography has a cost and mechanical advantage over using two separate cameras: one color and one monochrome (Black and White). Effective sensitivity reduction in the blue and green channels (FA) is approximately 30%. The resolution is reduced by 25% for the red pixels and an additional loss from the low exposure to the green pixels by up to 50%. When used in a monochromatic imaging situation (e.g., FA), color cameras will have less resolution (because of the extra pixels required to capture the color information for the same size chip) than their monochrome counterparts. Even considering these losses, there may be adequate sensitivity and resolution to use a color digital camera for angiography.

Working with the Digital Imaging System—Image Capture

Follow the ophthalmic photography procedures as outlined in Chapters 2, 3, and 5, modifying your technique for digital imaging as described below.

Computer software and hardware controls all the image acquisition steps as well as the mechanism by which the image is manipulated, printed, and stored. Let us first look at image acquisition (capture).

After patient data are entered and the camera is prepared for patient photography, you are ready to begin a dye study. Color fundus photographs are taken (film or digital), monochromatic green images are taken to document the area of the fluorescein study, and then the patient is prepared for the intravenous injection. Pressing the joystick button or foot switch signals the solenoid eyepiece to move the viewing mirror to send the image to the imaging chip (Figure 7-13).

A signal from the mirror is sent to the computer and, in combination with the control box, a signal is sent to the digital camera's CCU. The signal then travels to the computer's CPU with its image capture board, and finally to the fundus camera's flash tube trigger circuit to initiate the firing of the flash. If a digital camera is mounted on the video port on the fundus camera, the fundus camera synchronizes the image going to the video port and the triggering of the digital camera. When a digital camera back is used, as opposed to a digital camera mounted on a video port, then coordination of these signals is taken care of by the digital camera back, the same as with film.

Each of these components must be ready to record the image. On receiving instructions from the computer's CPU, the camera's CCU tells the imaging chip in the digital camera head to get ready to receive an

FIGURE 7-13
Digital camera eyepiece head and optical schematic. Note the position of the additional mirror and the relay lens. In this system, the viewing mirror moves into place to shift the image upward to the digital camera.

image. In older digital cameras the CCU was in a separate physical box. In newer cameras, the CCU is integral with the camera head. Adjustments may be physical knobs and switches or controlled through software. The chip is set up to receive a new image by clearing any image that may have been stored on it. The frame grabber is told to go through the same process: It is cleared and put into a ready state. After the imaging chip and the frame grabber are prepared, the fundus camera is signaled to fire the electronic flash, which illuminates the fundus. The image is received by the digital camera head and sent via its CCU to the imaging board in the computer, and the image is displayed on a monitor. The image is then off-loaded into the computer's RAM to free the capture board so that it can be cleared and made ready to acquire another image.

HOW MUCH RANDOM ACCESS MEMORY IS NEEDED?
HOW MANY IMAGES DO YOU WANT?
After a series of FA images are acquired, they must be moved from the RAM to make room for more images. Images are typically 1–4 MB in size. The amount of RAM can be the limiting factor as to how many images can be recorded quickly before some images must be saved. Some systems use fast HDs to save each image to the HD just after it is acquired. As computer processors and HDs become faster, it has become possible to write images in unlimited numbers directly to the HD. On the other hand, as image resolution, and therefore file size, increases we may still use RAM, lots of RAM.

No matter which system is used, check the minimum time for continuous image acquisition to make sure it meets your needs. Shorter is better.

CONCURRENT ANGIOGRAPHIC PROCEDURES
If a second patient requires an angiogram, and images of the first patient are desired beyond 10 or 15 minutes, most systems permit you to start a

second angiographic study. There is a second timer so that you can use the software to alternate between patients. The times are linked to the patients' database records. This capability has limited use in a high-quality photographic service but might be used to keep a timer running to document late images in a patient with suspected cystoid macular edema.

Dual timers are also useful for combined FA and ICG-A procedures to keep track of both injection start times. Make sure that your software will permit a single patient to have two timers running concurrently, and that the two studies will be placed into separate sets of thumbnail images or contact sheets. The software should also record filters that are used for an image.

Image Distribution

There are two basic ways to view an electronic image: on paper (or transparency) or on the computer screen. These methods may be referred to as *hard-copy* and *soft-copy*. Paper prints or film transparencies may be adequate for limited purposes, but monitors are required to show the images in their full brilliance and resolution. The image monitor has no substitute for its quality. Consider that computer monitor phosphors permit a great dynamic range, whereas a photographic print has a more limited dynamic range of a density range of 2.8 and an illuminance ratio of 1 to 160. Transparency material falls in the middle, with a tonal range of nearly that of the computer display monitor. Typically, we print only 35-mm contact sheet "positives," therefore the monitor has the advantage of easily increasing the viewing magnification.

Because the monitor is a light source unto itself, the available dynamic range is greater than that of a (reflective) print or transparency. Although the information contained in a high-quality print may contain the same tonal information as a computer monitor, it has a lower dynamic range—thus making the information harder to visualize. The computer image can be dynamically modified. The monitor allows the ability to enhance and zoom the image. While prints are convenient, interpretation or treatment of the patient should be performed only from the computer monitor image. In the film world, we "read the negatives." In the digital world, we "read the screen" (and not the print).

Before printing, you may choose to modify the images through enhancement techniques, imaging tools, or both. The imaging software and your computer are the workhorses of this phase. How you use these tools is discussed later in Using the Digital Imaging System.

THE DISPLAY MONITOR

Monitors are viewing devices for viewing images and for reading the menus from the computer software. Some systems have a separate monitor for the images, and some share one monitor screen between the images and the software menu. The advantages of using dual monitors are twofold. The first is that the angiography monitor can be black and white. Not only does this reduce the cost of the larger monitor, it also increases the sharpness of the black and white image. However, if the image monitor is in color, it can be used for color fundus images, and other imaging work is more convenient with a large monitor. Second, having a separate image monitor provides room for the software menus. Disadvantages of a two-monitor system include the greater cost and the additional space.

While monitors are typically of a resolution similar to that of the images that are to be displayed, the resolution of the image is not limited by monitor resolution. The stored image file should be kept on the computer at the highest resolution that the camera and optical system are

Table 7-4. Computer Monitor Resolution Standards

Computer Monitor Standards	Resolution (Pixels)
VGA	640 × 480
SVGA	800 × 600
XGA	1280 × 1024
UXGA	1600 × 1200
QXGA	2048 × 1536

capable of producing. The image can be displayed on computer monitors by using a software package that permits "zooming" the image to reveal the full resolution and the fine detail of the image (Table 7-4). This table shows this number of pixels (width and height) that are used to fill the monitor. This is separate from the physical size of the monitor.

CALIBRATION AND STANDARDIZATION

Color calibration of your system, from image to monitor(s) (including shared images) and on to the printer is important. Software to consider using includes Apple Computers, Inc.'s ColorSync and Pantone's Personal Color Calibrator (www.pantone.com and www.colorsync.apple.com). See the section Monitor Set-Up—Calibration.

IMAGE AND PRINTING RESOLUTION

Maintaining image quality is important in maximizing diagnostic information. If an image is reduced in tonal information or resolution, then there may be a decrease in the quality of the diagnostic interpretation. Ensuring that the full resolution of the captured image is maintained throughout the image storage, retrieval, and printing functions is sometimes difficult but is nonetheless paramount in preserving image quality.

When you are ready to print, the software will permit you to select the number of images to be included on a single sheet of paper. Typical formats are for one, four, nine, or 16 images to be printed on 8-$^1/_2$-in. × 11-in. paper or transparency. Note the decrease in viewable information as more images are put onto a single screen or print. Image resolution and image size should be appropriately balanced for cost and quality (Figure 7-14).

If four 1-MB images are printed on a single 8-$^1/_2$-in. × 11-in. page with a high-end printer, it is important to have the full resolution (information) in the images reproduced on the print. Taking a 1-MB screen image "screen dump" and sending it to the printer produces results different from those produced by taking four separate 1-MB images and sending them, with their full resolution, individually to the printer. Printing four 1-MB images as a 1-MB file produces four prints that are only one-fourth MB in size. This is less than the resolution of the original image and of the printer; the software is not giving you the quality image that you have worked so hard to produce. The manufacturer should be able to tell you if you are getting a "dump" from a 1-MB monitor image file or actually going back to the original image files and printing them as four separate 1-MB files.

Several printing technologies have been used in electronic ophthalmic imaging. Printers range in price from $500 to more than $10,000. Obviously, there are some differences in these printers. The right-hand column of Figure 7-15 shows a ×100 view of images from different printers.

ANALOG VERSUS DIGITAL PRINTERS

Some printers reproduce values with the appropriate tonal value. These photographic quality printers are referred to as *analog printers* because they reproduce tones on a continuous density scale.

FIGURE 7-14
Printing layouts: 1-up **(A)**, 4-up **(B)**, 9-up **(C)**, and 16-up **(D)**. These show the relations of image size and the final resolution of the image.

Other printers are capable of placing a black dot at a prescribed location on the paper to represent darkness in the image or the lack of a black dot to represent lightness. These are digital (output) printers (e.g., office laser printers). Between these two systems is the high-resolution inkjet printer, which, though digital in nature, attempts through increased resolution to simulate an analog print.

Printer specifications include the resolution in dots-per-inch (dpi). This is just one factor used to determine how well your image will be reproduced. If your image is 1024 pixels wide, and you want it to be

FIGURE 7-15
Prints from different technologies make a considerable difference in how your images are presented. Magnified views of sample prints of different printing technologies include **(A)** original file printed from the digital file; **(B)** photographic-quality laser, Fuji Pictographic 3000 laser printer (Edison, NJ); **(C)** inkjet printer, photo-grade inkjet paper, Epson 1200 printer (Long Beach, CA); and **(D)** laser printer at 600 dots-per-inch.

printed 4 in. wide, then you need a printer of at least 256 dpi (1024/4) if the printer is representing the value (0–255) of each pixel at its appropriate density (darkness). This is true for the higher cost dye sublimation and pictographic printers. However, it is not true for the laser printers or inkjet printers that can only place a dot of one density on the paper. To replicate or approximate the tonal information of these printers, their resolution would need to be 5–10 times greater than their analog counterparts. There is one caveat—inkjet printers with special software that can differentiate densities of ink (placed into the six ink compartments that are normally used for color inks) to increase tonal information on a printer with inherently lower resolution.

Printers create a likeness of the original image by replicating the image on a pixel-by-pixel basis. The value of each pixel is replicated on the paper. Scaling of the image may increase or reduce the number of pixel values actually needed to create the final image. Each pixel in a black and white image is assigned a brightness value between 0 and 255 (in an 8-bit system).

Let us look at how each works, starting first with a photographic grade printer.

Photographic Printers.   Higher-resolution digital printers (Agfa's MSC-200) can use a true photographic process with a computer-driven digital "front end." The output medium is color photographic paper, which is processed with conventional color photographic chemistry, RA-4. The image quality is not that of "digital imaging," but assuming the image file resolution is adequate, these printers achieve marvelous near-photographic quality images. These printers accept digital computer files or can directly scan a slide into the printer. My unit is networked to receive files from up to 65 computers as set up in the Wake Forest University Baptist Medical Center's Biomedical Communications Department.

The Pictography (Fuji) silver halide printing technology creates images without conventional photographic chemistry (see Figure 7-15A). A light-sensitive (silver halide) material, called the donor, is exposed simultaneously by three laser diodes, one for each pixel value of each of the three colors in the digital image file. The donor is then moistened with distilled water. This is the only wet part of the process. A receiver sheet is bonded to the damp donor with pressure, and heat is then applied to activate the thermal development process. The self-developing dyes from the donor migrate into the receiver paper. The donor is stripped away, revealing the photographic-quality image (see Figure 7-16B). Prints made with this technology are sharper than prints made with dye sublimation, because not only are all of the pixels transferred in a single pass but also the image is transferred into the receiver instead of onto it from the dye sublimation ribbon. At 400 dpi, the potential image sharpness is four times greater than that of a 200-dpi dye-sublimation printer (see Figure 7-15A). The residue silver in the donor material may be recovered.

Dye Sublimation Printers.   Dye sublimation printers can print true tonal (analog) information. The process takes a digital image comprised of shades of black from 0 to 255 and places a dot of the corresponding darkness on the paper. The paper (substrate) is not a light-sensitive material. These printers use a ribbon whose pigment is moved via a transfer roller to the paper or transparency. The ribbon passes across a 200-dpi linear laser print-head, the print-head heats the ribbon, causing the ribbon dyes to change directly from a solid to a gas. *Sublimation* is the term for this phase change, which skips the usual liquid stage. The gas is then condensed and diffused onto the paper's surface. The transferred image is then heated in the "finisher" to stabilize the image onto the substrate. Black and white prints can be ready in less than 3 minutes.

Dye sublimation printers at 200 dpi have greater apparent sharpness than office laser printers at 600 or even 1200 dpi, because they can reproduce dots of appropriate density, and they do not use any of their resolution for screening the image (see Figure 7-15B).

Color dye sublimation printers use a color ribbon that has three separate color transfer strips that are sequentially transferred onto the paper. The paper, which is attached to a transfer roller, sequentially receives each of the colors (Figure 7-16A). An additional clear ribbon may be used to overcoat the image to protect it from chemical contamination (chiefly formaldehyde), and the resultant fading.

Dye sublimation prints are very stable under a variety of test conditions. If the prints are left in contact with polyvinyl chloride (PVC),

A

B

FIGURE 7-16
Color digital printing processes. **A.** Dye sublimation process showing the image being transferred onto the paper. **B.** Fuji Pictographic process, roller transport. Pictographic one-pass dye transfer into the receiving paper. When selecting a printer, evaluate the image quality for sharpness, color accuracy, and image evenness (lack of image banding).

non-archival, slide pages or acidic paper (patient chart folders), there can be a dramatic shift in their print densities as well as a color shift toward a reddish brown. These effects can be seen within weeks of a polyvinyl chloride slide page being placed in a file folder. Newer printers reduce this problem by over-coating the print with plastic. However, two recommendations have merit: First and foremost, sleeve the dye sublimation prints in Mylar jackets, and second, use archival-quality pages to hold your 2-in. × 2-in. transparencies.

The heat and noise from older dye sublimation printers can be more than most camera room personnel (patients, physicians, and photographers) will tolerate. Unless it is a cool and quiet model, the printer should not be in the same room as the fundus camera. There are limitations as to how long the printer cable may be, so be sure to check before purchase.

Inkjet Printers.   On inkjet printers, printer paper must be matched to the amount of ink that is being sprayed onto the paper. High-quality glossy photographic style papers do not let the ink bleed. This keeps the ink where the computer instructs, thus using the full image quality of the printer (see Figure 7-15C).

Stepping up to a paper with photographic grade coatings increases the quality of the image. This technology is often used to create scientific posters. Long-roll printers produce prints 36-in. or 48-in. wide.

To add more tonal information in the color highlights, photographic-grade inkjet printers are outfitted with more than the standard configuration of three colored inks (CMY) along with a black ink (K) cartridge. Thus, the usual printer's colors of CMYK (*cyan, magenta, cyan,* and *black*) are augmented with a light cyan and light magenta ink, to total six ink colors. For black and white prints with more tonal range, these printers can often be outfitted with a special set of inks to give more tones of gray.

At resolutions of 2880 dpi × 720 dpi, photo-quality inkjet printers give you images of amazing quality. Printers use six color quick-drying photographic-quality ink cartridges. They can print an 8-in. × 10-in. in less than 2 minutes. 13-in. × 44-in. panoramas are also possible and can fill the entire paper with the image for a border-free print. Some printers use advanced Micro Piezo technology, AcuPhoto Halftoning, and 4 picoliter variable-sized ink droplets. Tiny droplets vary in size, resulting in finer shadow detail and amazing highlights across a wide spectrum of colors. Don't forget that smaller is better.

Office Laser Printers. Laser printers (office type) provide an economical, high-contrast and low-resolution (600–1200 dpi) solution to producing a chart copy of the digital image (see Figure 7-15D). A laser printer can be driven via the normal printer ports or with a special cable and a card, which, when placed inside the laser printer, increases the printing resolution and speed. When the laser is driven directly from the computer, images can have a resolution of 2400 dpi. However, there are limitations. The laser cannot create true tonal information, but rather produces the appearance of tones via a screening process. Screening creates black dots of different sizes, which, when placed close together (and seen at the proper viewing distance), create the illusion of an image with continuous tones. Computer-generated halftones can use either frequency-modulated screening or stochastic screening. The effect is to produce higher-resolution halftone representation of grayscale images with lower-cost printers. The results with these printers are very good considering both the initial cost and low per-print cost. Although the image is not of sufficient quality to diagnose or treat a disorder, it is sufficient for noting in the patient chart the diagnostic information that was read from the computer screen.[10]

Network Printing. Placing the image acquisition station and the printer on a network can allow multiple angiographic stations to print to one printer, as well as make the printer available for other applications. Printer software automatically prints any file when it is "dropped" into a designated directory on your computer. One software package is RasterPlus by Graphx (Woburn, MA). Investigate this type of software if you have more than a stand-alone digital camera.

Stereo Image Viewing

The ability to view stereo fundus and FA images has always been an important diagnostic tool. See Chapter 3 for information on the viewing of stereo images. Electronic stereo images can be viewed in the same way as conventionally produced images, as well as using several additional techniques. Sixteen- or 20-image contact sheets, when displayed on a 20-in. image monitor, produce images that may be a little too large for easy free viewing. Base-out prisms combined with a +4 diopter lens will help most viewers to view the stereo images on the monitor.

Viewers with four mirrors make viewing 4-up images easy (see Figure 3-25). Capabilities to display zoomed stereo images reduce limitations of screen resolution. This is an excellent feature for viewing stereo optic nerves or macular pathologies. Some people can use "cross-eyed view-ing" to look at a reversed stereo image pair. A photographer friend of mine who used this cross-eyed technique throughout his long career believed that this could have possibly been a cause of eye muscle imbalance problems later in life.

The software must be capable of rearranging the position of the images on the monitor and onto the print. Check the software you are thinking of purchasing and try to rearrange the images on both the screen and for printing. Software capable of marking the images as a stereo pair permits easy retrieval of the stereo pairs.

Of particular note are systems that can use the color image monitor to align stereo images and to display them simultaneously. An anaglyph is two superimposed images of different colors, such as red and cyan, representing slightly different angular views of the same subject.[11] When viewed through filters of the same colors, each eye sees the corresponding left or right image, but the viewer perceives a single fused three-dimensional image.[11] The left image is shown in red and the right image in cyan (blue and green).

The images are viewed with red-cyan glasses without requiring convergence or divergence from the viewer (see Figure 3-34). This technology can also be used to overlay hyperfluorescent lesions over a monochromatic green (post-treatment) image. It is important to know how much time it takes to prepare two stereo images for viewing. If a procedure is too lengthy, it may not be convenient to view a stereo image. After you have identified, aligned, and magnified a stereo pair, it is important to be able to save your work.

Visit-to-visit comparisons can be performed by alternately displaying two images that have been registered. This permits the clinician to track, for instance, the optic nerve changes subjectively. This technique is known as *flicker chromoscopy*.

Image Storage and Archiving

A photographer would never consider keeping only prints and throwing out the original negatives. Likewise, the digital angiographer needs to store the original digital (computer) image files and keep the images on a long-term storage medium. To keep using your imaging system, you will need to move and then delete images from the HD to make room for additional fluorescein studies. Later, you will need to make archival copies of the image files.

First, the images are recorded onto the computer's HD. This either happens as the images are taken or transferred from the computer RAM or shortly after the images are taken. Local HD "storage" is fine for the day's work. Some systems save duplicate image files on a second local HD. For easily accessible storage of images taken during the preceding weeks, a large HD on the acquisition system's computer or on a local area network (LAN) is needed. Multiple drives may be combined to form a drive array to provide image storage redundancy. Black and white images, in uncompressed form, are a minimum of 1 MB per image, and high-resolution angiograms are 6 MB and color images are 18 MB for each image. At 20 images per angiographic study, plus a few 18-MB color images, it does not take long to fill up even a large HD. Some form of less-expensive storage medium is needed for safely archiving the images.

CD-ROM (compact disk—read only memory) technology is usually used for this task because of its low error rate, standard format, and non-magnetic technology. CDs are much slower than HDs, but they are also much less expensive. The first CD-ROMs held 650 MB of data. The related technology of DVD (digital video disk) disks store 4.7 GB of data. Obviously, data storage systems will continue to provide greater amounts of data online with decreasing cost and space requirements.

COMPACT DISK—TECHNICAL DATA

Here are a few abbreviations to help you with the CD "techno-speak":

- CD 5 $^1/_4$-in. disk that holds 650 MB of data (images).
- CD-R is the recorder that can write the data onto a blank disk.
- CD-RW is the recorder that can write data onto a blank disk and onto a re-writeable disk. These disks are more expensive and not frequently used for archiving due to data instability and because file modification is possible.
- DVD 5 $^1/_4$-in. disk that holds 4.7 GB of data (approximately 7× the data of a standard CD).

Although commercial music CDs are mass-produced, our data are individually "burned" onto the coatings in the mid-layers of the CD. These "pits," or lack of pits contain the coded information that represents our images. Gold (a very thin layer) is one of the materials that is used to record the data. At this time, it appears that the gold disks may have better longevity, although under reasonable storage conditions, most technologies provide good archival qualities.

On CD-ROMs, the information is read through the bottom side of the disk, so it is important not to mark or scratch this surface. Flexing the disk could also produce separations of the layers and make the data unstable. Finally, don't subject your CDs to high temperatures by leaving them in a hot car.

WHEN TO ARCHIVE YOUR IMAGES

Storage of your images should be completed after printing so that any additional images (combinations, overlays, print groupings, etc.) may be saved with the original images. You need a smooth way to move images from the HD onto the storage media. You may use one of several types of media, but the way that you interact with them is similar.

Storing images is a two-part process: copying the original file onto a CD-ROM and then deleting the original file from the HD. The database is then updated to document the new location of the copied files. If the files are left on the HD—from the previous day's patient studies, for example—they will be accessible quickly. The software should make it easy for you to distinguish between the patient images that have already been archived and those that have not. When you want to erase the now duplicated copies of the files that are on your acquisition system's HD, your software should tell you that you have already made copies of the files. Well-designed software will not let you delete your only "copy" of your images. Your software should, when you ask for the images on any patient, tell you which disk it needs for access to the stored images.

Databases—Image Retrieval

After images have been acquired, the physician must review them for diagnostic information. To find a patient's images, you need an index of your patients and their images—on a computer this index is called a *database*. The database tracks patient information and the location of image files. Important information to be entered includes the patient's last name, first name, middle name, hospital number, insurance number, date of birth, sex, race, physician, referring physician, photographer, diagnosis, procedure, and camera. Also, some user-definable alpha fields and several logical fields should be included. The software should provide the date of the procedure, the location of the patient's images (disk, path, and directory), the time each image was taken, and, in the case of a fluorescein angiogram, a method of recording or calculating the lapsed time after the start of the angiographic injection. Additional information to record for each image includes which eye, magnification (X pixels = Y mm), filters used, injection time, and the lapsed time (relation to time of injection).

The ability to export the database to a network database will become more important as more ophthalmic practices use networks, both intranets and Internet, for patient information and patient records. Once new patient data are entered at the acquisition station, the ability to query the network for patient demographics not only saves time but also reduces data entry errors. Databases are discussed further in the section Equipment Selection.

Retrieving images should be easy. Typical requests that can be expected would be to recall the last (most recent) angiographic study, to recall all of the glaucoma patients for Dr. "X" for the past week, or to recall all of the photographs of a particular patient. Additional database considerations are included later in Image Retrieval via the Patient Database.

Which database fields are displayed on the screen or included on a print is important to your filing system and workflow. If you are to be involved in research projects or drug studies, you may be asked to not include items specific to a particular patient (e.g., patient name). Flexible database software allows you to set specific parameters for research projects.

DATABASE BASICS: FLAT FILE AND RELATIONAL

A simple list of patients' names, identification numbers (ID), and demographic information constitutes a database. As a single list, this is called a *flat file database*. The flat file could include the visit date, the type of photographic procedure, and the location of the images (image filenames).

If the same patient is photographed on a different day, a new patient record (repeating the name, identification number, etc.) would need to be entered to have a place to record the new date, procedure, and image file locations.

To reduce having to make duplicate entries of patient name, number, etc., the database system could use a relational database. In a relational database, a second database file "relates" to fields (e.g., the identification number) in the first database file. This lets you enter patient demographics once and then have the information for subsequent visits related back to the initial information (Table 7-5).

REVIEW STATIONS

Monitors show the images in their full detail and brilliance. Prints may be adequate for review purposes, but the image monitor literally has no substitute.

The simplest solution is to use the acquisition system to review your images. Although this is cost-effective for the initial cost of equipment, if the practice is busy, it may hinder the utilization both of the staff and the best use of the expensive image acquisition system.

If a physician is reviewing images on the fluorescein acquisition station, then the system may not be available for a study, and it cannot be put back into use until the review has been completed. Although some systems let you "step out" of an ongoing study and review a case, it is better to complete a fluorescein angiogram without interruption. If the practice is small and scheduling permits, a second image monitor may be installed in the laser suite if it is close to the angiography room. An

Table 7-5. Database Types

Flat file

Name	ID #	Date	Procedure	Dx	Disk-Study #
Jones, Mary	123-45-67	01/14/2005	FA	SRN	423-802
Smith, Jim	234-56-78	01/15/2005	ICG	ARMD	423-869
Jones, Mary	123-45-67	01/21/2005	FA	SRN	434-201

Relational database

Name	ID #
Jones, Mary	123-45-67
Smith, Jim	234-56-78

Visit

ID #	Date	Procedure	Dx	Disk-Study #
123-45-67	01/14/2005	FA	SRN	423-802
234-56-78	01/15/2005	ICG	ARMD	423-869
123-45-67	01/21/2005	FA	SRN	434-201

ARMD = age-related macular degeneration; Dx = diagnosis; FA = fluorescein angiography; ICG = indocyanine green; ID = identification;

Table 7-6. Image Review Systems Based on Size of Retina Practice

Size of Practice	Acquisition	Laser Room
Small	Acquire and review	Monitor only
Medium	Acquire and review	Simple computer review
Large	Acquire	Full review computer with network
Very large	Acquire	Network feed to laser and physician's office

A-B switch box would then send the signal to either monitor. A computer monitor line amplifier can be used to send signals to multiple computer monitors. Obviously, this solution would tie up the acquisition system for the duration of the laser procedure, but this arrangement may be appropriate for small ophthalmology practices. If the laser suite is too far away for the monitor signal to be sent, then another method of transferring the image(s) must be used.

In concert with the decision of how the images will be transferred, decide whether the review station will be a simple single-image station or a full-function review station (Table 7-6). If the photographer will enhance the images and prepare them for the physician in a manner similar to that in the darkroom, then the simple-image review computer may be sufficient. However, if the retinologist wants to enhance these images or to create his or her own image overlays, the review station should be a full-function system.

Images may be moved either by physically moving them with a floppy or an optical disk of images (the "sneaker-net"—physically running the disk down the hall) or with a cabled computer network. If the needs are simple, a single image that has been placed on a floppy disk can be loaded onto the floppy review station. Because there is limited or no image manipulation at this station, a low-end computer system with a single high-resolution monitor will provide an adequate system (Figure 7-17). Inexpensive software will permit you to view most formats of image files.

A peer-to-peer connection is faster but requires some additional initial expense for setting it up. Which to choose is purely an economic decision: time versus money (Figure 7-18).

FIGURE 7-17
Floppy review station. (1) Computer with 3.5-in. disk drive. (2) High-resolution multi-sync monitor. (3) Isolation transformer with hospital-grade plug. (4) Wheeled cart to hold components.

NETWORK IMAGE REVIEW SYSTEMS

The advantages to having diagnostic imaging systems connected to a computer network, with a centralized archiving system and images from many sources available at multiple workstations, are obvious. The hardware required to create the image archives can be a single system that provides archival and retrieval functions for imaging systems ranging from corneal topography to ICG-A. Access to such a system also means that more images can be kept online for use at multiple desktops and examination rooms. Networked computers reduce the need for multiple printers. Integration of color fundus photographs and other images is possible with the addition of a slide scanner or a color digital fundus camera. Images from corneal topography, visual field machines, and magnetic resonance imaging and computed tomography scans are just some of the possibilities. All of these images can be sent to printers and film recorders for slide making. Centralizing the image archiving can simplify procedures as well as reduce equipment duplication. The financial advantage in sharing expensive archiving and printing equipment is significant. With the introduction of online electronic medical records, the possibilities are literally infinite.

The ability to send images between offices in a timely manner may be useful. This is easier to accomplish when the images are already in electronic format. The Internet is a group of computer networks interconnected via high-speed data lines that forward information to a user's computer address. It permits transmission of text, or images, or both, anywhere in the world where the network goes. Additional offices can be connected—admittedly at slower transfer speeds—with computer modems via telephone lines or radio links. Internet service providers sell connections to the Internet. In addition to a connection to the Internet or the creation of your own intranet, software to make the patient information and the images is needed.

Intranet-(inside networks) and Internet-(many computers or networks) based systems that use Web browser software permit physicians

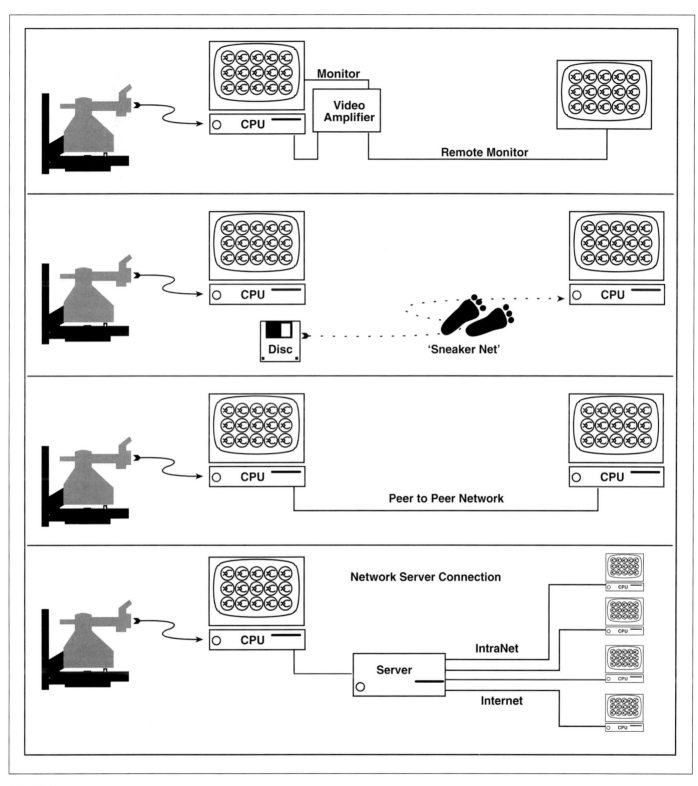

FIGURE 7-18
The appropriate network solution is one that meets your needs. (CPU = central processing unit.)

to see their images almost when and wherever they want. Systems that permit comparison of images from different dates, in stereo, and even with the office notes on a patient are emerging. The ability to give a referring physician access to their patients can make the patient care a seamless event. Obviously, security is an important feature to incorporate. One such system is OcuNet, which was developed by Joe Warnicki (Justice Ophthalmics, Inc., Memphis, TN) (Figure 7-19).

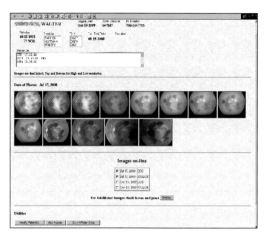

FIGURE 7-19
OcuNet Web-based image retrieval software (Memphis, TN).

Image Standards: DICOM

DICOM is the acronym for Digital Imaging and Communications in Medicine.[12] This standard was developed with an emphasis on diagnostic medical imaging as practiced in radiology and related disciplines; however, it is being expanded to all image-related information exchanged in a clinical environment. The DICOM standard pertains to the field of medical informatics. Presently, there are several manufacturers that are DICOM compliant, but the present standard is not very broad. Even if there is not a full implementation presently available, there are good qualities of DICOM that can be emulated by individual users until such time as the manufacturers of ophthalmic imaging equipment implement a more complete set of standards as applied to ophthalmology.

Information to be "attached" to each image could include, for instance, some of the following items: camera model, serial number, magnification (nominal and calibrated), sensor type, sensor manufacturer, software manufacturer, software version, eye, location of field of view (or attempted field of view), exposure setting (nominal and calibrated), filters used (manufacturer, type, identification number, spectral curve, and date of manufacture). See the sidebar DICOM History and PS 3.14.

Using the Digital Imaging System

There are a number of differences between digital imaging systems and film-based systems. Some of these differences are obvious, but some may not be at first. On all of the systems, the greatest benefit to you, as the photographer, is the instant feedback you receive when your images appear on the monitor. This assists you in understanding how the session is progressing. Focus, exposure, the dynamics of the dye flow, and patient cooperation are all easily monitored, so that you can clearly see and analyze the quality of the diagnostic information. Other participants in the team, physician, resident, or intravenous administrator, gain an insight into the angiographic process.

Although each imaging program and computer platform has its own way of doing things, all of the same steps should be included. In the same way, different photographers may do things in a different order or in a different style of working, but they must accomplish the same tasks (Table 7-7).

Exposing the Image— Digital Camera Sensitivity and Dynamic Range

Some (8-bit) digital cameras do not have the dynamic range of exposure that film cameras possess. The dynamic range (or exposure latitude) is the range of exposures from which the camera will produce information that represents the original subject.[13] The size of the pixel affects the dynamic range of the camera. A camera with a 6.8-micron square pixel (Kodak Megaplus, Model 1.4, M1 technology) will not be able to accept as many electrons as a camera with a 16-micron square pixel (DCS-100, M3 technology).

This ability to hold electrons is called the *well capacity*. The Megaplus 1.4 has a well capacity of 45,000 electrons, whereas a DCS-100 has a well capacity of 250,000 electrons. This gives the Megaplus 1.4 a dynamic range of 60 decibels and the DCS-100 a greater dynamic range—70 db. Kodak has some digital cameras with even better light-gathering capabilities that use more advanced (Kodak DCS-420 using M5 and the DCS-460 using M6 technology, etc.), and therefore, more expensive, technology. Time will bring the cost of these and other new technologies into the everyday practice of ophthalmology.

What are the implications of this potential limited exposure latitude? Where Tri-X photographic film gives a high-quality fluorescein angiogram without changing the relative exposure to the film, an M1 technology camera may not accept the large dynamic range of illumination that is required to image a fluorescein angiogram. To compensate for this limitation, you will need to adjust the flash output on the fundus camera's power supply and/or adjust the electrical gain (like film ISO) on the digital camera. If the flash is properly set, then there can be an adequate exposure range for a high-quality individual image during the fluorescein angiographic sequence. There are additional problems if the camera flash power supply does not allow the output to be adjusted in smaller than full f-stop increments. Images are either over- or underexposed (Figure 7-20). This situation occurs with older Zeiss fundus camera power supplies. A "workaround" is to use a half f-stop (0.15 log units) neutral-density filter in the flash light path. This is accomplished by placing a filter in the slider filter holder (Figure 7-21). Finer gain adjustments (e.g., 3 db) on the digital camera would also be helpful. It would be ideal if the changes in the amount of illumination on the fundus were documented with the digital image with each individual exposure.

If exposures are too great and the flash setting cannot be adequately reduced, then the gain control of the digital camera can be used to reduce the camera sensitivity. This is not usually needed during the fluorescein angiography but may be needed during monochromatic photography. If this maneuver does not reduce the light level sufficiently, such as you might need for monochromatic red images, it may be necessary to turn off the electronic flash and use only the viewing light. However, you might then need to add camera sensitivity by turning up the gain on the digital camera (+6 db to +12 db) and adjusting the viewing light to obtain a good exposure.

Table 7-7. Digital Angiography Steps

Getting ready for the patient
Power up equipment—internal computer system diagnostic checks
Monitor setup and adjustment—black level and contrast
Enter patient information into a database
Ready medical supplies for the angiography injection
With the patient
Review the procedure with the patient
Take color slides on photographic film, or color electronic images
Take monochrome and pre-injection digital images
Have the i.v. site made ready for the injection
Set the timer to start
Call for the injection and start the timer
Acquire the early angiography images
Delete blank images and duplicates (extras)
Save images to the hard drive
Acquire additional images
Patient may leave
Review images: enhance, combine, and print
Send images to laser suite or other physician-reviewing area
Archive images

The imaging software will give you tools (computer functions) for you to accomplish the needed tasks. The main categories are image acquisition, enhancement and printing, saving or archiving images, and utilities.

Comparison of Film and Electronic Imaging

Most of the components of digital fundus cameras are similar to those of photographic film cameras, but the former have additional components that replace the film and the processes that film usually undergoes. Film is first processed (developed, stopped, fixed, washed, dried, printed, and stored) and then the images are reviewed. This review may be directly from the film negative, contact transparencies, or prints. The digital camera replaces these "film steps" with electronic substitutes (amplified, digitized, enhanced, archived, and displayed).

Let us look at the flow of the electronic image through the computer system. Please note that exposure latitude and technical considerations of dynamic range are discussed in the sidebar Exposing the Image— Digital Camera Sensitivity and Dynamic Range.

After the digital camera's CCD is exposed to the image-forming light, the digital signal is created in the digital camera. Then the picture is translated into a digital image of a particular file format, which is then sent to the computer imaging board. This board acts as an interpolator of the electronic image and sends the image to the computer memory. The software controls where and how the image is stored in the temporary computer memory, called *random access memory* (RAM). After images are stored in the RAM, the software permits the user to delete any of the unwanted images and then save the desired images onto the HD.

The image stored in RAM is like the latent silver image on the film. It is volatile (nonpermanent) and, just like exposed but unprocessed film, it can be destroyed. If the computer loses its power (including any backup power supply), the images in the digital camera, on the image capture circuit board RAM, or in the computer RAM will be lost. Just as a film image is stable once the film is processed, once the digital image is copied onto the HD, it will be preserved even if the computer power is turned off. Images are copied from RAM to the HD by the end of the procedure. Some imaging systems write the images to the HD "immediately"

FIGURE 7-20
The exposure latitude of some digital cameras is limited. Three different fluorescein dye phases are shown on lines 1, 2, and 3. Each column represents a different exposure. The middle column **(B)** is properly exposed. The first column **(A)** is underexposed by ¹/₂ f-stop and shows a lack of shadow detail. The last column **(C)** is overexposed by only ¹/₂ f-stop and shows "blocking" in the highlights.

FIGURE 7-21
Filter slider for use in the Zeiss fundus camera with a 0.15-log neutral density filter, which provides a ¹/₂ f-stop exposure difference.

(well actually, continuously but shortly after the image is acquired). These stored images can then be enhanced, printed, reviewed, and finally archived.

For film images to be usable in the future, the film must be dried, labeled, and stored in a filing system. Likewise the digital image

FIGURE 7-22
A standard image is used to adjust your monitor. Your standard image should reflect the uses to which the monitor must be adjusted. In addition to the mid-tones in the grayscale, it should adjust for both shadow and highlight details. The "Shirley" should contain all the pictorial elements for which you might be using the monitor. For fluorescein angiography, a monochromatic green and a few key dye phases are the minimum. A color scale and additional color images can be useful if the system is also used for color image acquisition.

needs to be copied onto a mass storage device, typically CD-ROMs for archiving.

MONITOR SET-UP—CALIBRATION

Quality control is paramount in achieving an optimal quality fluorescein angiogram, whether shooting digital or film.[13] In a digital system, the first step is to adjust the image monitor with a standard image. This should be done under the same viewing conditions you will have when you actually acquire and review the images. This includes room light level, the amount the door is open, and so forth. You will be making decisions that require you to make a judgment call about brightness and contrast. For example, if the image monitor is adjusted to give too dark an image, then you might select images that appear totally black as images for deletion, when, in fact, they may be high-quality images of the early choroidal phases of the angiogram. The system integrator (manufacturer) should provide a "Shirley" (the trade nickname for a standard image), which includes a full tonal range image, a stepped grayscale tablet, as well as a continuous grayscale (0–100% illuminance). This image should be presented before every FA study, not just the first time the system is turned on for the day. Integrated into the "Shirley" should be squares of near white on a white field as well as near black squares on a black field. The standard image should be readily available at all times so that you can recheck the monitor (Figure 7-22).

To adjust the monitor, after setting the room illumination, I suggest the following procedure: First set the monitor black level using the brightness control so that the "black" background of the image is just ever so slightly above the true black of the non-image area around the test image. Then, using the monitor's contrast adjustment, change the highlights of the standard image so that they are just below the brightness level where these areas bloom—that is, blend together into a white mass. This will maximize the brightness dynamics of your monitor when it is used in that particular level of room illumination. Recheck the black level, as it may have been modified by the contrast adjustment. If the printer look-up table is properly calibrated, the print will closely approximate the image on your monitor. Keep in mind, however, that while there is a greater dynamic range (contrast) on the monitor than on a print or transparency, all of the tones should be maintained on the print.

DIGITAL CAMERA—SET-UP PARAMETERS

The fundus imaging system's manufacturer should always adjust the digital camera to create appropriate outputs on the particular individual fundus camera on which it will be used.

This section addresses how some of the initial settings are adjusted to create optimal imaging. Most systems should be adjusted (or checked) every 3–6 months to ensure that the camera is still in balance for the flash output and the optical system. Settings should also be checked after changing flash tubes, cleaning the optics, changing filters, or making other modifications to the system.

Before making any adjustments to the camera, insure that any unsaved images are first saved. Next, and this is most important, you must first adjust the image monitor (see previous section). After adjusting the monitor to your "Shirley," you may continue adjusting your camera.

In both black and white and color digital cameras, there is an adjustment/setting for the black level. This adjustment is used to set the sensitivity threshold at which the smallest amount of exposure will produce an output; a pixel value above "0." Depending on the technology of the camera that you have, you will use one of two methods to make this adjustment. In one system, you will use the camera set-up portion of the menu system. Following the manufacturer's directions, Black Level Calibration will be one of the first choices. Trigger an exposure without any flash with the lens cap in place. The system will automatically adjust the digital camera to provide appropriate sensitivity for shadow detail.

If your camera is an older model, you will need to set this adjustment manually. To do this, you must first readjust the brightness setting on your monitor. Increase the brightness to the point at which a black part of your standard (Shirley) image has black values that are just barely perceivably lighter than the black background of the monitor screen that is not being illuminated by the scan display (raster area). Next, make an exposure, without any flash and the lens cap on the fundus camera. Adjust the settings on the digital camera to achieve a black level that is just barely perceivable above black. This is a trial and error adjustment. Some photographers choose to set this at pure black. Although this will give you nice looking "blacks" in the image, you will be setting the system to potentially lose shadow detail. Now, don't forget to reconnect your flash sync (if you disconnected it for the "no-flash" exposure) and readjust your monitor to your standard image.

Color digital cameras need to be adjusted to present colors accurately. Most systems do this by imaging a known color test target, usually white or near white card, taking the color information from the test target and adjusting the system to create a good white. This is accomplished in a manner similar to setting the black level. This time, leave the flash sync cord connected and your monitor calibrated properly.

For color images, there are more complex procedures for calibrating the system. Pantone and Apple's ColorSync are some products to assist you in calibrating your system. Ask your vendor for the procedure that you need to follow.

DIGITAL ARTIFACTS

As with conventional photography, digital imaging has its own variation of image artifacts—items that appear in the final image that were not part of the original subject (Figure 7-23).

FIGURE 7-23
The complexity of a digital imaging system brings rise to a new set of ophthalmic imaging artifacts. Transient noise artifacts **(A)**, like the black lines near the bottom of this image, will disappear when the system and camera are restarted. **B.** White scan line artifacts (*white arrow*) are an indication that your digital camera is overheating or failing, whereas out-of-focus blobs (*black arrow*) indicate dust on the adapter relay lens. Always check with the manufacturer before attempting to clean your relay lens. Compression artifacts **(C)**, seen here in the blocky nature of the mid-tones, remind us that we should take special care not to distort information when we choose to electronically compress patient records. Failure to make the digital camera ready for the next image can create the capture of a partial image **(D)**.

Pixel defect is the failure of a pixel on the CCD sensor to respond to the light falling on it with an appropriate numeric value. Usually, the value reported is "0." Software can mask the deficiency by assigning the pixel a value based on the value, in an image, of the adjacent pixels.

PATIENT INFORMATION DATABASE

Enter the patient information into the imaging database. If the database is kept on a LAN, then you may only need to enter the patient hospital number, and then accept or modify the diagnosis for this visit because all of the other information is already on the LAN.

Working with the Patient

All of the preliminary photographic tasks, as well as the setting up of the medical supplies for the FA, should be completed before the patient enters the room. First, the system power must be turned on. This is done, just as for a fundus camera, with an electrical power switch. Because there are many components to the digital system, there may be a master power strip with a single power on-off switch. This could also be the on-off switch on an uninterruptable power supply (UPS).

Once turned on, the computer will go through its internal diagnostics and then load the computer OS from the HD. After it loads its OS, it will present an opening prompt or menu. If this is a dedicated digital system, this menu may be that of the digital imaging system. If not, you must enter the program name to start the imaging program. The imaging program will be loaded into RAM, and the imaging software menu will appear on the monitor.

Review the procedure with the patient. This provides time for the patient to obtain additional information and to ensure that the patient understands the procedure. It is important to establish good rapport to achieve the optimal clinical information. The conventional color slides or color electronic images, or both, are exposed first.

Some systems build a "proof sheet" of images to let you monitor the progress. Other systems permit you to view full screen images, allowing you to check focus or alignment. A system should allow you to choose between the large-picture mode and the contact-sheet mode. A hybrid system could show the most recent image as a large image with the previous four images being displayed as proof-sheet–sized images. With the press of a button (function key or mouse click), you can toggle between the two modes.

COLOR AND MONOCHROMATIC IMAGING

Perform color fundus photography either with film or digitally. Photographing nerve fiber layer images with blue light and choroidal images with red light may provide additional clinical information.[14,15] Digital systems lend themselves to imaging the fundus with monochromatic light. As with film systems, insert the appropriate filter into the optical path of the illuminating light of the fundus camera. Spectral sensitivity of the digital camera must be analyzed using the same considerations as for film to ensure compatibility with the selected color of the monochromatic filter. Make sure that the digital camera is sensitive to the color that you want to record by checking the spectral sensitivity curve of the camera. Also find out if the optics in the fundus camera, including any filters, will pass the desired color of light. IR and ultraviolet (UV) blocking filters may have been added to reduce exposure of the CCD by non-visible radiation. Later, you may use image enhancement techniques to provide additional information in these images.

FLUORESCEIN ANGIOGRAPHY AND INDOCYANINE GREEN ANGIOGRAPHY

Continue by making the patient ready in the same manner as you would for a film angiogram. There is the customary timer to record the lapsed time after the start of the injection of fluorescein sodium. To start the timer on a FA series, most computer-controlled systems use the same device as a film-based fluorescein system. This is typically either a button located on the camera-positioning joystick of the fundus camera or a foot pedal. Sometimes it is a computer keyboard function. The exciter and barrier filters are selected for insertion into the light path. The images are exposed as in a film fluorescein angiogram (Figure 7-24).

It is important to know how many images may be saved into the image buffer RAM before you must stop acquiring images and save the images to the HD. Unlike your routine with a 36-exposure roll of film, if you can only acquire 16 images (older digital systems), you must plan how to handle the early-image acquisition sequence. If you have a patient who has delayed filling and you are at frame 14 when you first see the dye, you may miss many of the required choroidal flush or arterio-venous images. One solution is to upgrade the imaging system to allow 30 or more images to be acquired. Each 1024×1024 pixel image will take 1 MB. High-resolution systems use more space (Table 7-8). With appropriate software and high-speed HDs, unlimited images can be written continuously and directly to the HD. The number of images is then limited only by the amount of available space on the HD. After the early frames are acquired, they can be examined, and the redundant or poor-quality images can be deleted.

After you acquire the early images, they can be examined, and redundant or poor-quality images can be deleted from the RAM (see the sidebar Exposing the Image—Digital Camera Sensitivity and Dynamic Range). The best systems have a method of editing images at each natural break in the procedure. A full-screen image displays image detail that is very helpful when choosing images to delete. You may use the proof-sheet mode to see if there are redundant frames and the full-screen mode to see which frames are the sharpest. Most systems also use a keyboard key (delete or backspace) to delete the last image. Some systems let you select multiple images in the proof-sheet mode and then delete the selected group of images. It is important to see, on the image monitor, the result of pressing this key—that is, continuously revealing the next image that you are about to delete. An "undo" function or an "image trash can" function is also useful.

STEREO IMAGING

Stereo fundus photography and stereo angiography are important imaging techniques in ophthalmic photography. The ability to select, view, register, and enlarge the image pairs is important for your software to make these processes easy to execute.

Selecting potential stereo pairs and having them appear on the monitor for your review should be simple. If reverse stereo is seen, then a function key or mouse click should reverse the image pair. After the stereo effect is seen correctly, vertical and horizontal alignment should be checked and modified if necessary. A grid overlay may assist some photographers in aligning similar points on both images. Rotation corrections can also help in making a more perfect image pair. Increasing magnification of the imaging may help to see important details in the image on the computer screen.

Locking down these adjustments to this image set permits the stereo image pair to quickly be viewed next time it is to be reviewed. Simultaneous stereo, taking both the left and right image of the stereo

FIGURE 7-24

Monitor your computer screen throughout the procedure to confirm that you are capturing all necessary phases of the angiogram: preinjection (A), transit phase (B), mids (C), lates (D), and images to print (E). Some systems will allow you to choose between the overview of a contact sheet (A–E) and the single image (F), which can be used for focus and detail check.

Table 7-8. File Size for Typical Charge-Coupled Device (CCD) Sizes

CCD	Monochrome (MB)	Color (MB)
1024 × 1024	1	3
2048 × 2048	4	12
2048 × 3096	6	18

MB = megabyte.

pair at one time, overcomes the preceding problems. Hopefully, more digital fundus cameras will implement simultaneous stereo imaging in the future.

Reviewing the Study

After the angiogram has been completed and the images have been saved from RAM onto the HD, it is time to review your work. There are several ways to view digital fluorescein angiograms. The computer monitor is the best way. Other output devices include paper prints, large transparencies, or slide-imaging equipment. The digital images also can be sent to other computers via removable media (floppy, zip, or CD-ROM) or a LAN, and to distant locations on commercial networks using modems and telephone lines or high-speed data lines.

There are several steps involved in getting the image to the person who will be reviewing the angiogram (see Table 7-6). The order of the steps may be different with each vendor's system.

PATIENT FLOW

Patient flow through the photography area is different with electronic imaging. In a film-based FA clinic, as soon as the patient is finished, the film can be removed from the camera and another patient study can be initiated. In a digital angiography clinic, this may not be the case. One reason is that, unless there is a full-featured review station available on a network, most of the printing process takes place on the acquisition camera workstation. This interferes with the ability to start another angiogram. In effect, the photographer is now performing darkroom work in the camera room. The implication of this change in timing one's work schedule is that, as the film does not get handed to the darkroom person, the camera is not available to photograph the next patient until the images are ready for the physician. There is time saved for the patient and the physician, but not necessarily for the photographer, who now must enhance and print the images in the camera room.

If there is a full-featured review and printing station, then the camera can quickly be used for another angiogram. The images can be transported either on removable media, e.g., a Zip disk (IOMEGA, Roy, UT) or over a network. It takes less time (a few minutes) to write these images onto the disk or to put them onto the network than to prepare a case for review by the physician.

IMAGE RETRIEVAL VIA THE PATIENT DATABASE

The patient database is your inroad to recalling (finding) the images you need. First, the patient and visit must be selected. A useful database features your most recently recorded patients without having to enter their names or identification numbers. Look for databases that display the informational fields you would find most helpful. Seeing the most recently photographed patient's name, diagnosis, date, and physician's name will let you work efficiently. Searching on multiple fields will let you find patient records based on other parameters. Select a database that addresses your needs.

Image Enhancement: An Educational Responsibility

The process of photography has always required the photographer to work with the light that falls onto the film, with the tonal information that is produced on the negative, and with the densities that are produced on the final print. These basic steps comprise a multitude of small processing steps, requiring decisions about how the image will be represented and being subject to the variabilities of the photographic processes.[17]

Technical limitations of the printing processes that are used in textbooks and journals have always required compromises in the tonal information that is reproduced. To maximize the limited tonal range, photographers work with their images to provide the maximal information to the viewer as presented on the final printed page.

The photographer who uses film has always had a variety of tools that can be used to modify the image. With the digital image, these tools are easier to access (see Table 7-7).

It is important for you, and for anyone who is reading diagnostic information, to be completely cognizant of the extent to which an image has been enhanced and the type of that enhancement. In addition to having the responsibility of maintaining image integrity, you have an "educational responsibility" when giving the physician an enhanced image.

We recommend that a complete imaging system record and display the type and magnitude of the enhancements that the original image has undergone. There are many types of image enhancement, so each system integrator or software manufacturer may have slight variations in its naming system for the enhancement tools. Nonetheless, some naming conventions and standards should be used. If an image is enhanced before publication, it could become common practice to include an explanatory statement on the type or extent, or both, of enhancement. That said, it is also the responsibility of the viewer to understand normal and accepted darkroom practices, which may now, via the computer, be used in printing the image.

Some image enhancement systems perform their functions quickly by letting you work on a low-resolution version of a larger image. The desired manipulation, when completed, performs those functions on the high-resolution image. This type of software produces a small script file that records the desired enhancement functions. This approach allows the original file to be maintained and the enhanced image to be re-created at any time.

The following statement should be obvious, but it must be made. Image enhancement and manipulation have always been within the working tools of the photographer. The ability to mislead has always been within the capabilities of the photographer and the photographic technology. New computer tools make it easier to create misleading images. The responsibility and integrity remain the same: Has an image been modified to clarify it for the viewer, or has it been changed to misrepresent reality (Figure 7-25)? An image, like other academic work, is the responsibility of the individual who represents the work as truthful.

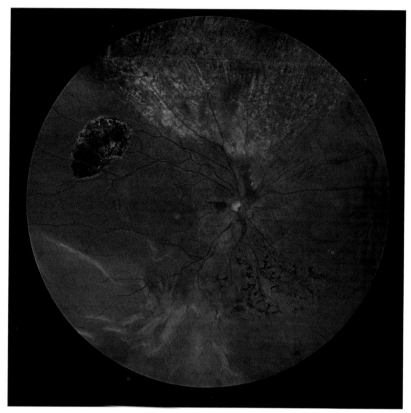

FIGURE 7-25
Computer-manipulated composite illustration from multiple fundi was created from photographs of multiple patients with multiple conditions. Although this combination image may be a useful teaching tool, it is not an accurate representation of a single patient's condition. (FundusMap courtesy of Richard E. Hackel, Kellogg Eye Center, University of Michigan, Ann Arbor, MI.)

After a patient and visit date are selected (the patient may have been photographed on more than one visit date), the software will display small (thumbnail) images. These are small versions of the images that were acquired during the photography session. Some manufacturers call the display of these small images a *proof sheet*, after the photographic counterpart. The number of thumbnail images the manufacturer chooses to display at one time is a function of the type and size of that manufacturer's monitor and software. Images should be sorted and marked to permit stereo images to be viewed on the monitor.

The selected patient file should display the thumbnail images of the procedure. Choosing an image will pull up a full-screen image on the monitor. In addition to viewing a single image, you may wish to group images using the appropriate choices from the software menus. These images may be enhanced and then printed.

Image Enhancement Software

Computers can change an image to reveal information in a photograph that could be difficult to see without the enhancements.[16] See the sidebar Image Enhancement: An Educational Responsibility. Some of these are similar to the enhancements we routinely perform in the darkroom, whereas others would be difficult or impossible to perform in the darkroom. Small local-area contrast enhancements are more complex if performed in the darkroom, and the image overlay functions are almost impossible to replicate in the darkroom.

After the images are safely stored on the HD, a copy of the image(s) can be loaded back into the computer RAM for manipulation. Once you select an image from the proof sheet, a full screen-sized image is displayed. You could, at this point, simply select one or more images and send them to a printer. Don't forget that if you (or someone else) mistakenly adjusted the brightness and contrast controls on the monitor, the print of the image would not reflect the changes you made to the monitor. Always adjust your monitor to a calibrated standard (see section on Monitor Set-Up—Calibration) before modifying or printing an image.

CONTRAST STRETCH

Some of the easiest manipulations are of the contrast and brightness ranges. This is equivalent to selecting different contrast grades of photographic paper and different enlarger exposure times, or to adjusting the brightness and contrast settings on a television. The results of your image manipulations are seen on the image monitor.

The variations of illuminance or brightness levels that a monitor displays are much greater than either reflective or transmission print materials can record and display. This is the same limitation that occurs between the information that is on a photographic film negative and the information that can be displayed on the photographic print. When the brightness range is compressed for producing a photographic print, the printed image may look flat (inadequate contrast) unless some photographic compensations are made.

Contrast expansion, or contrast stretch, is a helpful tool to allow rapid expansion of the available tonal information. The viewing of this image on the computer monitor may be adequate, as the dynamic process of expanding the contrast window allows you or the physician to expand a particular part of the "tonal window." To make better judgments about the density values in an image, refer to the histogram, which is discussed later in the section Advanced Image Enhancement Tools. If the computer equivalent of high-contrast paper is used to accentuate detail in one part of the image, then other parts of the image will suffer. This is an unacceptable method of manipulating an image for printing, because shadow or highlight detail, or both, will be compressed, resulting in the loss of information. This contrast- and density-shifting technique is fine for dynamic viewing of the information on the monitor. Local-area contrast expansion is helpful (Figure 7-26). See also Advanced Image Enhancement Tools for a discussion on the Photoshop versions of these tools.

LOCAL-AREA CONTRAST EXPANSION

Burning and dodging in the photographic darkroom allows the tonal information in a portion of the image to be expanded for easier viewing (Figure 7-27). In a fluorescein angiogram, the relatively dark area of the fovea is difficult to print while maintaining the detail of a hyperfluorescent disk or a neovascular complex. In the darkroom, when the negative is printed, there may be some burning and dodging of the appropriate light and dark areas to maintain tonal information in all areas of the print. Good imaging software allows you to perform the same type of manipulation that you would do in the darkroom. The computer's ability to take predefined mathematical algorithms and apply them to the image is very powerful.

Local-area contrast enhancements help to overcome the limitations of the dynamic range of the monitor and the printing media. Some of the parameters used are image resolution and magnification, the size of the dodging tool, the duration of dodging, and the range of contrast needed for the image. This computer technique is essentially an electronic burning and dodging tool kit.

FIGURE 7-26
Printing limitations and controls in fluorescein angiography. **A.** Image printed "straight" to retain all tonal information, but the print does not use the full tonal range of the print material (flat print). **B.** Image printed with the maximal contrast stretch without clipping either the shadows or the highlights. **C.** Image printed with a computer to simulate a higher-contrast paper and adjusted to expand highlight detail (shadows lost). **D.** Image printed with a computer to simulate a higher-contrast paper and adjusted to expand shadow detail (highlights lost).

FIGURE 7-27
Localized tonal enhancement. Burning and dodging in the computer can enhance the presentation of the image, providing additional information to the clinician. **A.** Original. **B.** The same image with burning and dodging in the computer (e.g., Adobe Photoshop). Then the image is adjusted to expand the image's tonal range to take full advantage of the printing medium (contrast stretch).

Local-area contrast expansion tools increase the tonal contrast throughout the image or in a selected rectangular area. There may only be one contrast enhancement tool to choose from, and all or most of the values are preset. It is important to understand how your image is being manipulated and the limitations of predefined tools. Some systems may have several predefined tools for use on different image magnifications.

There are multiple mathematical algorithms for determining this "average" value.[16] Some mathematical models use pixels within a horizontal and vertical distance of the base location or use a neighborhood pattern. Better models use values that attempt to approximate a radius distance, which reduces the squaring off of the image as it is enhanced (Figure 7-28).

Three basic values in the model can be changed: the area of neighborhood, the weighting of the values, and the amount of change. This strategy is called the *neighborhood area of influence*. The fall-off of the average value can also be changed. How the average brightness is calculated

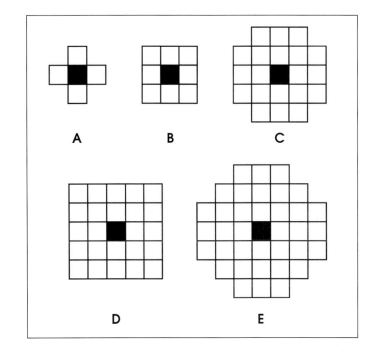

FIGURE 7-28
Neighborhood patterns are used for local contrast calculations. **A.** Nearest-neighbor cross. **B.** 3 × 3 square containing 9 pixels. **C.** 5 × 5 octagonal region containing 21 pixels. **D.** 5 × 5 square region containing 25 pixels. **E.** 7 × 7 octagonal region containing 37 pixels.

A   B   C

FIGURE 7-29
Enhanced images with neighborhood pixel level adjustments. **A.** Original image. **B.** Image enhanced with a radius-based algorithm. **C.** Image enhanced with contrast enhancement software, which uses a neighborhood square algorithm for increasing local area contrast. Notice also that the black "background" is reflected into the image area with this algorithm.

(center weighted, even distribution, etc.) is similar to the changes that are made in the relative distance between the enlarger lens and the photographic print paper. Finally, there is the degree of change or, in darkroom terms, how long the dodging tool blocked the light (Figure 7-29).

The first choice is how far from the pixel you wish the influence of the enhancement to extend. If there is a 1024 × 1024 pixel image, you could choose to influence an area 20–50 pixels to provide a pleasing smoothness of the tonal levels. If you were to apply this same algorithm to a page of 20 thumbnail images, the result would be reduced tonal shifts. The selection of this value is akin to the selection of a particular size of dodging tool and its distance from the paper used while printing a photographic print (Figure 7-30).

The software examines the average brightness at each point in the image. The brightness of pixels within, for instance, 16 pixels of the pixel

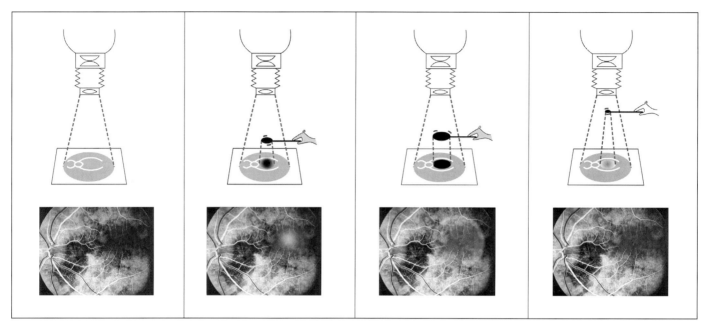

FIGURE 7-30
Computer software that is used for "burning and dodging" of our images is akin to the darkroom counterparts. The distance from the enlarger lens and the size of the dodging tool control the feathering of the effect and the relative size of the effect (think of the width of the image in pixels and select the tool size based on a percentage of the image size). The duration of how long the tool is in place is controlled in the software as a percentage.

A   B   C

FIGURE 7-31
Burning and dodging different sizes of images. **A.** Original image. **B.** Image enhancement performed on a contact-sheet–size image. Note the darker central foveal zone and the lighter choroidal flush visible in the branch of the supratemporal vein. The same enhancement routine was performed on the full-screen image **(C)** and shows less extreme changes in density in small areas.

at the top left-hand corner (pixel 0,0) is logged, averaged, and tabulated. The next pixel (0,1) is examined. The average brightness of pixels in the neighborhood of this pixel is also recorded. This is repeated for every pixel in the image.

Finally, the table of average values may be adjusted for the amount of increase or decrease in contrast that is desired. This will adjust the local contrast of the final image and is a measure of how severely the mask is applied. With these tools, an image's tonal information can be enhanced to show information that was not obvious (Figure 7-31).

SHARPENING

Increasing edge definition is a feature that would seem valuable, especially when trying to sharpen a blurry image. Sharpening routines define an edge by increasing the contrast when there is a small rapid shift in density. A mathematical model defines this edge. The computer then makes this transition from one tone to another in a fewer number of pixels. The result is an apparent increase in image sharpness. Sharpening actually reduces the information in the image while making the image more visually pleasing.[16] Sharpening should be used in moderation and with caution, as it is a destructive tool (Figure 7-32). Sharpening may be even more destructive on an original image without fine detail (see Figure 7-32, column C). This enhancement tool should be used last (just before viewing or printing) to prevent interference with other enhancement tools.

Check your system to see if the order of enhancing and sharpening makes a difference. Zoom in to check (Figure 7-33). Sharpening a destructively compressed image may yield unreliable results.

ZOOMING

Image enlargement by zooming the image on the monitor provides visualization of important details that might otherwise be difficult to see. A larger image will not provide additional pixels (unless your monitor shows you less resolution and detail than your image contains), but will make the image easier to see. This may be particularly helpful in the laser treatment area where the monitor may be placed more than a few feet from the physician. Scroll the window to position a zoomed image on the monitor so that the area of interest is centered. Printing the zoomed image is useful if you print with a lower-resolution printer.

IMAGE OVERLAYS

Computers can do things that are practically impossible in the darkroom. The image overlay is one example. These programs allow a lesion to be outlined on one image and to overlay that outline onto a second image. This can provide feedback to the physician about the relative position and size of the lesion and the area of treatment. To make sure that the image overlay is placed correctly on the image, the two images must be in identical registration. With this tool, you can manually trace the borders of a laser treatment area onto the FA image of a neovascular complex (Figure 7-34).[18]

With the manual method, the two images are usually presented next to each other on a single screen. You then alternately select similar points on each image to act as tie-points, points that will serve to register the images. If you are placing tie-points by the eye, make sure that you have enough magnification on the images so that you can place the points with certainty and precision. After between three to 10 pairs of tie-points are selected, the computer then offsets (moves), warps (stretches) and/or rotates one image to make a "best fit" with the other image. You then outline the lesion that you wish to be presented onto the other image.

In a semi-automated system, you assist the computer in finding similar tie-points on each image. The program then identifies the geometry of the points. These points are used to position the second image and to create the image overlay.

Selection of tie-points is important. Structures that are easy to see in both images are a prerequisite. Vessel crossings and bifurcations are usually the easiest structures for both a person and the computer to recognize. The best starting points are those located near the area of interest. Additional points should be selected throughout the image to give as much area between the tie-points. This will enhance the accuracy of the

FIGURE 7-32
The sharpening tool is used with increasing degrees. The original image is on the left. Three columns of images—full image and two sections of the image at ×8 magnification. The first column **(A)** shows the original with levels of sharpening (rows 2–6) and finally sharpening level 5 repeated two times (row 7). The second column of images **(B)** shows imaging sharpening on part of the image with fine detail. As sharpening is increased, it reaches a level at which the image becomes degraded. Imaging degradation appears earlier in an image that does not contain fine detail to be sharpened (column **C**). The image appears to be degraded at a lower level of sharpening.

A   **B**

C   **D**

FIGURE 7-33
Sharpening versus enhancement order. **A.** Original.
B. Enlargement of original. **C.** Image enhanced, then
sharpened. Note the accentuated highlights on the
larger vessels and a decrease in shadow detail.
D. Image sharpened, then enhanced. Note the
increased shadow detail.

warp and rotation. You can check the accuracy of alignment by using the overlay to check the branching area of vessels outside the area of interest.

If you are using automatic alignment software, it should be reliable enough to register with consistency even images of marginal quality. The software should have an option to display the number and location of tie-points that are matched on the two images. This information should be transferred to the print so that any future viewers of the image are informed of the quality of the overlay match. Running the local contrast enhancement tool on both images before starting the overlay function may increase the quality of the overlay "best fit."

MACULAR PHOTOCOAGULATION STUDY RINGS
Software that meets the Macular Photocoagulation Study protocol assists the clinician in judging the size of a lesion relative to the size standard of disk diameters.[18] This software permits circles of multiple disk diameter sizes to be placed over an area of subretinal neovascularization (SRNV). This allows the physician to measure the size of the lesion (Figure 7-35).

ADVANCED IMAGE ENHANCEMENT TOOLS
Advanced imaging tools as found in Adobe Photoshop are available with some imaging software.[19,20]

Using Histograms.   A histogram presents a graphical display based on an image of the number of pixels in each brightness level. Because most fundus or angiography images have a black background, there are many

FIGURE 7-34
Overlays are useful for evaluating treatment margins, following patient changes in time, and planning treatments such as photodynamic therapy and indocyanine green–guided laser. The user selects a starting point **(A)**, being careful to select centrally located points near the area of interest. The computer compares a vessel-enhanced version of the images **(B)**, rating the match from low to very high. The area a user traces on one image is transposed to the other **(C)**. Each image may then be enlarged **(D, E)** for careful scrutiny. The image with tracings should be saved to the patient's electronic record **(F)**.

Area1= 4.50   Spot Size=4304   GLD=3304

A   B

FIGURE 7-35
A. Macular photocoagulation study rings. A disk diameter ring overlying a subretinal neovascular complex (SRNV) assists the physician in assessing the size of an SRNV. Sizes can be adjusted: 1 disc diameter (1-DD), 1.5 DD, 2.0 DD, etc. **B.** Photodynamic therapy. Digital overlay technology simplifies calculation of the photo dynamic therapy treatment area. Typically, one outlines the lesion using a mouse to place dots, then selects calculate for a specific set of fundus camera parameters. The computer calculates the greatest linear dimension and suggests the treatment area. Calibrate each angle of view separately according to the manufacturer's instructions.

pixels with a value of 0 or very close to 0. This is displayed as a high spike on the left side (dark pixel side) of the histogram (Figure 7-36). On the histogram to the right of the black background will be the shadow detail of the image. In the middle of the histogram are the image mid-tones. The highlights are presented on the right side.

In a properly exposed image, there will be tones throughout the full range of values (see Figure 7-36A). If an image is underexposed, there will be more pixel values in the darker range (see Figure 7-36B). If an image is overexposed, it will be displayed in the lighter values (see Figure 7-36C). If tonal values are compressed or forced into a value of 0 or 255, then tonal information in the image will be lost forever.

Photoshop (v6.0+) permits these adjustments to be made in an adjustment layer. This maintains the original image and permits multiple adjustments without posterizing the original image. In Photoshop, the histogram tool permits you to move the shadow and highlight levels toward (don't go all the way) the ends of the graph. There is also an adjuster for mid-tone values that can push the mid-tones lighter or darker.

If an image is simply low in contrast, then its grayscale values may need to be expanded to display them with more contrast. In older programs, or if you do not use the adjustment layer, or you save the Photoshop file without the layer, readjusting an image a second time will force the gray levels into a new set of pixel values (Figure 7-37).

Using Photoshop "Curves."   After looking at the histogram to see the distribution of tonal values, you may wish to use Photoshop's "Curves" function to give you more control in making adjustments. Not only can you adjust the end points of the tonal scale and slide the midpoint brighter or darker, but you can adjust density points anywhere along the tonal scale.

The graphic for the "curves" function displays the brightness of original image along the x-axis and displays the resultant output on the y-axis.

FIGURE 7-36
Imaging tools in Photoshop. Original histogram (image **A** and image **D**) shows most of the pixel values are in the shadows. The black level of the background around the fundus image was adjusted to have the background set at approximately 12 (out of 256) levels above pure black. In the second histogram (**B**), sliders below the histogram are set to have the shadows represented slightly darker and the highlight detail to be represented much brighter. The final histogram (**C**) shows the expanded tonal information as seen in the adjusted image (**E**). The curves tool (**F**) permits the mid-tones to be adjusted. For this image, lightening the mid-tones permits the viewer to easily see more diagnostic information (**G**). Be aware that though this image has been made easier to view, there is—technically—no new information in the final image. Always expose the images for the maximum tonal information.

FIGURE 7-37
Multiple adjustments. The histogram reveals multiple adjustments to an image, creating a posterized image—an image without all of the values to make an image with continuous tones. The image becomes posterized (fewer levels of gray) and loses information.

FIGURE 7-38
Photoshop curves. **A.** Original image. **B.** Lifting the center-point of the curves tool will lighten the mid-tones without changing the levels at the white or black end of the tonal curve. Notice the shift of the histogram values of the mid-tones toward the white end of the scale. **C.** Bending the curve to a more vertical slope increases the contrast in the mid-tones. The histogram shows the spreading of the mid-tones over a wider range. **D.** Bending the curve to a more horizontal slope decreased the contrast in the mid-tones. The histogram shows the mid-tones pushed closer together in the center of the tonal range.

By adjusting this curve, one can control the resultant brightness for any brightness in the original image. This control permits you to vary the contrast of the mid-tones—either increasing the contrast or decreasing it (Figure 7-38). Photoshop permits the curves function to be performed in a layer—thus preserving the tonal information of the original image.[19,20]

Fundus Mapping.   Some software permits you to place the fundus images on a page or screen in the correct position relative to the original field of view in the patient's eye. This feature helps the clinician to understand, quickly, where each image was photographed. Some software takes images that were taken of overlapping fields and registers and overlaps the images when they are displayed. Additional compensation for brightness, contrast, color balance, and magnification are needed to make the resultant image seamless.

Manually mapping together the fundus images using Photoshop, as pioneered by Richard E. Hackel, CRA, and Marshall E. Tyler, CRA, FOPS,

FIGURE 7-39
FundusMap created by Marshall E. Tyler, CRA, FOPS, from twelve 50-degree fundus photographs. This image shows the postoperative result of a patient with a traumatic total retinal detachment. (Courtesy of C. Greven, MD.)

is a time-consuming process, but the rewards of their labors are unprecedented. These photo-illustrations are called *FundusMaps*. One of Mr. Hackel's images was used for the illustrations of standardized fundus fields used by the reading center. Figure 7-39 is Mr. Tyler's FundusMap of the postoperative appearance of a retinal detachment.

SAVING ENHANCED IMAGES
Once an image has been enhanced, you will want to save the results. The type and amount of enhancement the original image has undergone, or at a minimum, to have an indicator that the image is not an original but a modified image should be saved with the image file and indicated in the database.

SCRIPT FILES
A shorter way to save modified images is to record the program commands that are used to create the desired enhanced image. This file can be stored with the proof sheet (thumbnail) image of the enhanced image. This must also reference the original unmodified image file.

Advantages are threefold:

1. The script file is much smaller than a full image file and therefore transmits much faster over a network.
2. The original file is (and must be) kept unmodified.
3. Script files may be modified to change the outcome of the image appearance.

Disadvantages are twofold:

1. Imaging software is needed to re-create the modified image from the script file.
2. The re-creation process takes more time to re-create than it would take to display a saved image.

Image Archiving

The speed and frequency requirements of image access determine the technology appropriate for archiving your images. Just as patient charts that have not been accessed for many years may be stored in the basement, images that are not likely to be needed soon may be put onto a less expensive or less accessible medium for archiving. The creation of a CD-ROM can be a little problematic. When a CD is being "burned," there can be no interruption of the data (image files) that are being sent to it. If there is an interruption, then the disk becomes defective and none of the information that had been recorded on it will be available. There are two factors in maintaining this flow of data from the HD to the CD-ROM recorder (CD-R). The hard drive (HD), as well as the overall computer system, must be fast enough to keep up with the CD-R. Although the CD-Rs do have a file cache to hold a little information, basically the drive must be able to keep up with the writing process.

There will be data transfer delays whenever a file has been broken up and recorded onto different areas of the HD. This file breakup is called *file fragmentation*. Additionally, many small files need to be placed adjacent to each other on the HD to keep the data flowing quickly.

There are solutions for these problems. One option is to create, on a separate and clean HD partition, a single large file that will then be transferred all at one time to create the CD-ROM. The CD-R software (e.g., Easy CD-Pro by Adaptec, Milpitas, CA) assists you in this process. Because the data are now one continuous file, there will be no delays in data transfer.

Another transfer method is to simply copy all of the desired files onto a clean hard-drive partition. By moving the files and never erasing a file from this partition before making the CD-ROM "burn," there will not be any file fragmentation. With this method, one hopes to avoid any delays in the data transfer.

It is also important to only use HDs that use intelligent (and not thermal) recalibration. The intelligent recalibration feature ensures that the drive will not pause for self-diagnosis and align itself while data are being transferred.

Screen savers should not be used as they may create an interruption in the transfer of data when they start. Obviously, do not perform any other function on the computer while it is writing a CD-ROM. If the computer on which you are performing this CD-R function is on a network, don't forget to either take it off the network or make sure that any e-mail notices, for example, will not be posted to the machine and interrupt the flow of data.

As with any important file copying, make sure that you enable the software's "verify" function to ensure that the write was successful. Any interruption in the CD writing process can produce a "bad burn." Therefore, appending data to an existing CD could destroy the previous data.

Image Compression

There are both advantages and disadvantages to compressing (reducing the file size) of your image files. Obviously, they will take less space to store, and the ability to store more information in less space is important. The expense of image storage is not insignificant. A compressed file can be transferred more quickly over a computer network than an uncompressed file. Once the image has been transported, it must be uncompressed at the review station before you can view the image. It is faster to ship compressed images and to uncompress them after the transfer. Recent images that may require image enhancements should be kept online in an uncompressed format.

It is important to understand that if the size of the image file is made smaller, there is the possibility that information may also be reduced. Best of all are the loss-less compression programs, which make the file smaller and then bring it back to its original size without the loss of any information. The original and reconstructed files will be identical. Other file compression methods (e.g., lossey-compression) actually remove information from the file. This is not a desirable situation, but it does permit the file to be made much smaller. The degree to which the file is made smaller and the method of file compression determine the amount of image degradation.

PK-Ware's PK-Zip and Win-Zip (Brown Deer, WI) are commonly used compression programs. They work for all file types: images, text, spreadsheets, etc. How does a compression program make a file smaller without any loss of information? When characters, which may represent image densities, repeat themselves in the file structure, they are replaced in the compressed file with a code that states what the character is and the number of times the character is repeated. When the file is re-expanded, all of the original characters are re-created. The original and reconstructed files will be identical. Photoshop stores its images using a similar compression scheme so "PK-Zipping" a Photoshop image file will not reduce the size of the file.

One disadvantage of lossey-compressed images is that they are not identical to the original images. This may have medical-legal implications as well as being a practical diagnostic problem. Although they may be visually "close enough" for most clinical situations, there would be significant limitations to performing image enhancements and manipulations on a previously compressed image (Figure 7-40).

Photoshop produces quality compressed images by first analyzing the color pallet (the colors and tones used in the image) and creating a unique color pallet for each image. This system uses color efficiently to represent the original image. This maintains the highest quality image for any given file size. Photoshop can write image files into a JPG image file format. This method uses a scale of 1–10 or 1–12, depending on the version of Photoshop to indicate the amount of image compression desired. A compression level of "1" indicates the smallest image file and the greatest amount of compression. The largest number indicates the least amount of compression and a larger file (Figure 7-41).

It is important medically, legally, diagnostically, and photographically to maintain high-quality, uncompressed original images. There may be a time when images are so large that compressing them will not significantly reduce the image integrity. One way to manage the vast quantity of data that images comprise would be to have 3–6 months of patient data on the network at full resolution. Older records could be kept online in a compressed format to permit viewing without manipulation. If manipulation were to be required of an older image, then the original archive disk could be manually loaded onto the network to give access to the uncompressed file.

PRINTING: THE HARD COPY

Printing makes the digital information contained in a computer file available for interpretation without computer hardware. The digital computer images are put onto paper or transparencies for the patient's chart or to be sent to the referring physician, or both. These copies can be used to indicate diagnostic notes or to accompany interpretation of the FA. Keep in mind that the original image is the digital file, and the print is only a representative copy. Because the tonal range of the monitor is greater than the print, local-area contrast expansion tools assist in creating a printed image of the best quality.

FIGURE 7-40
Image compression (destructive). Compressed images may not tolerate simple image enhancement techniques. **A.** Original with close-up. **B-1.** Image sharpened. **B-2.** Image compressed and decompressed. **C-1.** Image compressed and decompressed, and then sharpened **(C-2)**. Notice how detail of the fine perifoveal vascularization does not tolerate image enhancement after an image has been compressed.

Although prints are convenient, quality interpretation or treatment, or both, of the patient should be performed only from the computer monitor image. Because the monitor is a light source unto itself, the available dynamic range is greater than that of a (reflective) print. The information contained in even a high-quality print conveys less tonal information than a computer monitor. This is analogous to directly reading the film negatives on a FA study or reading the positives: The negatives always contain more information. Also, the ability to enhance and zoom an image permits the highest quality of diagnostic information to be shown.

Prints from office-type laser printers may be an extremely cost-effective "chart copy" of the photograph. However, it is important that these lower-quality images not be used for diagnosis or treatment; they should be used for reference only. For responsible treatment, a computer for image review must always be accessible in the laser suite.

A   B   C

FIGURE 7-41
Levels of JPG (Joint Photographic Group) file compression affect the clarity of the image. The magnified section of a fluorescein image **(A)** is shown with different levels of compression. JPGed to level "10" **(B)** shows little degradation of image quality, whereas shrinking the file size to only one-fourth the size of the previous image, JPG compression level "0," shows a greatly compromised image **(C)**.

Although stacks of full image prints are impressive, sometimes the ability to put multiple images onto one sheet of paper may be not only more economical but also more convenient. The choice of the number of images to be printed on the paper is related to the final image size and the printer resolution. Additional selection factors include the cost of the print material, storage costs, ease of handling (if there are fewer sheets of paper), and, most important, size and printer resolution of the final image. Considering that there is a 56% increase in image area from the 16-up (16 images to the page) to the 9-up page, I find the 9-up printing format to be very useful. Nine images are often adequate to represent both eyes of most studies. Also useful are 4-up images, one for each eye, which give greater magnification, but obviously use twice the paper as a single 9-up set of images (see Figure 7-14).

Some software even permits an "enlarged version" by magnifying the image while trimming the edges of the circular fundus image. The ability to magnify and re-center images is important, particularly for stereo imaging (see Figure 3-25). The image area is typically less than the full size of the paper, so that patient data can be printed on the paper as well. In addition to the desired images, database information, such as patient name, number, visit date, physician name, and photographer's name will make the print more useful. Examine how your clinic functions when determining which database fields are to be included on the print.

Manufacturers should permit you to print the database information that you want. Some information is from data that is the same for all prints (e.g., the name of the institution). Other information is taken from the database and is unique to that patient (e.g., the patient's name). Some databases permit the fields to be changed for each patient visit or photography session (e.g., the diagnosis for different sessions can change from macular degeneration to SRNV to status post-laser treatment with an overlaid image). Be cautious when a manufacturer tells you that the physician's name can be put on the print if what you really need is for the physician's name for that patient visit to be on the print. Having the correct physician name on the prints may make it easy to sort and deliver the prints, and recording the diagnosis for each session permits accurate photographic records.

DISTRIBUTING VIA A NETWORK

When there are many studies to be reviewed, LAN can be set-up to facilitate image distribution. The LAN can use computer programs from the ophthalmic imaging company or the ophthalmology department may choose to distribute the images via either specialized ophthalmic software or generic software. This task should be executed by professional computer network personnel (Figure 7-42).

Presentation Output: Onscreen Slide Shows and Web Pages

With the creation of more digital images, using these images for presentations and publication is becoming routine. PowerPoint presentations, web pages, and desktop publishing on both the intranet and Internet all require expertise in handling digital images.[21]

Images that are to be used for presentations in PowerPoint slide shows and in web pages need to be made "lean-and-mean"—or, photographically speaking, "small-and-quick" so that that the images load quickly. Balancing the amount of detail and file size is challenging. Let's look at the compromises that we will need to make.[21]

As with all resolution questions, we first start with the output device and then work backward to calculate the appropriate image size. In this case, we are looking at computer screen resolution. There is quite a range of possibilities. Early computers started at video resolution and then moved up to 640×480. It is assumed that now a computer will have at least 1024 pixels in the horizontal dimension. Even laptop computers can have 1024 or 1280 pixel-wide screens. Desktop computers will run the range from 1024, 1280, to even 1600 horizontal pixels. Computer projectors will have 1024 or perhaps 1280 horizontal pixels. Film recorders will be far beyond the typical computer resolutions, going from 2048 to 4096 pixels for the width of a 35-mm slide.

If you are creating full-screen images, think about converting your images down to 1024 pixels-wide. Photoshop is the most widely used program for image enhancement and manipulation. By selecting the image and from the menu the following: Image, Image Size, and then clicking on both Constrain Proportions and Resample Image, you may modify the size of the image—after selecting Pixels in the upper part of the dialogue box, enter the new width of the image. Then press OK to resize the image. The image will be subjected to the least amount of image interpolation if you can select a resizing parameter at an even division of the pixel count (e.g., $1024/2 = 512$ pixels, $1024/4 = 256$ pixels). If the original image has an odd number of pixels in either dimension, this can be corrected by either adding or removing a single row of pixels, thus creating an even number of pixels. This is done in Photoshop with the Canvas Size command. Place the image in one corner (within this command) to force the deleted (or additional) row of pixels to be placed on one side of the image.

Image compression is the next consideration, once the image is correctly sized. Image compression will impact the file size of the image as well as contribute to loss of detail. A color image of 1024×768 pixels will be 2,359,296 bytes ($1024 \times 768 \times 3$ color layers). Reducing the file to 512 pixels wide will reduce the file to one-fourth the size (589,824 bytes). This is still more than $1/2$ MB. If the image is to be inserted into a PowerPoint slide with a title, this is a good resolution for the image. Adding JPG compression when saving the file will reduce the color palette, the number of colors used in the image, and wasted image file space by compressing the information required to store redundant pixels. Additionally, with greater compression, fine details are lost. The

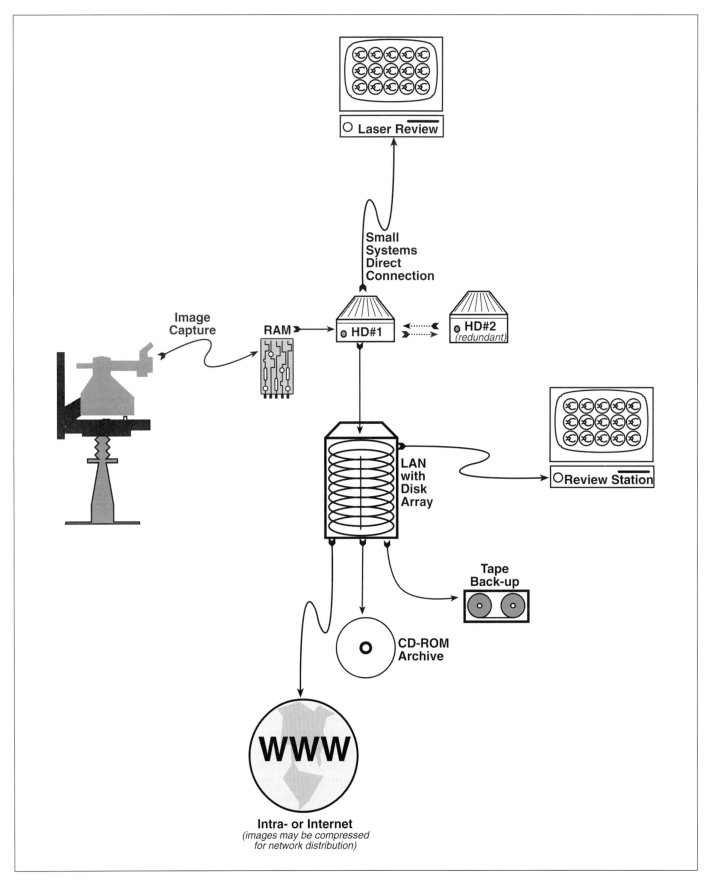

FIGURE 7-42
The method of and features of the interconnection of computer components is paramount in the distribution of images beyond the camera room. (CD-ROM = compact-disk–read only memory; HD = hard drive; RAM = random access memory.)

amount of lost information you can tolerate depends on the purpose of the image. If it is only to stay on the screen for a few seconds in a PowerPoint presentation, then it could be compressed to, perhaps, less than 100k. This would save storage space and image loading time when viewing the presentation. I find that shooting for a file size of 250k is a reasonable compromise for large-screen images that you use in PowerPoint presentations.

When setting the images for use in PowerPoint you should select the Resolution (pixels/inch) setting at 72 or 150. This sizes the image on the screen when you insert the picture from file in PowerPoint to a reasonable size. To change the image size in PowerPoint, grab the corner of the image with your mouse cursor and drag it to the desired position. Do not drag the side handles unless you wish to change the aspect ratio (width to height) of the image. Make sure that you selected the desired Page Set-up (On-screen show, 35-mm Slides, etc.) before you import images. If you redo the Page Set-up after you insert images, the aspect ratio of all of the slides and, therefore, images will also be modified.

Web page images are often smaller. I find that an image of 256-pixel width gives reasonable image detail, but is low enough image resolution to discourage image theft. JPGing the image to an image size of 30–60k will provide fast image loading and reasonable image clarity. Thumbnail images at 64 pixel width in the GIF image format makes the image files size at 2–3k. Reducing the bit depth to 4- or 5-bit color can create extra contrast and simplification of the image as well as smaller images. To create the GIF images in Photoshop, you first need to change the image mode to index color.

Equipment Selection

Digital ophthalmic imaging systems are expensive. Before you purchase one, we suggest you think about how your system is to be used in the clinic. Ask yourself purchasing questions about the entire system (Table 7-9).

Image quality is the prime concern of the retinologist as well as the photographer. Before choosing a digital ophthalmic imaging system, evaluate the image sharpness, both central and peripheral, as well as the tonal information, remembering that the manufacturers' promotional material will provide only the highest-grade images from the best patients. Ask other photographers about their experiences with the system you are considering, which fundus camera is used, and how it performs on patients with poor media.

Hardware

The digital camera is central to the control of image quality that you will receive from your system. Imaging qualities that will be important to your clinical practice include exposure latitude, image saturation thresholds, tonal information (bit-depth), and resolution.

Computers—their processor speed, amount of RAM, size of HD, video card, and monitor specifications will be specified by the imaging system's manufacturer. If you also plan to use Photoshop on the system, allow 10–20 MB of RAM for the OS plus three to six times the RAM of the largest image on which you plan to work. U.S. Food and Drug Administration regulations may not permit other software to be loaded onto diagnostic equipment, so don't be surprised to find that the manufacturer balks at your desire to multi-task your new computer.

Table 7-9. Choosing a Digital Angiography System

Follow these 10 steps when evaluating a new digital system.

1. Perform a needs assessment.
   Consult with both practitioners and photographers.
   Characterize your practice and your patient population.
   Sample questions:
   Will you need ICG?
   Will you need to see the FAZ on a regular basis?
   Will users need computer training?
   Telemedicine opportunities?
   Color digital images?

2. Is your staff computer literate?
   Will your photographer need additional technical training?
   Will your practitioners read angiograms from the monitor?
   Other training issues?

3. Is new system compatible with your current system/network?
   File size/network speed issues
   Electronic medical records integration?
   Security?
   Multiple offices?
   Network integration issues?

4. Evaluate the hardware aspects of each system.
   Bit depth: 8/10/12?
   Pixel resolution? 2048 vs.1024 vs. 640 vs. 512 vs. 256.
   Digital color imaging of acceptable quality?
   ICG capable?
   Fundus camera fields of view?
   Fundus camera based vs. SLO (still versus motion).
   Extra wide angle?
   Look at images from multiple patients to evaluate sharpness, contrast, and resolution.
   Note: Evaluate the imaging aspects of the fundus camera separately from the digital system!

5. Evaluate the software aspects of each system.
   Ease of use?
   Macros?
   Overlay: convenient and accurate?
   Archive media? (see below)
   How do image manipulation controls change the picture? How easy is it to manipulate the images? Are the original or the manipulated images saved in the patient record?
   Software stability and compatibility with other standard software
   DICOM compliant?

6. Fundus camera?
   Your current fundus camera
   Modifications needed?
   Will this save money?
   Is it ICG capable?
   A new fundus camera
   Image quality at each angle of view?
   What is the photographers' choice?
   Is it ICG capable?

7. Archive media?
   Proprietary vs. generic?
   Cost/MB?
   Compression quality?
   Life span?

8. Printer?
   Image quality?
   Cost/print (paper and ink and ribbons)
   Film recorder?

9. Cost?
   Buy/lease?
   Warranty?
   Payback?

10. Purchase your digital imaging system!

DICOM = Digital Imaging and Communications in Medicine; FAZ = foveal avascular zone; ICG = indocyanine green; MB = megabyte; SLO = scanning laser ophthalmoscope.

Of Mice and Photographers

In working with images on computers, it is mandatory to use some type of pointing device. The most commonly used one is the computer mouse. This is a bar-of-soap-sized device that is held under the hand, palm down, and moved over a flat surface. There are one or more buttons on the top of the mouse so positioned that they can be pressed by the fingers. There is usually a wire connecting the computer and the mouse—hence the name, as the wire looks like a mouse's tail. Inside the mouse is a small ball, which is slightly exposed on the lower side of the mouse. This ball rolls on the desktop and sends rotation information to the computer. You see the results of this movement with the display of an arrow or cross-hairs on the computer monitor screen. With the mouse you can point at something on the screen and tell the computer that you wish to do something by pressing the appropriate mouse button. The computer can also understand the rapid pressing of a button twice as a request different from that made when the button is slowly pressed twice.

Another pointing device is a trackball. This is simply mouse technology that is turned upside down and lets you move the exposed ball with your thumb, while you use your fingers to press buttons.

Tablets use a mouse-like device that does not have a positioning ball but has a physical cross-hair on a plastic window. The tablet can sense where the cross-hair is. Tablets can also use a pencil-like pointer.

A light pen is a pencil-like light sensor that can recognize the spot on the monitor screen to which you are pointing. It has a switch built into the tip that, when pressed onto the screen, tells the computer that you wish to select the choice at which you pointed.

Touch screens are special monitors with built-in sensors that know where a finger is in contact with the screen. Touch screens do not have the precision of other pointing devices.

Consider the throughput of angiographic images—how fast can you take how many images. Beware of saving money by purchasing an under-powered system.

Obviously, the optical components are also important. See Chapter 2 for guidelines on selecting a fundus camera. In analyzing the optical interface between the fundus camera and the digital camera, review the image quality for sharpness and evenness of illumination.

Monochrome monitors are typically sharper than color monitors. Check the image for fine detail in the macula. Don't forget that the time data that is contained within an image on these small images can be difficult to read on a poor monitor. Typical presentation of contact sheets on a 20-in. monitor is four rows of images by five columns of images. Some manufacturers use display boards that create a square display that, of course, would not use the entire horizontal width of the monitor. Their boards typically display only 16 images.

An uninterruptable power supply (UPS) keeps the digital camera and the computer system powered in the event of an electrical power failure. The UPS has a battery strong enough to keep the computer running for 5–10 minutes if the main power goes off. Images in the RAM are volatile; thus, if the RAM loses power, the images will be lost. With a UPS, there is enough time for you to copy the images from the computer RAM onto the HD. Without a UPS, a power outage of less than a second would cause a loss of all the recently acquired images and would also require the image acquisition program to be reloaded from the HD before additional images could be exposed. The UPS is usually left plugged into the wall power outlet so that the internal battery remains charged and ready for use. If the power remains off, then the problems of taking additional frames are the same as those of conventional photography, as without power—lots of it—the camera flash cannot operate.

Evaluate the imaging software by attempting some of the tasks on the checklist in Table 7-10. Talk with other photographers who use digital systems. Be wary of photographers who have worked on, or even looked at, only one manufacturer's system. Remember the software needs to be a good tool—logical, user friendly, and provide the tools and functions unique to our work.

The user interface (fancy words for the software you must use to get the system to work) is the key to productivity. Your software should give you little interference in getting the images to assist the physician with high-quality diagnostic information. The interface should be logical and should make it convenient to complete frequently performed tasks. Menus should not require you to go through more than two levels to access these sections of the program. Drop-down menus make it easy to look at most of the choices. The program should respond to both mouse and keyboard for every command—see sidebar Of Mice and Photographers.

Good computer software should be intuitive and have clear menus. It is important to understand the strengths and weaknesses of the different systems you are considering. The menu is the road map to the imaging system's computer program. It will become either your friend and assistant or your antagonist and downfall. Pick your imaging system only after carefully analyzing its software.

Evaluate the software by considering the specific jobs that need to be accomplished. With some of the early imaging software, one could accomplish a task but it required multiple steps and was not intuitive. One could have to memorize arcane terms and remember the purpose of function keys without references even being included on the menu. Make sure that the system you choose does not have these kinds of problems.

Table 7-10. Imaging Software Task Check List

System startup
    Startup and monitor calibration.
    Check date and time.
    Enter patient information. Check for information fields specific to your practice.
Image acquisition
    What is the resolution of captured image?
    Is resolution stored?
Image enhancement
    Is there contrast stretching capability?
    Is there sharpening capability?
    Is there contrast enhancement (auto-burn and dodging)?
    Can enhanced images be saved to the disk?
    What imaging tools are available? Overlay, zoom, macular photocoagulation study rings, etc.?
Printing
    What are the options for image layouts on a page?
    Is adequate tonality recorded on the print?
    Does tonality match the screen?
    Is full-image resolution maintained to the printer?
    Are the prints archivable?
    What is the cost of the printer and prints?
Storage and archiving
    Does software ensure that images are not deleted without first archiving them?
    Does software ensure that duplicate images are not created (unless you want them)?
    What do the media cost?
    What is the speed of the media, writing, and reading?
    For image retrieval, which fields can you look up?
Other considerations
    Is there slidemaking capability?
    Can the image file be exported to other computer programs?
    Can you export the patient database?
    Is the UL-544 listed? Or is there a letter from manufacturer stating that the system is built to meet or exceed the UL-544 standard? In
        part, the standard requires that hospital grade cord caps (plugs) be used and that the total ungrounded ground leakage be less
        than 100 μA (microampere).
    Is the equipment layout clean and neat?
    Will it fit into your room?
    Are two phone lines available (one for the computer-modem, and one for the voice)?
    Are the air conditioning and air flow adequate to condition the space into which this heat-producing equipment is going?
    Are there two separate power circuits available for the imaging system with a computer and the fundus camera power supply?
    Is the equipment energy efficient? Do the computer and the monitors go into a sleep mode to save electrical energy when they are
        not being used? Can I set the time of the sleep mode so that it will not interfere with angiography?

Attention should be paid to reviewing sample ICG-angiogram late images to ensure that the system has adequate flash power, optics, and camera sensitivity images of these late phases. This also applies to SLO systems.

Patient Database

The date and time should be automatically entered from the computer's internal clock. It is good to have the date displayed so that you can check that the computer's internal clock and calendar are accurate.

Entering data should be simple and make sense. The database should help you fill in the blank fields (e.g., diagnosis) by making "suggestions" from an alphabetical list of possible diagnoses. The same system could be used for patient names, unit numbers, physician names, etc. This will not only save time, but also increase the accuracy of the entries.

The types of information that a photographer wants to enter into the database record may include the database fields (Table 7-11). Make sure that the diagnosis and the physicians can be changed to match a changing diagnosis on subsequent studies if that is important for your practice. Additional capability could include the automatic recording of eye, field of view, filters, flash output, digital camera gain, and so forth.

Table 7-11. Database Field List with Field Lengths

11	Patient identification number
11	Social Security number (automatically placing dashes)
20	Last name (Patient)
20	First name (Patient)
15	Middle name (Patient)
6	Date of birth (DOB)
1	Sex
1	Race
15	Diagnosis (primary); *ICD-9*
15	Diagnosis (secondary); *ICD-9*
15	Diagnosis (systemic disease)
10	Study (drug)
6	Date of procedure
5	Type of procedure: FA, ICG angiography, monochromatic, color, NFL
15	Physician (staff)
15	Physician (resident/fellow)
15	Physician (referring)
15	Referring source (group/practice name)
15	Photographer
1	Teaching quality T/F
72–254	Memo

ICD-9 = *International Classification of Diseases, Ninth Revision;* FA = fluorescein angiography; ICG = indocyanine green; NFL = nerve fiber layer; T/F = true/false.

Table 7-12. Factors to Consider When Transitioning to Digital

Economic factors
Time factors
Test availability (e.g., indocyanine green angiography)
New office, consider instead of a darkroom
You want the newest technology
Networking of images
Telemedicine (remote clinics, Internet access)
Patient convenience and education
Marketing

Each field should be long enough to ensure that the data your practice needs are sufficient to retrieve the patient's record. Keep in mind that this database may be the only computer database you have for retrieving patients or their images, or both, for teaching purposes, so discuss this with potential vendors before you purchase, buying only if the system will meet your needs. Another question to ask is whether the database can be used for other non-angiographic digital images you may acquire (e.g., a hand-held digital camera or even your color film fundus images).

Cost Considerations

Technical equipment continues to be more sophisticated and powerful, although the prices have become more competitive. The original purchase price is only one of the factors in deciding if and when to "go digital" (Table 7-12). The (electronic) job functions in the photography area may be different, but the desired results are the same—quality images in a timely fashion. The photographer in the digital world typically edits, enhances, and prints his or her own images.

Cost considerations can be divided into categories: initial costs and training, yearly costs, and operating and updating expenses. The initial cost is the most obvious. Systems may include a fundus camera, or the digital system may be adaptable to your existing fundus camera. Systems can come as a bundled package complete with a digital camera, the computer system (computer, imaging board, monitors, mass storage for images, and network connection), software, and specialized hardware (optical and computer interface), as well as a printer. There is usually an image review station in the laser suite.

Training by the vendor is important to quality and productivity, so do not ignore the need for, and the cost of, personnel training. Make sure that the training program will provide a specified amount of training at a time when the photographers are available. Installation time should not be included in the promised training time. One schedule might be to spend an evening learning about the system and its software before training with patients on another day.

Yearly costs include two major areas: the cost of the physical space for the equipment and depreciation of the software and hardware portions of the system. Your space costs may be less with an electronic system because you will not need to maintain the space for a darkroom. Computer equipment should be depreciated in 3–5 years. Software upgrades will help keep your system and photographers running at peak performance and capability. Hardware keeps getting better and will always need updating to provide the patients with access to the current imaging technology. Do not expect your digital system to be a one-time capital expense, but rather a system that will need regular upgrades.

Per-patient costs consist of the usual angiography supplies plus the cost of the archiving media (CD-ROMs) and the cost of reference prints for the patient chart and perhaps the referring physician. Color fundus and stereo images should be considered in the number and size of the images that are to be printed. Networking available images could reduce printing costs but will increase the time needs and the cost of a network server (computer). Analysis of your patient workload will assist you in selecting printers and storage or archiving methods for your imaging system.

Scanning Laser Ophthalmoscopes

Thomas M. Clark

Introduction

This section begins with an overview of the history of the scanning laser ophthalmoscope (SLO), then continues with a description of instrumentation and technique.

In the early 1970s, Yuhasz[9] demonstrated a technique in which he used video FA with fundus cameras of the time. This extended the work pioneered by Dallow[2] and van Heuven et al.[3] by showing a more dynamic view of the entire flow of dye. The quality of the images he achieved were fair, but the high illumination level required for good images didn't allow this technique to be commercially viable until the early 1980s.[22] At that time, electronic fundus camera systems adopted the more sensitive class of silicon CCD imaging tubes. In addition, CCDs used in conjunction with newly developed video frame grabbers allowed for digitized color and fluorescein images, which could be readily viewed, stored, and manipulated by computers.

In 1980, Robert Webb, PhD, et al. described the Flying Spot TV Ophthalmoscope, and illustrated for the first time a fluorescein angiogram, imaged from a laser scanned across the retina.[23] Webb's intent was to develop a system that would allow for extreme low-light imaging of the ocular fundus. In conventional fundus cameras, the retina is illuminated with a large amount of light through a dilated pupil. The imaged light

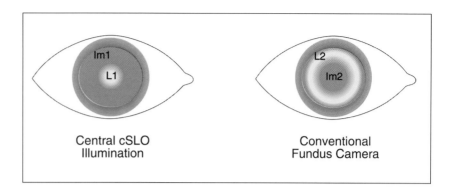

Central cSLO
Illumination

Conventional
Fundus Camera

FIGURE 7-43
The reallocation of the imaging pupils. On the left is the central illumination (L1) of a confocal scanning laser ophthalmoscope (cSLO) with the image being formed from the larger area (Im1) outside of the illumination beam. On the right is a fundus camera illumination with the familiar doughnut ring illumination (L2) and image being formed from the smaller area inside the ring (Im2).

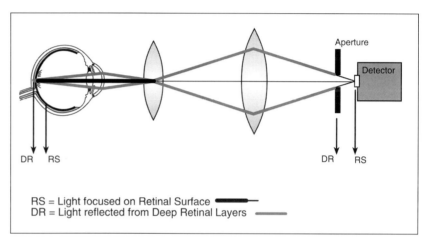

RS = Light focused on Retinal Surface
DR = Light reflected from Deep Retinal Layers

FIGURE 7-44
A confocal aperture placed in front of the detector will pass light that is focused on the retinal surface while blocking light that is scattered from structures in the deeper retinal layers.

returning to the film or video camera must pass through a small central area. Webb realized he could use a 20 µW focused laser beam and scanning mirrors to project a 20 µm spot on the fundus through the center 0.9 mm of the pupil, thereby utilizing the remaining area to collect the light. This reallocation of the imaging pupils would greatly increase collection efficiency (Figure 7-43).[24,25]

By 1981, the Scanning Laser Ophthalmoscope (SLO) was being used as a clinical research tool for FA. The quantity of light necessary for dye fluorescence was ~1% of the light used by fundus cameras of the time, depth of field was greatly extended, and it required 90% less dye for successful FA.[25] One year later in 1982, Martin A. Mainster, MD, working with Robert Flower, described enhancements to their SLO and demonstrated additional clinical applications. Because the laser beam could be modulated to project images, Mainster used it for retinal function testing of scotomas, to test visual acuity of the fovea, and also Amsler grid measurements.[25]

In 1987, Webb described the confocal SLO (cSLO). The modification consisted of placing an aperture at the retinal conjugate in front of the photo multiplier, which was a 1 mm, avalanche diode with internal amplification. This aperture had the effect of greatly enhancing the contrast of the retinal image by reducing light scatter from other ocular structures (Figure 7-44). The aperture stop was adjustable to allow for three types of views. Used in conjunction with different wavelength lasers, the smallest aperture gave a tightly confocal view with the highest contrast whereas the large aperture allowed for scattered light to reach the detector reducing the contrast and allowing for a better differentiation of pigmented structures (Figures 7-45 and 7-46). Finally, a central occluding stop provided a Tyndall view.[23,24,26–28]

In 1986, Heidelberg Instruments (HI) GmbH of West Germany introduced the first commercially available SLO for ophthalmic use. It was a

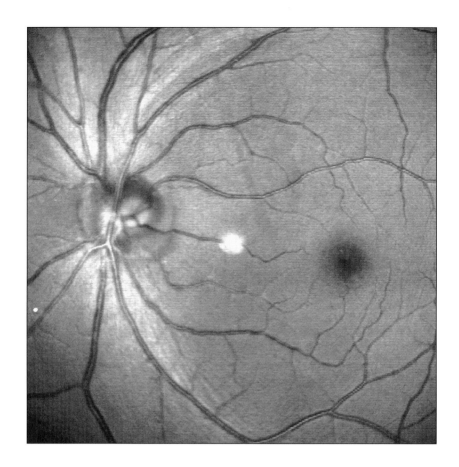

FIGURE 7-45
A moderately tight confocal red-free 514-nm image illustrating good contrast and separation of the nerve fiber layer.

A   B

FIGURE 7-46
Compare the posterior pole of a 514-nm red-free image **(A)**, with that of an 830-nm infrared reflectance image **(B)**, both utilizing the same size confocal aperture. Notice the deeper choroidal layers showing through the blood and an apparent deep circular retinal pigment epithelium defect not seen in the standard red-free image.

topographic scanning laser system, which illustrated dimensional structures by creating three-dimensional wire frame constructs. The device received scientific acclaim but failed commercially for multiple reasons: the high cost of $200,000, the large size, and, speaking from personal experience, the difficulty in use. The company closed their ophthalmic instruments division in 1990, and later that year sold their research equipment and software rights to one of two separate partnerships, comprised of researchers and scientists from the original project, who would go on to form their own independent companies.[29,30]

There are now several devices that use SLO technology within the eye. Current ophthalmic applications include the measurement of fluorescence of fluorescein and ICG dye, topography and tomography of struc-

FIGURE 7-47
This 10-degree fluorescein angiogram clearly shows the foveal avascular zone with even the finest capillaries visible. When viewed as a movie, the image twinkles as the fluorescein-stained cells can be seen coursing through the veins (*arrow*).

tures, the rate of blood flow within vessels, the degree of polarimetry exhibited by the nerve fiber bundle, and for microperimetry of scotomas and visual function. Additionally, development is under way to apply this technology to optical coherence tomography scanners.

In 1989, Scheider and Schroedel published an article entitled "High Resolution Indocyanine Green Angiography With a Scanning Laser Ophthalmoscope."[31] The fundus has a reflectance of 5%, and ICG has a low fluorescence of only 4% as compared to sodium fluorescein. It previously required 200 mW/cm^2 illumination to achieve a fair quality image with the current camera systems. However, with the use of an SLO equipped with a 780-nm laser diode running at 2.4 mW/cm^2 and the appropriate 820-nm barrier filter, a high-resolution and moderately high-contrast set of ICG images were achieved. In the years to follow, filtration and resolution improved.

In 1991, Heidelberg Engineering Inc. (HE), Carlsbad, California, was formed and introduced the HRT Heidelberg Retinal Tomograph, which was the first commercially available SLO for routine glaucoma examinations.[32]

In 1992, the second partnership formed Laser Diagnostic Technologies (LDT), San Diego, California. They would demonstrate their first devices at the 1992 American Academy of Ophthalmology meeting in Dallas, Texas. These included the TopSS Topographic Scanning System and the NFA Nerve Fiber Analyzer.[33]

From that point on to the present day, SLOs (in conjunction with digital fundus cameras) refined ICG-A understanding much as the fundus cameras of the 1960s defined FAs. We have seen improvements on resolution, sensitivity, and storage options, and an expanded understanding of the eye's diseases and methods of treatment. Figures 7-47 and 7-48 are examples of the current state of the art in SLO angiography.

FIGURE 7-48
In this case of two foveal/juxtafoveal membranes, a fluorescein angiogram does not provide clear information for laser treatment **(A, B, C)**. However, the arterial phase **(D)**, of the indocyanine green angiogram clearly show several ascending feeder vessels, which can be differentiated from the choroidal veins in the venous phase **(E)**. In the arterial view **(D)** and the late phase **(F)** at least two plaques are seen.

Current Instrumentation

There have been six manufacturers to commercially market some form of SLO since 1980: HI (LTS), Rodenstock Instruments (Rodenstock SLO 101), HE (HRT, Heidelberg Retinal Angiograph [HRA], HRF, HRII), LDT (TopSS, GDx-NFA, AngioScan, GDx Access), Carl Zeiss (SM 30-4024), and Optos (Panoramic 200).[26,28,32–34]

Of the six companies, only three currently produce SLO instruments. HI was the first manufacturer to release its unit in 1986. The LTS was not an angiographic device, and they closed the ophthalmic division in 1990. Rodenstock released their SLO 101 unit around 1988, and, as of this writing, they are still providing service to its original devices. No new instruments are currently being produced, but the company is reportedly working on a totally new model with an undetermined release date.[35] Carl Zeiss, now Zeiss Humphrey Systems, produced several prototypes and marketed their device in the late 1990s. Zeiss is currently producing the Optical Coherence Tomography Scanner, which may replace angiography for some retinal pathologies.[36] Optos is not an angiographic system, but rather an ultra-wide 200-degree angle-of-view system leased to individuals and organizations as an ophthalmic screening device.[34]

HE and LDT have several systems, including some that perform optic nerve head analysis, though in completely different ways. In addition, HE offers the HRF, which is a scanning laser Doppler flowmetry system that measures blood flow through specific sights on the retina. Both com-

Scanning Laser Ophthalmoscope Detection Devices

The photomultiplier tube and avalanche photodiode are similar low-light gathering devices. They differ in the size of their light-sensitive aperture, spectral sensitivity, operating voltage, and amplification scheme.

The photomultiplier is a zigzag-shaped cylindrical tube on which one end is coated a photoabsorbing semiconductor. This light-sensitive surface measures up to 1 in. and is most sensitive in the visible light spectrum. The operating voltage is approximately 1,000 volts, and the amplification scheme is as follows:

As photons fall on the semiconductor surface, an electron charge is emitted inside the tube and is directed to the first amplifying dynode. This amplifying dynode then emits several more electrons in response, which fall on the subsequent dynode and so on, each time multiplying the numbers of electrons, which fall on the next dynode. The potential total amplification may reach 1,000,000 with nine dynodes customarily being used.

The avalanche photodiode by contrast is a small solid-state diode chip with a photoabsorbing semiconductor light aperture of approximately 0.5 mm and is sensitive into the non-visible light spectrum. The operating voltage is approximately 5 volts, and its amplification scheme is based on a process called *impact ionization* and works as follows:

As photons fall on the semiconductor surface, an electron is emitted into an electrical field with a standing potential of electrons. As the emitted electron collides with adjacent electrons, they form hole-electron pairs, which in turn collide with other electrons forming more hole-electron pairs, building up a charge until an avalanche voltage is reached. As the name implies one electron affecting others creates an avalanche of electrons or a voltage.

FIGURE 7-49

Diagram of a basic confocal scanning laser ophthalmoscope set-up, loosely based on the Heidelberg Engineering, Inc. (Carlsbad, CA) and Laser Diagnostic Technologies (San Diego, CA) devices. (AD = analog digital converter; BS = beam splitter; CD-ROM = compact-disk–read only memory; CPU = central processing unit; HD = hard drive; PBS = polarized beam splitter; QWP = quarter wave plate.)

panies also produce devices to perform angiography. HE makes the HRA that performs simultaneous FA and ICG-A. LDT makes the AngioScan that performs only ICG-A while simultaneously recording a retinal reflectance image.[29,32,33]

Understanding the Scanning Laser Ophthalmoscope Mechanism

In the simplest sense, all SLOs operate by focusing a laser to one spot on the retina. As this beam is scanned across the retina, the reflected or emitted light travels back though the optics, is separated from the incident beam, and recorded on a light detector. Scanning is achieved either by a set of dual galvanometric mirrors or by a combination of a rotating polygon mirror and a single galvanometric mirror. The detection devices could be either a photomultiplier tube or an avalanche photodiode (see sidebar Scanning Laser Ophthalmoscope Detection Devices).

The Rodenstock SLO 101 used the spinning polygon mirror system for the scan and a photo-multiplier tube as the detector. It had a standard 20-degree and 40-degree imaging field with a 30-degree and 60-degree option. The device produced a video signal that was recorded on tape.[28,35]

The Heidelberg HRA and LDT AngioScan are similar in size and operation and use much of the same basic type of parts. These devices incorporate dual galvanometric mirrors, polarized light, and PhotoDiodes. A basic illustration of how these systems work in the angiographic mode is illustrated in Figure 7-49.

First, light is emitted from a laser source (L1, L2) and passes through a polarizing beam splitter. This beam splitter redirects light from the different wavelength lasers, polarizes it, and places it on the same optical path to the second beam splitter (BS). BS directs the light to a scanning unit (SU) that converts the light into a horizontal and vertical scanning beam. As the light leaves the SU, it is projected through a set of lenses (LN1) that modify the size of the beam to an entrance pupil from 1–3 mm. The light that enters the eye through the cornea and crystalline lens is focused to a spot in the range of 10–35 µm on the retina.

If this light is in the range of either 488 nm (FA) or 795 nm (ICG-A), it will excite dye that is present in the eye. The emitted light will pass back through the pupil to the SU and a quarter wave plate, where it will be isolated from the incident beam. This split-off excited light will be directed through BS and SU for a second time, pass through a barrier filter and be focused through another set of lenses (LN2) to an avalanche diode. The actual positions of these optical devices differ from one manufacturer to the other, but the principle holds true. If the system is set up for confocal scanning, a light-stopping pinhole aperture will be placed at the retinal conjugate in front of the diode, thereby blocking scattered non-image light.

The resulting signal is processed with a personal computer, and a dot-for-pixel representation appears on the monitor. A single laser image at a scan rate of 256×256 or 512×512 spots make up an image of more than 65,000 or 262,000 pixels of 256 individual light values. This is said to have 256 or 512 lines of resolution at an 8-bit depth. The field of view can be adjusted 10 degrees, 20 degrees, or 30 degrees (42 degrees diagonal) to produce a view of the retina.[26,28–30,32,35,36]

cSLOs have certain advantages, which include higher contrast due to the confocal aperture, lasers with highly monochromatic light sources that yield high radiance only at the peak excitation wavelength, small depth of field to allow for discrete z-axis imaging, and extremely sensitive detection devices. This whole package allows for a system that can produce an image better than what the eye's optics will allow at a much lower light intensity than a conventional fundus camera.[26,28,29,32,33,37,38] Current models cannot perform full color photography. Examples of SLOs are seen in Figure 7-50.

Scanning Laser Ophthalmoscope Technique

Current SLOs offer a combination high resolution and contrast. When outfitted with the appropriate laser and filter combinations, SLOs are capable of providing images high in temporal and spatial resolution with detail equal to or superior to that achieved by video fundus cameras. Owing to the extremely small entrance pupil, pure monochromatic light source, and highly efficient light collector, these devices can function through undilated pupils and around opacities in the optical media all with immediate results.[39,40] The confocal design allows for discrete separation of the individual layers of the retina and optic nerve (Figure 7-51).

Angiography is used for the study of many diseases such as age-related macular degeneration (ARMD). Of particular interest, FA and ICG-A are used in the study of choroidal neovascularization,[42–44] simultaneous FA/ICG dye flow,[39–41] central serous chorioretinopathy,[39] choroidal melanomas,[46,47] SRNV and occult choroidal neovascularization,[42,45] feeder vessels of occult choroidal neovascularization,[48] autofluorescence of macular holes and nerve fibers,[49] and oral FAs[50] and automated wide-field montages of chorioretinal diseases.[51]

Though there are differences in the specific SLO designs, the acquisition of images is performed very much the same way. With that said, I

FIGURE 7-50
Composite picture of Laser Diagnostic Technologies (San Diego, CA) AngioScan **(A)**, Rodenstock's Scanning Laser Ophthalmoscope 101 (Danbury, CT) **(B)**, and Heidelberg Engineering, Inc. (Carlsbad, CA) Heidelberg Retinal Angiograph **(C)**.

will concentrate on HE HRA, which is one of the currently available angiographic models.

The following section is a step-by-step review of the basic procedures that are necessary to photograph a patient.

1. Turn on the power. When lasers are used in critical measurement situations, it is important to allow them to stabilize once the power has been turned on. Thirty minutes is typically sufficient time for these systems to warm up and stabilize.
2. Determine what is to be photographed, as it will determine the protocol to follow.
3. Ensure that there is enough RAM and hard disk memory available to acquire the full image set.
4. Enter demographic data in to the database. All systems require certain demographic data to be entered to go to the next step.
5. Make sure the device is clean and all mechanical adjustments are in their neutral position.
6. Position patient for comfort and ease of operation of the device.
7. If your system allows it, preset the device for the patient refractive data found in the patient chart. This sets the instrument to the approximate focusing adjustment for the patient.
8. Adjust the laser intensity and detector sensitivity to its base setting.
9. It is often desirable to have an establishing image before administration of dye. Depending on the type of image required, it may not be necessary to use dye as in the case of imaging the nerve fiber layer, looking for optic nerve head drusen, performing wide-field montages, or looking at macular or pseudo macular holes.[49,51] These establishing images can use any of the lasers (488 nm, 514 nm, 830 nm) and all three imaging modes.
10. Determine what dye injection technique is to be used for the angiographic procedure. The commonly used methods are a single dye

FIGURE 7-51
This composite image shows four of the possible 32 z-axis images that can be sampled during a focal series scan. The most anterior image **(A)** focuses on the surface retinal vessels, whereas **(B)**, **(C)**, and **(D)** focus more posteriorly, bringing the choroidal vessels and a chorioretinal scar into focus.

injection of either FS or ICG, simultaneous injection of mixed FS and ICG, sequential injections of unmixed FS and ICG, and a pulsed injection method of administering the dye.[52–55] The reader is encouraged to find these references and establish his or her procedures accordingly.

11. Mix dye for the particular procedure and technique that is to be performed. It doesn't matter if the injections are individual, simultaneous, or sequential. It is important to consider all of the exhaustive studies that have investigated dye formulations and injection techniques of FA and ICG-A. Take all of the literature and the referring physician's desires into account to come up with a system that works best for the patient. Once the dye injection has begun, all photographic techniques follow the same basic set of steps. The differences in timing and injections are determined by the patient and pathology to be illustrated.

12. Start the timer and follow a predetermined timing sequence while adjusting the laser's focus, intensity, and sensitivity to achieve the best possible images. As a point of difference, the LDT AngioScan is used for only ICG-A and has a monitor in the camera head. This allows for focus and continuous viewing of the eye. It also has the option of automatic triggering so that once the dye arrives in the eye it starts acquiring images automatically. The Heidelberg HRA

on the other hand allows for simultaneous FA and ICG-A acquisition. In this mode, you can see the eye when the FA mode sensitivity is turned up to detect autofluorescence of the retina.[32,56] The HRA has an adjustable frame buffer that allows the system to record images up to 2 seconds before the series-acquire button is pushed. This allows the system to record the start of the dye before the operator has a chance to react.

13. One of the most important and most overlooked steps in the acquisition process with any electronic system is to save data from the volatile temporary RAM to the more stable HD after each step of your timing sequence. The processing power required to manipulate the tremendous amounts of data almost assures that the system will at some time crash. If this data is left in RAM, it will be permanently lost.

14. Edit out the substandard image files to save electronic storage space. If the system is connected to a server, transferring the files will allow others to have access to the images for review and treatment.

15. A hard copy is often required, and an unlimited number of identical original prints can be made from the digital data.

16. Copy the data from the relatively stable HD and transfer it to at least two sets of permanent archive media. It is best to keep these permanent files in separate locations to safeguard from a fire or like disaster. By doing this, the image data can be returned to the HD if it should fail.

With the development of electronic measurement systems in every area of ophthalmology, the need exists to have a method that allows a patient to have several different tests performed on unrelated devices and for the physician to have access to these all in one location.

As a means to accomplish this goal, the DICOM standard has been adopted by many of these devices.[57] This standard allows for patient demographic information to be entered on different devices and their information shared between all devices that are connected and comply to this standard. Once the testing is completed for the day, the system locks the information at midnight and it cannot be added to or changed for that particular day. If a practice is using a records management system that also supports this standard, all of the test data and patient statistics are available to the physician when he or she sees the patient.

Trouble Shooting

As with any dynamic imaging situation, difficulties can arise. Some of these can be attributed to the patient's physical condition, some to patient management issues, whereas others stem from the materials and equipment used. The following is a discussion of some of these issues and, if they cannot be avoided, how best to manage them.

Patient fatigue should always be of paramount concern because of the length of the procedure. The simplest way to reduce fatigue is to have the patient sitting properly at the camera and have all of the necessary materials available before imaging begins.

Adjusting for image quality is the second most important issue and is dependent on the camera and eye being aligned properly. The illumination and viewing pathways are opposite those of fundus cameras and must be handled accordingly. The excitation light entering the eye is the center 1–3 mm of the pupil, whereas the light returning accounts for the rest of the pupil. The camera head and eye should be perpendicular to one another and the axis formed should be parallel to the camera table. This allows for good illumination and viewing. If this arrangement is not followed, the illumination beam de-centers from the eye as the camera head is moved forward and back. With a narrow illumination beam, it is easier to lose the image on the monitor. The best method to regain alignment is to pull the camera head back and position the glowing pupil in the center of the field and push the camera straight forward until the monitor's view is of an evenly illuminated fundus. Slight adjustments may be necessary.

Bleaching of the image is due to improper adjustment of the intensity and sensitivity controls. This occurs in the arterial and early venous phases when concentrations of dye are highest. The controls must be aggressively adjusted to avoid loss of useful image data. During a simultaneous FA/ICG procedure during the arterial and early venous phases, the ICG laser intensity should be turned down and sensitivity up to acquire properly exposed images. The 488-nm FA laser intensity is fixed so the image is adjusted with the sensitivity dial. The 795 ICG laser is adjustable and can be used to limit the amount of IR light entering the eye and balance the image intensities.

On occasion, the pathology to be imaged is too anterior for the camera's built-in refractive controls to handle. In the case of a choroidal melanoma it is sometimes necessary to add an additional +10 or +20 diopter lens on the front of the camera lens. This can be from a trial lens set, or occasionally, the patient can wear his or her own glasses. It must be noted that this will compromise the image somewhat, but this arrangement should work well enough to obtain clinically useful images.

Media opacities are typically less of an issue with SLOs. This is primarily due to their small illumination pathway and pure monochromatic lasers. However, a dark swirling image from the dye at the vitreous retinal interface can sometimes be seen in the later phases. It is best to have the patient rapidly divert his or her gaze to get this to move enough to take a clear image.

Advanced Techniques

Finally, it is important to mention that today cSLOs are not cameras and, by comparison, they have been used in ophthalmology for a relatively short time. Additional computer processing strides will expand their capabilities. It is not within the scope of this writing to fully explore these latest techniques. What follows is a description of some of the more useful techniques for a clinical practice. References are provided to encourage readers to explore on their own.

One of the biggest problems encountered in angiographic imaging is the loss of detail due to leakage of dye. The resulting images are typically of low contrast, and structure detail is limited. The HRA has the ability to mean average images. The technique begins with the acquisition of a rapid temporal series of images. Manually select five frames and then allow the computer to display an average intensity for all of the 262,000 conjugate points of that 512 × 512 image.[58] This technique can be further extended to aid in the detection of optic nerve head drusen (ONHD).

ONHD, or the lack of, have been associated with several pathologies. Typically, the patient would be photographed at the fundus camera with just an exciter filter in the light path. Using an SLO with the 488-nm laser has the distinct advantage of a more pure light source, and the immediately available images can then be further processed as described above.

Wide-field views of the retina add another dimension to the understanding and follow-up of retinal diseases. In the past, a cut and paste method was used with paper photographs. Today, computers can be used to produce a seamless representation of the retina but usually require several human-hours of additional processing time. With the HRA, an

FIGURE 7-52
This montage is an oral fluorescein angiogram of a diabetic patient and is made up of 12 individual frames. Once the individual images were selected, it took approximately 45 seconds of total processing time to create the final image with a 533-MHz processor.

operator can acquire a series of images from the back of the eye by directing the field of view from side to side and from top to bottom. A series of perhaps 25 images would then be selected and, with the standard software available, be merged into a single image within a matter of minutes[51] (Figure 7-52). An even faster wide-field image can be obtained by the use of a supplemental contact lens placed on the eye. This has been reported by several people, but was first described by Webb, Hughes, and Pomerantzeff in their 1980 article, "Flying Spot TV Ophthalmoscope."[23]

A new method of laser treatment uses ICG-A to identify and treat feeder vessels that supply a choroidal neovascular membrane. Because of their high contrast and ability to separate layers of the retina, SLOs show great promise imaging these vessels (see Figure 7-49).[46,48]

The unique characteristics of cSLO show promise in helping diagnose melanomas. ICG-A is used to look at the choroidal circulation, and, as the cSLO can discreetly separate layers, the microvascular structures of melanomas can be imaged. The appearance of characteristic vessel patterns can help to guide the physician in determining the exact type of melanoma present (Figure 7-53).[46,47]

Finally, a technique that has been around for more years than the flash fundus cameras is oral FA. Though not a new technique, it is sometimes the only way to administer the dye and has received renewed interest when used with a SLO. Once again, it is the single wavelength laser that allows enough light to enter the eye to show all but the arterial filling and venous laminar phases. Images typically begin to appear within the first 7 minutes and at leakage can be seen as early as 12 minutes after ingestion. This technique has been demonstrated to be useful for cystoid macular edema and branch retinal vein occlusion in which leakage occurs. In diabetes, it can demonstrate

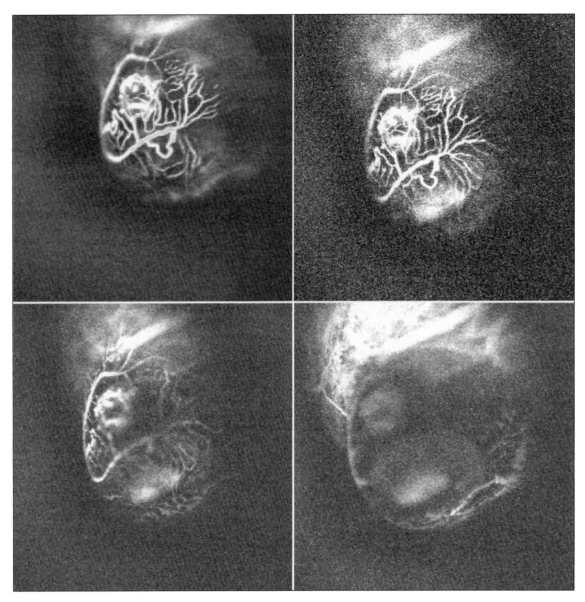

FIGURE 7-53
An indocyanine green angiogram was performed on this choroidal melanoma patient before nucleation. The Heidelberg Retinal Angiograph (Heidelberg Engineering, Inc., Carlsbad, CA) focal series mode was used to optically section the melanoma in the z-axis. These four selected images from a series demonstrate characteristic vessel pattern of concern in this particular type of lesion.

microaneurysms and capillary dropout. It has also been shown be useful in central serous retinopathy and retinal pigment epithelial detachments, but in none of these cases does it surpass that which can be achieved with injected dye.[50]

In conclusion, SLOs are useful ophthalmic tools that will continue to grow in popularity and in their ability to image retinal diseases.

Summary and Perspective

The advances in electronic imaging should not overpower the task that the ophthalmic photographer must accomplish. Deriving accurate and meaningful clinical and diagnostic information must be kept foremost in the mind of the photographer. Our ability to create images through a different modality should not lead to the instant demise of current technology. If, however, the new technology provides more diagnostic information and improves timeliness, then so much the better. The ability to use computers to perform electronic imaging is a function of your aptitude for technical devices, your training with computers, the user interface of the imaging system you select, and, most important, your ability to integrate your knowledge of ophthalmic photography with new technology.

In the age of digital imaging, to be a proficient photographer you should expand your knowledge base to include computers. This does not mean that you will need to know how to program them, but rather be able to use these tools to accomplish your goals. That basic understanding will put you in a better position to aid your practice in the efficient use of electronic images. Courses in computer theory and how to use applications will help. Remember that in today's ever-changing world, employees "get a new job every 10 years." This may not mean that you have a different title or that you will work somewhere else, but that your responsibilities will change. If you learn and understand these and future new tools, you will be well served through the years to come.

Because the user interface is so important, it is paramount that the photographer be actively involved in selecting the system that will be used. It is well worth it to allow the major players who will be using the imaging system to actually see the functioning of the system and perhaps even to use it in a clinical setting before a selection is made.

With digital imaging systems, the flow of work through the photography unit will be different. How different will depend on how the system is configured. These are some of the factors: Where and by whom are the images selected for printing? Where are the components networked? Is the review station full-featured? Are you moving images via floppy disks, prints, CD-ROMs, or a network? An electronic angiography system may make dramatic changes in how the ophthalmologist and the office staff function. Integration of computerized patient records and other diagnostic equipment is a serious consideration in how an office will handle image storage and retrieval systems. New fundus cameras that are designed specifically for CCD imaging devices will create higher-quality imaging systems. Hopefully, simultaneous stereo image capture will be incorporated in new cameras. These will aid the health care team in delivering even higher quality ophthalmic care.

One of the best positive outcomes that I have found is that patient communication and understanding of the ophthalmic situation are greatly increased. Instead of showing a patient a photograph of someone else's eye, the patient is able to see his or her own eye. The comprehension level that goes with the seeing of an image of one's own eye is monumental. Patients become participants in their health care and are able to better communicate with their physician. With an informed patient, there is better understanding and increased compliance, resulting in better patient outcomes.

References

1. Ridley H. Television in ophthalmology. Presented at the Sixteenth International Ophthalmological Congress (London). Acta Ophthalmol (Kobenhavn) 1951;2:1397.
2. Dallow RL. Television Ophthalmoscopy: Instrumentation and Medical Applications. Springfield: Charles C Thomas, 1970;1.
3. van Heuven WAJ, Schafer C, Mehu M. The use of low light level television in fundus imaging. Mod Probl Ophthalmol 1971;9:6.
4. van Heuven WAJ, Schafer C, Mehu M. The evolution of electronic recording systems for FA. Presented at the Twenty-Fifth Anniversary Congress, Retina Service, Boston, Massachusetts, 1972.

5. van Heuven WAJ, Schafer C. Televised FA. In K Shimizu (ed), FA. Tokyo: Igako Shoin, 1974;10–14.

6. van Heuven WAJ, Schafer C. Electronic imaging systems for FA. Internat Ophthalmol Clin 1974;14:31.

7. van Heuven WAJ, Mehu, M. The clinical applications of televised FA. In JJ Justice (ed), Ophthalmic Photography: International Ophthalmology Clinics. Boston: Little, Brown, 1976.

8. Kodak Megaplus Camera, Model 1.4 Users' Manual. Eastman Kodak Co., Inc., Digital Imaging.

9. Yuhasz Z, Akashi RH, Urban JC, Mueller MMH. A new apparatus for videotape recording of fluorescein angiograms. Arch Ophthalmol 1973;90:481.

10. Beer PM. A laser printing option for digital angiography systems. [Letter to the Editor]. Am J Ophthalmol 1994;118:535.

11. Stroebel L, Zakia R. The Focal Encyclopedia of Photography, 3rd Edition. ISBN: 0-240-80059-1.1993. Focal Press, an imprint of Butterworth–Heinemann, p. 26.

12. DICOM information from http://NEMA.com 3/2001.

13. Todd H, Zakia RD. Photographic Sensitometry. In JM Sturge (ed), Neblette's Handbook of Photography and Reprography; Materials, Processes, and Systems. New York: Van Nostrand Reinhold, 1977;165–196.

14. Behrendt T, Wilson LA. Spectral reflectance photography of the retina. Am J Ophthalmol 1965;59:1079.

15. Behrendt T, Duane TD. Investigation of fundus oculi with spectral reflectance photography. Arch Ophthalmol 1966;75:375.

16. Russ JC. The Image Processing Handbook. Boca Raton, FL: CRC Press, 1992.

17. Todd HN, Zakia RD. Photographic Sensitometry. The Study of Tone Reproduction. Hastings-on-Hudson, NY: Morgan and Morgan, 1969.

18. Macular Photocoagulation Study Group. Subfoveal neovascular lesions in age-related macular degeneration: guidelines for evaluation and treatment in the macular photocoagulation study. Arch Ophthalmol 1991;109:1242.

19. Adobe Photoshop 6.0 for Photographers, Martin Evening, 2001, Focal Press.

20. Photoshop 6 for Windows Bible, Deke McClelland, 2000, New York, Hungry Minds, Inc.

21. Microsoft PowerPoint 2000 Bible, May 1999, Hungry Minds, Inc; ISBN: 0764532529.

22. Saine PJ, Tyler ME. Ophthalmic Photography. A Textbook of Fundus Photography, Angiography, and Electronic Imaging. Boston: Butterworth–Heinemann, MA, 1996.

23. Webb RH, Hughes GW, Pomerantzeff O. Flying spot TV ophthalmoscope. Applied Optics 1980;19:2991.

24. Webb RH, Hughes GW. Scanning Laser Ophthalmoscope. IEE Translations on Biomedical Engineering. 1981;BME-28:488.

25. Mainster MA, Timberlake GT, Webb RH, Hughes GW. Scanning Laser Ophthalmoscopy, Clinical Applications. Ophthalmol 1982;89:852.

26. Webb RH, Hughes GW, Delori FC. Confocal scanning laser ophthalmoscope. Applied Optics 1987;26:1492.

27. Frambach DA, Dacey MP, Sadun A. Stereoscopic photography with a scanning laser ophthalmoscope. Am J Ophthalmol 1993;116:484.

28. Plesch A, Klingbeil U, Rappl W, Schrodel C. Scanning ophthalmic imaging. In RE Nasemann, ROW Burke (eds), Scanning Laser Ophthalmoscopy and Tomography. Munich, Germany: Quintessenz, 1990;23–32.

29. Zinser G. Heidelberg Retina Angiograph: Confocal digital fluorescein and indocyanine green angiography. Lecture presented at American Academy of Ophthalmology annual meeting, 1999.

30. Bartsch DU. Scanning Laser Imaging in Ophthalmology. Lecture presented at Ophthalmic Photographers Society 2000, mid-year meeting.

31. Scheider A, Schroede C. High resolution indocyanine green angiography with a scanning laser ophthalmoscope. Am J Ophthalmol 1989;108:458.

32. Heidelberg Engineering, Inc. Manuals of Operation, Advertising brochures and Web site http://www.heidelbergengineering.com/10/2000.

33. Laser Diagnostic Technologies, Inc. Manuals of Operation P/N 251-0047A, Advertising brochures and Web site @ http://www.laserdiagnostic.com/ 2000–2001.

34. Optos, Scotland, UK. Advertising brochures and Web site http://www.optos.com/ 2001.

35. G. Rodenstock Instrumente GmbH, Rodenstock Scanning Laser Ophthalmoscope, SLO Handbook P/N 3056.002-886–7, Advertising brochures 5/1999 and phone interview.

36. Zeiss Humphrey Systems. Dublin, USA. Advertising brochures and Web site http://www.humphrey.com/ 1999.

37. Dreher AW, Reiter K, Weinreb RN. Spatially resolved birefringence of the retinal nerve fiber layer assessed with a retinal laser ellipsometer. Applied Optics 1992;31:3730.

38. American National Standards for the Safe Use of Lasers. ANSI Z136.1 (1993).
39. Bischoff PM, Niederberger HJ, Torok B, Speiser P. Simultaneous indocyanine green and FA. Retina 1995;15:91.
40. Holz FG, Bellman C, Rohrschneider K, et al. Simultaneous confocal scanning laser fluorescein and indocyanine green angiography. Am J Ophthalmol 1998;125:277.
41. Freeman WR, Bartsch DU, Mueller AJ, et al. Simultaneous indocyanine green and FA using a confocal scanning laser ophthalmoscope. Arch Ophthalmol 1998;116:415.
42. Yannuzzi LA, Slakter JS, Sorenson JA, et al. Digital indocyanine green videoangiography and choroidal neovascularization. Retina 1992;12:191.
43. Monahan PM, Gitter KA, Eichler DJ, et al. Use of digitized fluorescein angiogram system to evaluate laser treatment for subretinal neovascularization: technique. Retina 1993;13:187.
44. Monahan PM, Gitter KA, Eichler DJ, Cohen G. Evaluation of persistence of subretinal neovascular membranes using digitized angiographic analysis. Retina 1993;13:196.
45. Gelisken F, Inhoffen W, Schneider U, et al. Indocyanine green videoangiography of occult choroidal neovascularization, A comparison of scanning laser ophthalmoscope with high-resolution digital fundus camera. Retina 1998;18:37.
46. Mueller AJ, Bartsch DU, Folberg R, et al. Imaging the microvasculature of the choroidal melanomas with confocal indocyanine green scanning laser ophthalmoscopy. Arch Ophthalmol 1998;116:31.
47. Mueller AJ, Folberg R, Freeman WR, et al. Evaluation of the human choroidal melanoma rabbit model for studying microcirculation patterns with confocal ICG and histology. Exp Eye Res 1999;68:671.
48. Flower RW. Experimental studies of ICG dye enhanced photocoagulation of CNV feeder vessels. Am J Ophthalmol 2000;501:512.
49. Desatnik H, Treister G, Alhalel A, et al. ICGA-Guided laser photocoagulation of feeder vessels of choroidal neovascular membranes in age-related macular degeneration. Retina 2000;20:143.
50. Ruckmann A, Fitzke FW, Gregor ZJ. Fundus autofluorescence in patients with macular holes imaged with a scanning laser ophthalmoscope. Br J Ophthalmol 1998;82:346.
51. Garcia CR, Rivero ME, Bartsch DU, et al. Oral FA with the confocal scanning laser ophthalmoscope. Ophthalmol 1999;106:1114.
52. Rivero ME, Bartsch DU, Otto T, Freeman WR. Automated scanning laser ophthalmoscope image montages of retinal diseases. Ophthalmol 1999;106:2296.
53. Miller K. Protocols for the efficacious use of indocyanine green/sodium FA. J Ophthal Photog 1993;15:63.
54. Flower RW. Injection technique for indocyanine green and sodium fluorescein dye angiography of the eye. Invest Ophthalmol 1973;12:881.
55. Nyberg WC. Re-injection technique for establishing landmarks in late phase ICG-A. J Ophthal Photog 1993;15:65.
56. Saine PJ, Stevens RA, Cavender JC. A new technique for administering ICG during choroidal angiography. J Ophthal Photog 1999;21:44.
57. von Ruckmann A, Fitzke FW, Bird AC. In vivo fundus autofluorescence in macular dystrophy. Arch Ophthalmol 1997;115(5):609–15.
58. Fritz SL. Filmless Radiology: DICOM Standardization. New York: Springer-Verlag, 1999;311.

Chapter 8

Ophthalmic Photography: Maximizing Diagnostic Information

Stephen J. Sramek

Introduction

Ophthalmic photography provides information critical to the diagnosis and treatment of eye diseases. Although the concept is simple (take a picture), the process is complex. The different characteristics of equipment and patients significantly affect your ability to provide the needed information to the clinician. To accomplish this goal, the photographer needs technical training, knowledge of ocular anatomy, and an understanding of how images are used by the clinician in the management of ocular disease. Earlier chapters in this book discuss technical aspects of ophthalmic photography and angiography. The goals of this chapter are to review pertinent ocular anatomy and to help the photographer recognize the clinical information required by the clinician. Photographers who comprehend the reason for an image can assess the usefulness of their work, not just the technical quality. The more you understand about the process and the needs of the clinician, the better you are able to contribute to and be part of the patient care team. This chapter does not attempt to provide a comprehensive discussion of the clinical interpretation of ophthalmic photography. Several excellent reviews written from the perspective of the clinician are available.[1-3]

The elements of the useful clinical image include the correct eye, focused at the correct level in the anteroposterior plane, at the correct location, with optimal field size and magnification, and, if an angiogram, at the correct time. The correct eye and general location may or may not be apparent—and how does one determine what is "correct," "appropriate," or "optimal" for the other parameters? That is, how does one provide the maximum amount of information? Communication between the photographer and the clinician is key in this process. A large portion of the first 2 years of medical school is spent developing a vocabulary to allow further development of medical skills. Although the photographer is not responsible for using clinical knowledge for diagnosis, treatment, or interpretation, at least a portion of this vocabulary is necessary to have a common ground for discussion. Information provided by the clinician is required by the photographer to best prepare to obtain the image. In this framework, basic clinical knowledge is as essential for the photographer as knowing the correct flash setting. Both are required for the most useful images.

There are several possible models of differing complexity within which the photographer may operate. One may use all of the following models at different times. The simplest framework (and the one inexperienced photographers use most), is to photograph the eye at the location that the clinician requests, always at the same magnification, focused on the retina, with angiograms imaged in the same way—end of task. Following instructions from the person responsible for the medical care of the patient certainly cannot be faulted and should result in acceptable photographs most of the time. However, it makes the photographer a part of the camera—a button pushed by the clinician. Besides being less challenging and perhaps less satisfying for the photographer, it results in sub-optimal images more often than one might think. For example, a colleague from another clinic complained to me after reviewing a set of photographs of a glaucoma patient that only included the macula. The physician marked "glaucoma" for the diagnosis, but during a busy clinic mistakenly circled the macula instead of the discs on the photograph request form. The physician was quite upset that the photographer did not realize what was really needed, or did not at least question the request, even though the form was filled out incorrectly. Who hasn't heard, "Give me what I need, not what I ask for?" Further discussion revealed that the person was a part-time photographer with no experience and essentially no training at a satellite clinic. Education for both the physician and the photographer is an obvious solution to this kind of problem. This level of education and communication is the most basic, sort of the "Me Tarzan, you Jane" level—that is, glaucoma = nerve, diabetes = retina, etc.—and is the minimum that should be accepted by clinician or photographer.

Perhaps a more practical example is one in which a patient with proliferative diabetic retinopathy is sent to the photography department for photographs of the disc and macula, but neovascularization elsewhere is present in field 3. The clinician may have missed the change or erroneously believed it to be within the field selected for photography. If the photographer can recognize the abnormality, he or she can choose to document the change. Recognition of what is abnormal is a model frequently used as a beginning strategy in medical education. It is based on the concept of a firm knowledge of what is normal to be able to recognize "anything else" as abnormal. Photographing whatever is identified as abnormal is a reasonably good strategy for a clinical photographer because it increases the chances that the image provides the necessary information. An added advantage for the beginning photographer is that it does not require extensive clinical knowledge. Although one is working at a more sophisticated level within this framework, the technique has an inherent lack of sensitivity.

An unprepared mind (or one that is "unfocused") is limited in its ability to examine a problem or to find the appropriate steps needed for its

FIGURE 8-1
Information loss due to "improper" focus, not "poor" focus. The stereo pair in **A** is focused at the level of the optic nerve. However, the clinician will not be able to adequately assess elevated neovascularization, which requires a different level of focus, shown in stereo pair **B**.

solution. The concept is recognized in a number of areas. In psychology, the principle surfaces in Stephen Covey's book, *The Seven Habits of Highly Effective People*, as habit number two: "Begin with the end in mind." "To begin with the end in mind means to start with a clear understanding of your destination. It means to know where you're going so that you better understand where you are now and so that the steps you take are always in the right direction."[4] The medical student encounters the principle in the second year during an introduction to physical diagnosis or similar course. A philosophy of examination from such a course that I have always remembered comes from a widely used textbook on internal medicine: "The detection of a few scattered petechiae, a faint diastolic murmur, or a small mass in the abdomen is not a question of keener eyes and ears or more sensitive fingers, but of a mind directed to be alert to these findings. Skill in physical diagnosis reflects a way of thinking more than a way of doing."[5] Detection of subtle changes—that is, maximizing information—increases with preparation of the mind before the task. The photographer needs to develop a "way of thinking" to complement the technical training to help prepare for the photograph.

The paradigm proposed in this chapter is based on the clinical use of the photograph. Remember the perfect photograph of the macula when the physician was interested in the optic nerve? Perhaps not as obvious, but just as important, is the technically perfect photograph focused at the level of the optic disc when the clinician is interested in documenting elevated neovascularization of the disc (NVD) in proliferative diabetic retinopathy. The blood vessels may be sufficiently elevated to be out of the plane of sharpest focus, and the photograph is not as useful to the physician 4 weeks later when assessing the response of the NVD to panretinal photocoagulation (Figure 8-1). The photographer needs to have this information before taking the photograph. Therefore, a useful framework for preparing for a photograph is a categorization of its purpose— that is, why was the photograph ordered? Table 8-1 lists three common

Table 8-1. Purposes of Ophthalmic Photography and Angiography

Reason	Purpose
Documentation	Current status of a disease process
Diagnosis	Diagnostic pattern
	Rule out a diagnosis
Treatment	Localize the area to treat
	Assess the response to treatment

reasons clinicians order fundus photographs: documentation, diagnosis, and treatment. Briefly considering this table before actually taking a photograph is useful, especially for the inexperienced photographer. In the following examples, we review these situations to demonstrate how the purpose of a photograph might affect the thinking of the photographer.

Documentation

A common reason to order fundus photography is for documentation of the current status of a disease process. The images do not provide information in addition to the clinical examination, but are to be used for later comparison to assess change. In many cases of retinal disease, treatment is guided by the results of national, multicenter randomized trials.[6] In these trials, a certain level of change or "threshold" was necessary to allow the patient to enter the study. The common practice now is to wait until a patient has sufficient worsening of the ocular disease to the level of the initial study criteria. At that point, the risks and benefits of treatment are clearly better than no treatment. The national studies pertinent to fundus photography and fluorescein angiography are the Diabetic Retinopathy Study,[7] the Early Treatment of Diabetic Retinopathy Study (ETDRS),[8] the Macular Photocoagulation Study,[9,10] and the Branch Vein Occlusion Study.[11,12] For example, the criteria of treatment for macular edema from the ETDRS describes retinal thickening (edema) threatening or involving the foveal avascular zone (FAZ), or hard exudate associated with retinal thickening threatening or involving the FAZ. Large areas of thickening or hard exudate that do not directly threaten the FAZ, often in field 3, also are an indication for treatment. What does this mean for the photographer? The most useful photographs within the context of the ETDRS are 30-degree stereo pairs that include the FAZ and any large areas of retinal thickening in field 3. The clinician reviewing the photographs asks if retinal thickening or hard exudate with thickening that threatens the FAZ was underestimated or missed during clinical examination, or if, on comparison of photographs taken over a period of months, there has been progression in a borderline case. Clinically useful photographs hold the answers to these questions (Figure 8-2).

In addition to retinal and choroidal vascular diseases as examined in the national studies, another common situation requiring documentation involves a mass or pigmented lesion of the choroid. A choroidal nevus may be difficult to distinguish from a small choroidal melanoma. Documentation of growth on fundus photographs can be essential to management. In reviewing the photographs, one feature the clinician examines is lateral extension of the lesion; therefore, he or she needs to see all the margins of the lesion, and wide-field photographs may be useful (Figure 8-3). Failure to include the margins greatly decreases the usefulness of the image. Stereo is helpful for an indication of thickening, although usually the clinician relies on ultrasound measurements to make this determination.

FIGURE 8-2

Documentation of disease progression and need for treatment. **A.** Fundus photograph of the left macula of a patient with diabetes at the initial consultation. Although numerous retinal hemorrhages are present, hard exudate is minimal, and no thickening of the retina was apparent on contact lens examination. The patient was not a candidate for laser treatment based on Early Treatment of Diabetic Retinopathy Study criteria. **B.** Two months later, although there has been some decrease in retinal hemorrhage (*large arrow*), there has been an increase in hard exudate (*small arrow*), and definite retinal thickening could be seen on clinical examination. **C.** Early-phase fluorescein angiogram used as a guide for focal laser treatment demonstrates numerous microaneurysms that leak in the late phase **(D)**. Clinical photographs are essential to follow subtle but important changes, especially in patients with extensive disease.

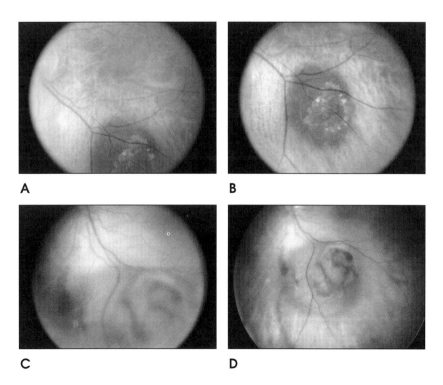

FIGURE 8-3

Document current status. Where's the edge? **A, B.** 30-degree fields showing a choroidal nevus/small melanoma. The image in **A** (field 5) is inadequate to follow this lesion for possible growth. Photographer needs to recognize importance of shifting fields to allow visualization of the entire margin **(B)**. **C, D.** Large melanoma with subretinal hemorrhage. **C.** Entire lesion will not fit in a 30-degree field and is quite elevated, making focus difficult. **D.** A wide-angle photograph not only allows the entire lesion to be visualized, but the increase in depth of field provides more detail overall.

A

B

C

FIGURE 8-4
Localize area to treat. **A.** Fundus photograph of a 74-year-old patient who presented with metamorphopsia in her left eye shows a deep pigment ring and subretinal fluid. **B.** Stereo pair of early phase of fluorescein angiogram reveals a fan-shaped, deep hyperfluorescent lesion that leaks in the late phase **(C)**. Early frame **(B)** was used to guide focal laser treatment.

Diagnosis and Treatment

In some circumstances, the diagnosis is apparent on clinical examination, and the clinician uses fluorescein angiography in combination with fundus photography for the treatment of disease. For example, an elderly patient may present with vision loss, drusen, pigmentary changes, subretinal fluid, and hemorrhage on examination. The diagnosis is exudative age-related macular degeneration (ARMD), and the purpose of the angiogram is to locate the source of the leakage and to determine if the leakage is treatable based on the guidelines developed in the national studies. Three elements are essential for adequate assessment and treatment. They include the relationship of the leakage to the FAZ, the relationship of the leakage to the retina (intraretinal or deep to the retina), and the change with time in the intensity and pattern of leakage. Again, the purpose of the angiogram dictates the photographic technique. The standard angiographic technique described in earlier chapters fulfills these requirements, providing stereo images in which the FAZ is visualized with high-quality early photographs (choroidal, early arterial). Imaging the early phase is crucial in this clinical setting because it is one of the frames in the early phase that guides laser treatment (Figure 8-4). Immediate post-treatment photographs are often used to assess the adequacy of coverage of the treated area. Finally, it is standard practice to repeat an angiogram several weeks after laser treatment to evaluate the response.

In other situations, the diagnosis may not be apparent on clinical examination. For example, a patient presented with unexplained vision

A   **B**   **C**

FIGURE 8-5
Diagnostic patterns in fluorescein angiography. Post-cataract surgery cystoid macular edema. **A.** Red-free photograph. **B.** Early venous phase of fluorescein angiogram demonstrates irregular hyperfluorescence at the level of the retinal vasculature. **C.** Late phase reveals typical pattern of cystoid edema and slight hyperfluorescence of disc.

loss 3 months after uncomplicated cataract surgery. Visual acuity decreased from 20/20 to 20/80. Macular edema was present on clinical examination. Common diagnostic possibilities include the Irvine-Gass syndrome,[13] occult choroidal neovascularization (CNV), or a macular branch vein occlusion. The angiogram is essential to determine the diagnosis. Figure 8-5 shows a macular photograph of the patient. Although the clinical photograph is fairly unremarkable, the fluorescein angiogram demonstrates late intraretinal dye leakage and leakage from the disc (see Figure 8-5). These angiographic characteristics suggest post-cataract cystoid macular edema, or Irvine-Gass syndrome, which occurs in a small percentage of patients after uneventful cataract surgery. This situation is different from the previous example in that the late photographs are extremely important, as are photographs of the optic discs both for comparison and to assess leakage from the disc. An excellent arterial-phase photograph of a well-defined FAZ may be technically perfect, but is not very helpful in the absence of 10-minute late photographs and late bilateral optic disc photographs when assessing this patient.

Color Fundus Photography

Understanding the purpose for which the image is to be used prepares the photographer to anticipate the outcome and allows the basic technique to be varied to obtain optimal results. In deciding where and how to obtain an image of the fundus, the photographer must, of course, begin with the request form sent by the clinician. At a minimum, the request should include a diagnosis and a location. If the request is unclear, the photographer should have the freedom to obtain additional information from the physician. By reviewing the purpose (see Table 8-1) and expected changes for the diagnosis, the photographer can then consider whether variations in basic technique might be required. For example, are additional images required at different levels of focus, or perhaps different locations than on the request? Are 30- or 60-degree fields more appropriate? It may be helpful for the inexperienced photographer to develop a mental checklist to ensure that all technical aspects of the photograph are considered and logically chosen or excluded based on the clinical need as determined by the diagnosis. Table 8-2 is one possible

Table 8-2. Photographer Checklist

Angle of view	Normal, narrow, or wide-angle?
Field of view	Macula or disc? Mid- or far-periphery?
Level of focus	Vitreous, nerve fiber layer, retina, retinal pigment epithelium, or choroid?
Stereo	Is stereo technique helpful? Is it possible?
Filters	For angiography? For monochromatic photography?
Patient	Comfort? Lids? Cornea? Media?
Exposure	Standard? Or increase/decrease?
Advanced techniques	Slit fundus photographs with auxiliary lenses? Monochromatic fundus photography?
	Always ask yourself: How can I make these pictures better?

FIGURE 8-6
Simplified model of the posterior eye wall demonstrating the layering of retina, retinal pigment epithelium (RPE), and choroid.

guide. Review of the diagnosis, location, purpose (see Table 8-1) and technique should provide reasonable preparation to increase the probability of obtaining a photograph with maximum clinical value. A solid foundation in ocular anatomy and an understanding of the fundamentals of angiography are needed for this process. The next section reviews pertinent aspects of ocular anatomy.

Retinal and Choroidal Anatomy

Fundus photographs and angiography provide information about ocular anatomy and ocular blood flow. Photographers need a working knowledge of ocular structures and blood circulation to assess the suitability of fundus photographs and fluorescein or indocyanine green (ICG) angiograms.

When interpreting fluorescein patterns, it is helpful to think of the posterior eye wall as a three-layered structure consisting of retina, retinal pigment epithelium (RPE), and choroid (Figure 8-6). Just behind these layers is the sclera, the opaque, tough, white, outer covering of the eye, while immediately in front of them is the optically clear vitreous. The blood supply to the eye can be divided into two distinct elements: the choroidal and retinal circulations. The central retinal artery supplies the retinal circulation, while the ciliary arteries supply the choroid. It also is useful to consider that these two compartments are separated anatomically and functionally by the RPE, a barrier layer between the retina and choroid (Figure 8-7). The microanatomy of these compartments is different and determines the appearance of fluorescein or ICG images. The

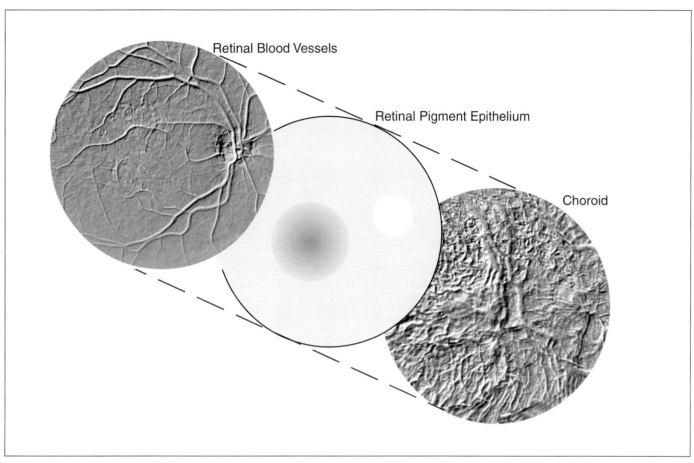

FIGURE 8-7
Retinal and choroidal circulation separated by the retinal pigment epithelium.

layering of the eye, differences in blood vessel anatomy, and characteristics of fluorescein or ICG dye result in the different patterns as dye passes through the eye.

The retinal layer consists of the light-sensitive photoreceptors, other nerve cells, support cells, and the retinal circulation. The source of the blood in the retina is the ophthalmic artery, a branch of the carotid. The blood vessels in the retina share a property with other blood vessels in the central nervous system. There is only minimal leakage of blood components, fluid, drugs, and chemicals such as fluorescein through the blood vessel wall. Specialized anatomic structures between cells called *tight junctions* (Figure 8-8A) are thought to be responsible for the blood-brain barrier, as well as a blood-retinal barrier. The retinal circulation behaves as a traditional vascular bed, with decreasing diameters of arterioles to the capillary level, and subsequent increasing diameters of the venous circulation.

Posterior to the retina is the RPE (see Figure 8-6), a single layer of pigment-containing specialized cells that perform a vital role in maintaining the health of the retina, particularly the adjacent photoreceptors. Bruch's membrane is a complex structure immediately posterior to the RPE that consists of the basement membranes of the RPE cells and cells from the choroid, as well as the layers between these cells. Damage to Bruch's membrane and the overlying RPE is important in the mechanism of vision loss in a number of diseases, including ARMD. The RPE, because it contains pigment, prevents visualization by fluorescein of the underlying choroid to varying degrees, depending on the pigment den-

A   **B**

FIGURE 8-8
Electron micrographs of ocular blood vessels. **A.** Tight junction in a retinal capillary that forms part of a blood-retinal barrier. **B.** Fenestrations in a choroidal vessel that allow passage of small molecules into the extracellular space. (Courtesy of I. Wallow, University of Wisconsin, Madison, WI.)

FIGURE 8-9
Photomicrograph demonstrating compartmentalization of fluorescein within the retinal blood vessel. (Courtesy of Ralph C. Eagle, Wills Eye Hospital, Philadelphia, PA.)

sity. In the center of the normal macula there is increased pigmentation in the RPE cells, recognized by the early pathologists and responsible for the name *macula lutea*.[14] The increased pigmentation in this area masks the underlying choroidal vessels. In contrast, in lightly pigmented individuals or individuals without pigment, such as in an albino, the choroid may be easily visualized.

The choroid is the layer of blood vessels between the RPE and the sclera. In addition to location, the anatomy of the choroidal circulation differs from that of the retinal circulation in several important ways. First, the choroidal vessels do not have tight junctions. In fact, the choriocapillaris or small choroidal vessels are fenestrated—they are built to leak (see Figure 8-8B). As a result, small molecules, such as fluorescein, freely diffuse into the extravascular space. Substances that leak out of the choroid are prevented from entering the retina by the outer blood-retinal barrier, the RPE. Figure 8-9 is an image that elegantly demonstrates reten-

FIGURE 8-10
Classic drawing demonstrating the lobular structure of the choroid. (A = artery; V = vein.) (Courtesy of Lee Allen, University of Iowa, Iowa City, IA.)

tion of fluorescein within the retinal circulation, diffusion of fluorescein in the choroid, and separation of the two circulations by the RPE.[15] ICG is highly protein bound, and therefore remains within both the retinal and choroidal circulation to a much greater degree than fluorescein. Rather than a single arterial source as in the retina, the choroid is supplied by multiple long and short posterior ciliary arteries, which are branches of the ophthalmic artery. In an angiogram, the choroidal circulation fills earlier than the retinal circulation because of the supply from the posterior ciliary arteries. Finally, the choroid is not a simple, progressive-branching type of vascular bed as is the retina, but consists of an interlocking network (anastomosis) of blood vessels that function as lobules (Figure 8-10).[16] The lobular arrangement of the choroid can sometimes be seen in the early phases of a fluorescein angiogram or in certain pathologic situations, but the pattern is rapidly lost because of dye diffusion through the fenestrated capillaries. Because of the multiple sources of arterial supply to the choroid, it is not as susceptible to occlusion by embolic disease as is the retinal circulation; however, a diffuse process can interrupt the choroidal blood supply. In fact, choroidal ischemia due to occlusion of posterior ciliary arteries can be an important angiographic finding in temporal arteritis, an inflammation that generally causes occlusion of a number of different arteries.

Except for the blood vessels, normal retina is optically clear. It has to be, as the photoreceptors are at the "bottom" of the retina, and light must pass through the retina to these cells. The fundus appearance, then, is a combination of what is seen by looking through the retina and various amounts of pigment in the RPE, to the choroid. Differences in these layers are enhanced with the dyes fluorescein and ICG. In the next sections, knowledge of ocular anatomy is applied to help understand the patterns seen in fluorescein and ICG angiograms.

Normal Fluorescein Angiogram

A fluorescein angiogram documents a dynamic process in which fluorescein moves into the eye from the arterial circulation, interacts with anatomic structures both normal and abnormal, and leaves the eye via the venous circulation. It is important to recognize the patterns of fluorescence that emerge in a normal eye. The phases of the normal fluores-

Table 8-3. Phases of the Normal Fluorescein Angiogram

Phase	Description
Prearterial	Earliest recording of dye
	Choroid fills
	Retina relatively quiet except with cilioretinal artery
Arterial	Dye in arteries only
	Very short: less than 1–2 seconds
Arteriovenous	Arteries still contain fluorescein
	Laminar flow in veins
Venous	Generally veins brighter than arteries
	Veins are filled with fluorescein
Recirculation	Arteries and veins of equal brightness
	Decrease in overall intensity of fluorescence
	Reduction of contrast and detail

cein angiogram are discussed in the following section and are briefly summarized for quick reference in Table 8-3.

Monochromatic green filter photographs document in black and white the appearance of the retina just before injection of fluorescein (Figure 8-11A). After injection, fluorescence begins to appear in 10–20 seconds, depending on the individual. The fluorescence that first appears in the eye is from the choroidal circulation. A diffuse or patchy choroidal filling can sometimes be seen immediately before the appearance of dye in the retinal circulation (see Figure 8-11B). A retinal artery supplied from the choroid ("cilioretinal artery") provides blood to a portion of the macula as a normal bilateral anatomic variation in 15% of individuals.[17] If present, cilioretinal vessels fill with the choroidal circulation (see Figure 8-11B). Any sense of structure in the choroid is quickly lost as dye rapidly diffuses from the choriocapillaris into the surrounding tissue matrix (see Figure 8-11B, C, D).

After the appearance of dye in the choroid, it next enters the retinal arteries (arterial phase, see Figure 8-11C), followed very rapidly by the veins over the next 1–2 seconds (the arteriovenous phase, see Figure 8-11D, E). Initially, dye does not fill the veins but is visible along the edge of the vessel walls in a very characteristic pattern (Figure 8-11D). This pattern is a result of laminar flow of blood in the vessel. As anyone who fishes for trout knows, water (or blood) flows through a stream (or blood vessel) in one of two patterns—either laminar or turbulent. "In laminar flow, all the molecules of water move parallel to each other in a single direction. In turbulent flow, there are countless little eddies and whirlpools that move the water in all directions as the main current moves downstream."[18] When dye moves from the smaller venous branches into the peripheral "lamina" of fluid along the wall of the larger veins, it tends to move in a position that stays in constant relation to the vessel wall. After a short period, however, there is sufficient mixing of dye (turbulence) to cause the entire vessel to fluoresce, whereas the arteries begin to empty. This is the venous phase.

In a normal eye, the central macula appears to be less fluorescent than surrounding tissue (Figure 8-12A). The decreased fluorescence is a consequence of two features of normal anatomy shown schematically in Figure 8-12B. First, retinal blood vessels are not found in a circular area approximately 500 microns (0.5 mm) in size in the center of the macula. This region is called the *foveal avascular zone* (FAZ) and includes the fovea, a specialized retinal section that contains a higher concentration of cones. The FAZ is responsible for the sharpest vision and is important to the clinician because it is a guide in laser treatment. In some individuals, the perifoveal capillaries cannot be well visual-

FIGURE 8-11
Normal fluorescein angiogram. **A.** Red-free photograph. **B.** Prearterial phase. "Patchy," deep (on stereo) fluorescence characteristic of choroidal filling can be seen in the posterior pole. In the cup of the optic nerve, an arteriole fills with the choroid and is a "cilioretinal" artery. Although the choroidal circulation is the first to fill, the delay in dye appearance in the retinal circulation is very short. Fluorescein is already present in other retinal arterioles but is not yet present in the venous system. **C.** Arterial phase. **D.** Arteriovenous phase. Dye is now beginning to enter the veins and shows a laminar type of flow pattern. **E.** Early venous phase. **F, G.** Recirculation phase. Overall fluorescence decreases in intensity and tends to be equal in arteries and veins.

A

B

FIGURE 8-12
A. Early venous phase fluorescein photograph from a normal patient in which the perifoveal capillaries are well visualized. The dark central area is normal—the foveal avascular zone (FAZ). (Normal fluorescein angiogram provided by Ophthalmic Imaging Systems.) **B.** Line drawing illustrating the reason for the hypofluorescent central area in the normal macula. Retinal blood vessels are absent in this area, and there is an increase in pigment in the retinal pigment epithelium (RPE).

ized, but failure to do so does not necessarily indicate an abnormality. In addition to an absence of dye in retinal vessels in the FAZ, fluorescein in the underlying choroid is not well visualized because the RPE contains a higher amount of pigment here compared to other regions.

The *transit phase* refers to the first circulation of dye through the eye, and consists of the arterial, arteriovenous, and venous phases. In the recirculation phase, dye that has already exited the eye through the venous system reenters. The overall intensity of fluorescence decreases and is approximately equal in the arteries and veins (see Figure 8-11F). Subsequently, the overall intensity of fluorescence continues to decrease as dye is further diluted and excreted (see Figure 8-11G).

Table 8-4. Abnormal Fluorescein Angiogram Patterns

Hyperfluorescence	Window defect	Hyperfluorescence early, then slow decrease in intensity
		No change in shape or size over time
	Staining	Hyperfluorescence late
		No change in shape or size over time
	Leakage	Early hyperfluorescence with late increased intensity, diffusion, and enlargement of dye
	Pooling	Slowly developing hyperfluorescence with sharply demarcated borders
Hypofluorescence	Filling defects	Results from decreased vessel perfusion; red-free and color photographs may be normal
	Blockage	Material (usually blood) often visible on red-free or color photographs; with shape or size corresponding to the area of decreased fluorescence

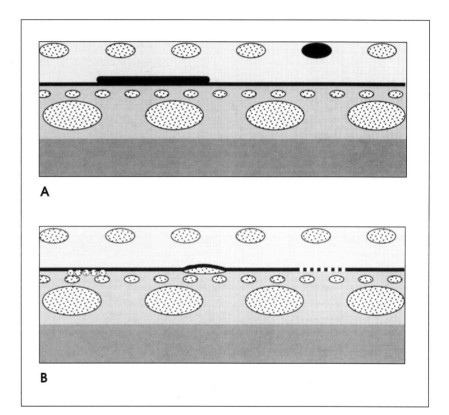

FIGURE 8-13
Line drawing illustrating hypofluorescent (**A**) and hyperfluorescent (**B**) areas. **A.** Opaque material, such as blood, prevents visualization of underlying fluorescein and is described as *blocked fluorescence*. Absence of dye in normal structures can occur with closure or obstruction of blood vessels. **B.** Three reasons for hyperfluorescence: absorption of dye by drusen (staining), pooling of dye, and window defect.

Abnormal Fluorescein Angiogram

Initially it is useful to characterize the findings in the abnormal fluorescein angiogram using the "second level" of clinical information discussed previously—concentrate on what differs from normal. With this starting point for analyzing a fluorescein angiogram, one must learn to recognize variations from the normal patterns as areas of either decreased fluorescence (hypofluorescent) or increased fluorescence (hyperfluorescent) (Table 8-4). A hypofluorescent area may be due either to an absence of dye or blockage of the dye by some other material such as blood (see Figure 8-13A). A hyperfluorescent area compared to a normal eye can be due to an increase in the amount of dye, termed *staining*, *pooling*, or *leakage*, or due to better visualization of a "normal" amount of dye (window defects) (Figure 8-13B). These patterns are shown in the following clinical examples.

A common cause of a window defect is loss of pigment in the RPE in ARMD. The pigment loss allows visualization of the normal amount of dye in the choroid as it moves beneath the RPE. A window defect is characterized by early hyperfluorescence during the choroidal phase, fol-

FIGURE 8-14
Clinical examples of hyperfluorescence. **A.** Fundus photograph of right macula of patient with macular degeneration. **B.** Early phase of angiogram shows a wide area of hyperfluoresence. **C.** In the midphase, hyperfluorescence decreases in the center and increases at the edges. Punctate hyperfluorescence outside the central lesion develops due to staining of drusen. **D.** In the late phase, hyperfluorescence at the nasal edge diffuses and increases in intensity (leakage). Hyperfluorescence continues to decrease temporal to this, behaving as a window defect.

lowed by a progressive decrease in fluorescence through the later phases of the angiogram as the choroid empties. An important characteristic is that the shape of the defect is unchanged. Another cause of hyperfluorescence is referred to as *staining*. Staining is the uptake of dye by a structure, usually drusen that are abnormal deposits in Bruch's membrane common in ARMD. Objects that stain behave the opposite of window defects—that is, drusen are not particularly hyperfluorescent in early stages, but as the angiogram progresses they become increasingly brighter. They are similar to a window defect in that their size and shape generally do not change. Figure 8-14 shows examples of staining, window defect, and leakage.

Remember that normal retinal blood vessels do not leak fluorescein, and that although the choriocapillaries normally leak, the RPE is a barrier that prevents dye from entering the retina (see Figure 8-10). Retinal blood vessels or RPE that have been damaged by disease and abnormal blood vessels that grow in response to certain disease processes (neovascularization) leak fluorescein, which then accumulates in the tissue space. *Leakage* and *pooling* are somewhat similar terms, as both refer to hyperfluorescence caused by an increased amount of dye. Leakage is used in any situation in which dye appears in an area where it is not normally observed. Fluorescence increases in intensity and spreads diffusely during the angiogram. The change in size and shape of the hyperfluorescence is important in distinguishing this abnormal pattern from window defects or staining where the pattern does not change, only the intensity. Leakage may be from normal retinal blood vessels that have been damaged, abnormal blood vessels that have grown (retinal or subretinal neovascularization), or from damage to the RPE. Pooling is a type of leakage in which dye accumulates in a confined anatomic space (e.g., intraretinal [cystoid

FIGURE 8-15
Clinical example of leakage and pooling.
A. Photograph of the right disc and macula of a patient with macular degeneration and decreased visual acuity. Hard exudate is apparent. Clinical examination revealed subretinal fluid and a solid elevation of the choroid consistent with a retinal pigment epithelial detachment (PED). **B.** In the early phase of the angiogram, the PED is visualized as a round hypofluorescent area, the result of blockage of choroidal fluorescence by fluid within the detachment. Between the PED and the disc is an irregular area of early hyperfluorescence. **C.** A few seconds later, the hyperfluorescence adjacent to the disc increases significantly, while only slightly in the PED. **D.** Late phase. The PED is a sharply demarcated, slowly filling area of hyperfluorescence due to pooling of dye within the confined space of the detachment. The adjacent choroidal neovascularization is visualized as an area of early hyperfluorescence and diffuse leakage in the subretinal and intraretinal space late in the angiogram.

A　　　　　　B

C　　　　　　D

macular edema], subretinal, or sub-RPE space). Because of the physical confinement of the dye, the edges of the hyperfluorescent area tend to be more sharply defined, and the fluorescence increases slowly because the dye is moving into a reservoir of fluid. The case presented in Figure 8-15 is interesting, because it demonstrates leakage from subretinal neovascularization, as well as pooling in an adjacent RPE detachment.

Hyperfluorescence due to dynamic stress on pre-existing normal pathways is often seen in vein occlusions. Figure 8-16 demonstrates dilated, normal vessels secondary to a central vein occlusion resulting in macular edema. In this particular case, perfusion is fairly good, and the patient is classified as having a non-ischemic vein occlusion. In other cases, the retina may be poorly perfused, resulting in hypofluorescent areas, indicating an ischemic vein occlusion. Retinal or anterior segment neovascularization (rubeosis) is a potential complication of an ischemic vein occlusion.

Earlier in the chapter, we examined two cases of hyperfluorescence due to the growth of abnormal vessels under the retina in ARMD—that is, CNV, sometimes also called *subretinal neovascularization*. The example also showed the progressive increase in fluorescein intensity and spread characteristic of leaky vessels. Another type of hyperfluorescence and leakage due to the growth of abnormal blood vessels occurs when the vessels grow from the retinal circulation as in proliferative diabetic retinopathy. Figure 8-17 is an example of diffusion of dye into the vitreous due to leakage from NVD and neovascularization elsewhere.

Hypofluorescence, an absence of the normal amount of fluorescence, is due to either a decrease in the amount of dye or to an obstacle that prevents visualization of the dye underneath. An example of hypofluorescence due to absence of dye is seen in capillary dropout or ischemia secondary to diabetic retinopathy (see Figure 8-17; Figure 8-18). In ischemia, the capillaries are closed, and there simply is no dye to fluoresce. In blocked fluorescence, however, the dye is present but cannot be visualized because of the intervening material (see Figures 8-13A, 8-16B, C, and 8-20).

FIGURE 8-16
Clinical example of leakage from stressed "normal" retinal vessels. **A.** Clinical photograph of a central retinal vein occlusion, showing intraretinal hemorrhage and venous tortuosity. **B.** No evidence of capillary nonperfusion is seen at 21 seconds. **C.** Late-stage fluorescein demonstrates fluorescein leakage from retinal vasculature and development of cystoid macular edema. Also note blocked fluorescence by scattered intraretinal hemorrhages.

FIGURE 8-17
Clinical example of leakage from abnormal vessels. Retinal neovascularization secondary to ischemia. **A.** Stereo fundus photograph showing elevated neovascularization of the disc (NVD). **B.** Stereo pair from fluorescein demonstrates hypofluorescence due to severe loss of perifoveal capillaries—that is, ischemia. Elevated neovascularization elsewhere (NVE) areas are visible in the lower left and are beginning to leak into the vitreous. **C.** Single image showing late fluorescein leakage from NVE and NVD. Fundus photographs and the fluorescein angiogram all play an important role in assessing the amount of damage to the eye from the disease process and in following the response to treatment.

FIGURE 8-18
Clinical examples of hypofluorescence due to non-perfusion. **A.** Arteriovenous phase of fluorescein angiogram in a diabetic patient demonstrating capillary closure/nonperfusion in field 3 (temporal to foveal avascular zone). Arrows point to stumps of closed vessels on several dilated capillaries. **B.** Early frame from a patient with a superotemporal branch vein occlusion shows a large area of retinal nonperfusion distal to a section of blockage by retinal hemorrhage. **C, D, E.** Because of the multiple ciliary arteries supplying the choroid and the interconnection of lobules, choroidal nonperfusion is uncommon. A diffuse process may, however, affect the choroidal circulation. The three frames here are from a patient who complained of "blotchy" vision and was referred with a diagnosis of impending macular hole. However, the fundus photograph shows several cotton-wool spots, indicating ischemia. The early phase of the fluorescein angiogram is remarkable for severe delay in filling of the choroid. On further questioning, the patient did admit to recent headaches, which led to an evaluation for and confirmation of temporal arteritis. Temporal arteritis results in closure of vessels due to inflammation and is a diffuse process.

Indocyanine Green Angiography

Fluorescein angiography has become the standard for evaluating the retinal and choroidal circulation; however, the information obtained can be limited in some circumstances because fluorescein's absorption and emission characteristics are in the visible spectrum. Fluorescence in the visible range is blocked by normal ocular pigment and by blood. ICG becomes bound to blood proteins once injected and has an absorption peak of 805 nm, with a peak emission at 835 nm. The absorption and fluorescence emission by ICG in the near infrared spectrum more readily penetrate ocular pigment. Another consequence of the infrared wavelength is that Mie scatter, or forward scatter, ameliorates blockage of ICG fluorescence by blood. Because ICG is bound to blood proteins, it does not leak as readily from the choroidal circulation as fluorescein.[2] Differences in the patterns obtained with these two dyes are due to the

Table 8-5. Phases of the Indocyanine Green Angiogram

Arterial	First appearance of dye in choroidal arteries; watershed zones may be identified; retinal arteries and veins dark; generally less than 2 seconds
Early venous phase	Appearance of dye in the choroidal veins; choriocapillaris filling complete though weak and difficult to visualize
Late venous phase	More uniform appearance to dye in the vessels; isofluorescence; approximately 10 minutes
Inversion phase	Dark vessels on a light background; late; 15–30 minutes

Source: RW Flower, BF Hochheimer. A clinical technique and apparatus for simultaneous angiography of the separate retinal and choroidal circulation. Invest Ophthalmol 1973;12:248–261.

highly protein-bound nature and infrared emission of ICG compared to non-protein–bound fluorescein, which emits in the visible spectrum. In general, ICG angiography is used to investigate choroidal abnormalities.

Robert Flower and Bernard Hochheimer were among the first to introduce ICG angiography.[19] However, it was not in widespread clinical use until digital imaging systems became available early in the 1980s. The angiograms that can be obtained with ICG are highly dependent on the type of equipment, which continues to evolve. It is useful to consider two major categories of imaging equipment for ICG angiography.[2] Systems based on the scanning laser ophthalmoscope provide rapid image acquisition up to 30 images per second and are well suited for delineating the early rapid passage of dye through the choroidal vasculature. Systems based on a fundus camera linked to a video-imaging device generally have higher spatial resolution but acquire approximately one image per second. The phases of the ICG angiogram are similar to that of fluorescein angiography (Table 8-5,[20] Figure 8-19). However, image acquisition rates of at least 10 per second are required to adequately visualize dye movement through the choroidal vasculature in the early phases of the ICG angiogram. The initial clinical applications of ICG angiography were based on relatively late events recorded on the lower speed digital fundus camera.[21] For the purposes of discussion in this chapter, we review examples of ICG patterns that are typical of the lower speed digital fundus cameras.

The following examples illustrate how ICG angiography adds clinically useful information in the presence of retinal or subretinal hemorrhage, and in delineating occult CNV in a patient with a pigment epithelial detachment. Note that in these examples inversion-phase ICG images are used to aid in the clinical decision.

In the first case (Figure 8-20), the fluorescein angiogram demonstrates blockage of fluorescence by subretinal hemorrhage in a patient with exudative ARMD. There is late fluorescein leakage of uncertain origin. The ICG angiogram on the other hand identifies a discrete lesion.

Figure 8-21 illustrates how ICG angiography may be useful in the identification of CNV in a patient with a pigment epithelial detachment. Two cases are shown in which clinical examination and fluorescein angiography demonstrate a pigment epithelial detachment. The fluorescein angiograms suggest CNV. However, ICG demonstrates CNV in only one patient, who may then be considered for ICG-guided laser treatment.[22]

Summary

The purpose of this chapter is to provide a framework within which photographers may apply their technical training to help the physician solve a clinical problem. The framework is based on the concept that pho-

FIGURE 8-19
Phases of the indocyanine green angiogram. **A, B, C.** Initial appearance of dye (<5 seconds) in three different patients. Arterial/early venous phases. In **A**, dye has not yet appeared in retinal vessels. In **B** and **C**, dye is in retinal arteries not the retinal veins, which appear as dark lines over disc in **B**, above center of macula in **C**. Area of delayed choroidal filling below the disc is normal and referred to as a *watershed area*. Round area of obscured choroidal vessels in **C** is due to scatter by fluid in a pigment epithelial detachment (see Figure 8-21G). **D, E.** Venous phase. Note filling of watershed areas seen in **A** and **B**. **F.** Late venous phase demonstrating isofluorescence in choroid. **G.** Late or inversion phase.

tographs are useful more often when the photographer is aware of the purpose of the photograph and is actively seeking specific changes, not passively recording events. The ability to apply photographic technique in this manner requires an understanding of normal ocular anatomy, normal and abnormal fluorescein and ICG patterns, and clinical information and experience. Table 8-6 is included as a "jump start" for beginning and intermediate photographers who want to achieve this goal. It truly is a pleasure to have the photographer as an active participant on the medical care team.

FIGURE 8-20
Age-related macular degeneration, subretinal hemorrhage. **A.** Red-free image showing subretinal hemorrhage and numerous drusen. **B.** Arteriovenous-phase fluorescein characterized primarily by blockage of fluorescence by hemorrhage. **C.** In a recirculation phase image, there has been some diffusion of dye, as well as staining of drusen. **D.** In contrast, inversion-phase indocyanine green image demonstrates a discrete lesion.

Reading Center Overview

Michael Neider

Ophthalmic photography reading centers play several roles in research studies. They serve as a central laboratory for the evaluation of study photographs and use trained graders working with standard grading protocols developed to evaluate different ocular conditions. A reading center uses several different grading protocols if it's involved in multiple areas of research, such as diabetic retinopathy, ARMD, acquired immune deficiency syndrome–related retinitis (cytomegalovirus [CMV] retinitis), or lens assessments. These grading protocols are designed to evaluate sets of photographs taken in a standardized manner by photographers working at many different sites. In some cases, as many as 75 sites, involving more than 200 photographers may participate in one study, and it is essential that all photographers follow similar photography procedures to allow the most accurate assessment of the photographic sets.

To standardize the photography procedures across multiple sites, the reading center develops photography protocols for different studies that contain a wide variety of photography elements important to image standardization. The reading center partners with photographers to help orient photography staff to the photography procedures and requirements. Photographer certification procedures, cameras and film types, and the specific fields of view required are outlined in the photography protocols. Among other elements, stereo photography requirements (with tips for obtaining good stereo images) may be included, as well as image han-

FIGURE 8-21
Age-related macular degeneration, pigment epithelial detachment (PED). **A, B.** Red-free images of two
different patients with PEDs. **C, D.** Arteriovenous fluorescein images at 16 and 20 seconds, respectively. In
both cases, the PED is beginning to fill with fluorescein. At the superior and nasal edge of the PED
there is an early, deep, speckled hyperfluorescence
suggesting choroidal neovascularization (CNV). **E,
F.** Recirculation-phase fluorescein images (7:50 and
7:49, respectively) show filling of the PED. In the first
patient **(E)** but not the second **(F)** there is also accu-
mulation of dye at the superior edge of the PED. **G,
H.** Inversion-phase indocyanine green (ICG) images.
No ICG fluorescence noted in the first patient **(G)**,
but the study supports occult CNV in the second **(H)**.
Subfoveal fluorescence not confirmed with ICG in
first patient, therefore, patient was not treated.
Photocoagulation was offered to second patient
with extrafoveal ICG fluorescence.

Table 8-6. Disease-Specific Fundus Photography and Fluorescein Angiography

Age-related macular degeneration (ARMD)

Nonexudative	Colors	Drusen, pigment change. Severity of disease, absence of fluid or hemorrhage, change with time.
	Location	RPE disease; macula.
	FA	May be required to ensure the absence of CNV.
	ICG	Not helpful.
Exudative	Colors	Document subretinal fluid or hemorrhage in macula, response to treatment.
	Location	RPE disease; macula.
	FA	Demonstrate CNV, imaging of FAZ important for treatment. Used to decide if treatable and then to guide laser treatment. Occasionally diagnostic.
	ICG	Particularly helpful with subretinal blood, pigment epithelial detachments, or occult disease on FA.[2,3,21] Early work with high-speed ICG video promising for feeder vessel treatment.[23]
	Other	Stereo FA is very important: required for accurate diagnosis of CNV. The pattern alone is insufficient.

Acute multifocal posterior placoid pigment epitheliopathy (AMPPE)

	Colors	Acute lesions typically multiple, post-equatorial, circumscribed, flat, gray-white. Resolve with mild pigment changes. (See serpiginous choroiditis.)
	Location	RPE/choroid; posterior pole.
	FA	Acute lesions block early in the study with late staining.
	ICG	Lesion hypofluorescent in early and late phases.[22,24]
	Other	Usually bilateral, recurrences rare.

Artery occlusion

	Colors	Pale, white appearance to retina acutely due to edema. Emboli may be visible in an arteriole. May look normal weeks after the event.
	Location	Retinal vascular disease; any field depending on central or branch artery occlusion.
	FA	To assess restoration of perfusion, ischemia, prognosis. Include disc in field.
	ICG	Not helpful.

Birdshot chorioretinitis

	Colors	Multifocal, round to oval, orange or yellow depigmented lesions with poorly defined borders associated with varying amounts of retinal edema, optic nerve edema, vitreous cells. Progress to deeply depigmented patches showing choroidal vessels.
	Location	RPE/choroid. Depigmentation scattered in posterior pole, often sparing macula.
	FA	Early choroidal lesions not visible. Resolved lesions appear as window defects. May exhibit fluorescein leakage from retinal vessels, optic nerve acutely.
	ICG	Multiple hypofluorescent lesions corresponding to acute lesions distributed along the larger choroidal vessels.[22,25]

Central serous retinopathy

	Colors	Fluid under RPE or retina, or both.
	Location	RPE; macula.
	FA	Hyperfluorescent, sharply demarcated lesion late if PED only. Edges less well-defined if serous RD present. May be multiple. Variable early-phase images. Some show early pinpoint hyperfluorescent lesions ("smokestack"). May be done to rule out choroidal neovascularization or to guide treatment in recurrent, persistent, or bilateral cases.
	Other	Stereo is important since leak is deep. Also can show elevation of retina. Document with green filter.

Choroidal nevus/tumor

	Colors	Document extent of lesion. Assessment of growth. Assist diagnosis in some cases. Red filter may help define borders and assist in focusing.
	Location	Choroid. Any field. A choroidal lesion but may be highly elevated; focus on base of lesion for extent, apex of lesion to indicate depth. Wide-angle view may be useful.
	FA	May be used to image tumor vascularization.
	ICG	Helpful in distinguishing choroidal melanoma from choroidal hemangioma (speckled pattern, stellate borders, progressive hyperfluorescence) and osteomas.[21]
	Other	Stereo helpful to give some indication of elevation, differential focusing for stereo.

Coats' disease

	Colors	Unilateral, serous retinal detachment, often massive amounts of hard exudate.
	Location	Retinal vascular disease; macula or periphery.
	FA	Diagnostic. Demonstrate areas of involvement with irregular vessel dilation, leakage, and nonperfusion.
	Other	Wide angle may be useful. May require FA during EUA for young children.

Cytomegalovirus retinitis

	Colors	Retinal hemorrhage, multiple gray and white retinal lesions in active disease. Progresses to area of atrophic retina with underlying RPE disturbance.
	Location	Retinitis; any field.

Diabetic retinopathy

Nonproliferative	Colors	Microaneurysms, retinal hemorrhage, hard exudate, cotton-wool spots, edema. Assists in determining progression of change, decision to proceed with focal laser treatment of macula, assess response to treatment.
	Location	Retinal vascular disease. FAZ most important because indication for treatment is HE or thickening that involves or threatens it. May utilize other fields to document severe NPDR and IRMAs, which indicate a higher progression to PDR.
	FA	Important in distinguishing edema from other causes or vision loss due to ischemia. Imaging of FAZ important to guide treatment.
	Other	Stereo very important in colors and FA to help assessment of thickening.
Proliferative	Colors	Status of NV, progression, response to retinal photocoagulation. Condition of macula can be crucial, because traction by fibrous tissue important in proceeding to surgery.
	Location	Retinal vascular disease. Can be any field, at the edge of a field, elevated or obscured by hemorrhage.
	FA	May demonstrate unsuspected NV. Occasionally used to assess amount of ischemia.
	Other	Stereo can be important for evaluation of NV or macula.

Glaucoma

	Colors	Cupping, disc notches, splinter hemorrhages.
	Location	Stereo pairs of optic discs.
	FA	Not applicable.
	Other	Clinician following cup to disc ratio.

Harada's disease

	Colors	Multifocal gray-white patches (similar to AMPPE). Vitreous cells.
	Location	RPE
	FA	Characteristic early, numerous, pinpoint areas of hyperfluorescence that gradually increase in size.
	ICG	Multiple hypofluorescent lesions.[26]
	Other	Vogt-Koyanagi-Harada syndrome: Patients that develop anterior uveitis, alopecia, poliosis, vitiligo, and dysacusis.

Idiopathic polypoidal choroidal vasculopathy (IPCV)

	Colors	Subretinal orange, red-orange polypoidal lesions. May see serous or hemorrhagic PED, serous retinal detachments, hard exudates.
	Location	Initially described as arising from peripapillary choroidal circulation, but can also arise from macular choroidal circulation.
	FA	Poorly defined leakage.
	ICG	Diagnostic. Branching choroidal vessels initially hypofluorescent due to apparent delay in filling that develop multiple, dilated, hyperfluorescent terminals or "polyps."[21]
	Other	Important to distinguish from choroidal neovascularization due to ARMD. IPCV more common in nonwhites, drusen not found in fellow eye.

Juvenile macular degeneration/flecked retina

	Colors	Deep RPE changes or deposits.
	Location	Macula, mid-periphery.
	FA	Silent choroid in Stargardt's and fundus flavimaculatus, diagnostic.
	ICG	"Flecks" hypofluorescent, edges stain late.[27]

Macroaneurysm

	Colors	Serous retinal detachment, retinal edema, hard exudate, retinal, subretinal, or vitreous hemorrhage.
	Location	Retinal vascular disease. Posterior pole.
	FA	May leak, be occluded, or obscured by hemorrhage.
	ICG	Can be useful differentiating macroaneurysm vs. exudative ARMD.[28]
	Other	May or may not be treated with laser depending on evidence of bleeding or progressive hard exudate in macula.

Macular holes

	Colors	Status, response to treatment.
	Location	Vitreoretinal interface, but generally with RPE changes. Macula.
	FA	Pattern characteristically a deep window defect. Occasionally mild, late leakage in retina surrounding the hole.
	Other	Stereo, higher magnification, slit-beam photography often useful to demonstrate a full-thickness hole. Occasionally an operculum.

Multiple evanescent white dot syndrome

	Colors	Multiple small, gray-white patches composed of tiny white dots.
	Location	RPE. Posterior pole.
	FA	Late staining, possible disc leakage.
	ICG	Hypofluorescent spots larger and more numerous than the clinically visible lesions.[21]
	Other	Dots resolve without residual RPE changes.

Table 8-6. (continued)

Myopic macular degeneration

Colors	Pigment disturbance, lacquer cracks, possible hemorrhage, document severity of changes.
Location	Macula.
FA	Rule out choroidal neovascularization in a patient with hemorrhage.
ICG	Linear hypofluorescence often more numerous and longer than seen with FA.[29]
Other	Important for level of leakage. May need plus diopter focusing range.

Ocular histoplasmosis syndrome
(and simulating disorders: multifocal choroiditis (MFC) and panuveitis, punctate inner choroidopathy)

Colors	Document deep RPE changes, chorioretinal scar.
Location	Choroid; macula, mid-periphery.
FA	Imaging of FAZ with suspected choroidal neovascularization. Guide treatment of choroidal neovascularization if present.
ICG	Hypo- and hyperfluorescent lesions described in MFC.[21]

Post-cataract cystoid macular edema

Colors	Mild macular edema may be difficult to show.
Location	Retinal vascular disease; macula.
FA	Diagnostic. Rule out CNV, other patterns of leakage in FAZ. Bilateral late disc photos helpful.
Other	Stereo important to demonstrate leakage from the retina.

Preretinal membrane

Colors	Demonstrate amount of retinal vascular distortion. Used to study anatomy in pre-surgical evaluation.
Location	Vitreoretinal interface; macula. Blue or green filters may highlight NFL changes.
FA	Helpful to assess amount of retinal vascular distortion, and presence of edema. Rarely will demonstrate another diagnosis such as occult choroidal neovascularization or branch vein occlusion.
Other	Stereo extremely helpful. High magnification may be useful.

Pseudoxanthoma elasticum

Colors	Angioid streaks.
Location	Choroid; posterior pole.
FA	May be needed for CNV.

Sarcoidosis

Colors	Anterior segment: skin nodules, conjunctival nodules, keratitic precipitates, iris nodules, synechiae. Posterior segment: vitreous cells (string of pearls nodules), disc edema, phlebitis-perivenous exudation (candle-wax dripping), solitary choroidal granuloma.
Location	Anterior and posterior segment.
FA	Perivenous and disc leakage.
ICG	Hypo- and hyperfluorescent spots and segmental choroidal vascular wall staining reported.[30]

Serpiginous choroiditis

Colors	Acute lesions are flat, white, resolve with extensive RPE changes. (See AMPPE.)
Location	RPE/choroid; peripapillary.
FA	CNV not infrequent.
ICG	Acute lesions block, fluorescence returns with resolution of lesion.[21]

Temporal arteritis

Colors	Show swollen or pale disc in optic neuropathy.
Location	Disc, posterior pole.
FA	Delayed filling of choroid helpful in diagnosis in absence of prior ischemic optic neuritis.[31]

Trauma/RD/choroidal detachment

Colors	May be photographed for documentation.
Location	May require external or slit-lamp photography.

Vein occlusion

Colors	Document quadrants involved with retinal hemorrhage, evidence of ischemia (e.g., cotton-wool spots), macular edema, presence of NV or vitreous hemorrhage. Treatment decision for macular edema based on FA and visual acuity. Patients with visual acuity of 20/40 or worse due to macular edema with good perfusion are candidates for focal laser in BRVO.
Location	Retinal vascular disease; any field. NV may be elevated.
FA	Imaging of FAZ for treatment. In BRVO, wide-angle or "survey FA" to assess ischemia in central vein occlusion. Blockage by intraretinal hemorrhage, hypofluorescence due to capillary nonperfusion, late fluorescein leakage from retinal vessels.

BRVO = branch vein occlusion; CNV = choroidal neovascularization; EUA = examination under anesthesia; FA = fluorescein angiography; FAZ = foveal avascular zone; HE = hard exudate; ICG = indocyanine green; IRMAs = intraretinal microvascular anomalies; IPCV = idiopathic polypoidal choroidal vasculopathy; MFC = multi-focal choroiditis; NV = neovascularization; NFL = nerve fiber layer; NPDR = nonproliferative diabetic retinopathy; PDR = proliferative diabetic retinopathy; PED = pigment epithelial detachment; RD = retinal detachment; RPE = retinal pigment epithelium.

dling procedures and digital system requirements. What follows is a closer look at some of these elements.

Photographer Certification

Photographers taking photographs evaluated by reading centers need to become certified for the relevant photography procedure(s) before submitting actual patient photographs. These certifications are typically reading-center specific, although one reading center may accept the certification of another reading center. Clinical sites are strongly encouraged to have a minimum of two certified photographers to allow for adequate back-up and to handle the additional photography volume that studies can bring to sites.

Certification may consist of (1) review of the study synopsis and photography protocol and (2) demonstrated ability to perform the photographic procedure by submission of photographs of acceptable quality. This could involve, for example, color photographs of four eyes for color photography certification or two fluorescein angiograms for angiographer certification. In some cases, lens photography certification requires the submission of separate slit-lamp or retro-illumination photographs. The second requirement may be waived if the photographer is currently certified for the identical procedure by the reading center. For example, The University of Wisconsin Fundus Photograph Reading Center (UW-FPRC) waives the requirement if the photographer has prior certification with the UW-FPRC using the same procedure, and the photographic quality of pictures taken within the past year has been good.

Camera and Film Requirements

Reading centers typically require specific camera types and image magnification for different studies. For example, studies evaluating diabetic retinopathy require the use of a 30-degree or 35-degree camera or one producing images with similar magnification. For the nine-field procedure used to document CMV retinitis, a 50-degree or 60-degree camera is required. In some cases, specific camera types are listed as acceptable choices, and sometimes camera approval must be obtained in advance from the reading center. Camera approval is obtained by submitting sample photographs for reading center review.

For color photography, professional films with an emulsion speed of less than or equal to ISO 100 are typically required. A reputable processing laboratory should always be used to process films. Study films are often archived for many years, and good quality film processing is essential, ensuring archival image stability.

Kodak T-Max, Tri-X, or Ilford 400 speed films are recommended for fluorescein angiography. The film may be processed by the clinic staff or at a local processing laboratory. The use of a particular developer may be specified. Any processing procedure that yields good quality negatives may be used. A reading center may recommend modification of film-processing procedures to ensure good quality negatives for evaluation. Proper care must be taken to adequately fix the film to ensure archival image stability.

Required Photographs and Standardized Photography Procedures

Standardized photography procedures are produced by the reading center to describe photographs required for a research study. Some of the most common fundus photography procedures include the modified seven standard stereo fields for diabetic retinopathy and the three fields for ARMD. Additionally, ARMD research studies often include a fluorescein angiography component, and the reading center may produce both film-based and digital angiography procedures. Procedures for documentation of acquired immunodeficiency syndrome–related retinopathy, such as CMV retinitis, using a nine wide-angle field procedure, have also been developed. What follows is a look at two of these procedures in much greater detail.

MODIFIED SEVEN STANDARD FIELDS FOR DIABETIC RETINOPATHY

The modified seven standard fields of the fundus of both eyes are taken in stereo. These fields differ from the traditional seven standard fields of the fundus taken in the ETDRS and other diabetic retinopathy studies in the position of two fields: Field 1M and field 3M are both modified to include the macula, in field 1M near the edge of the field and in field 3M midway between the edge and center of the field. Field 1M is centered on the temporal edge of the optic disc. Field 3M is positioned so that the center of the macula is halfway between the center and the nasal edge of the field. In this position, the camera's cross-hair is located approximately 1.0–1.5 disc diameter temporal to the macula. The modified seven standard fields are described below. The descriptions of the standard fields assume that there are two cross-hairs in the camera ocular, one vertical and the other horizontal (Figure 8-22).

Field 1M—Disc. Center the temporal edge of the optic disc at the intersection of the cross hairs in the ocular.

Field 2—Macula. Center the macula near the intersection of the cross hairs in the ocular. To keep the central gray artifact created by some cameras from obscuring the center of the macula, the intersection of the cross hairs should be placed approximately $1/8$–$1/4$ disc diameter above (or nasal to) the center of the macula.

Field 3M—Temporal to macula. Position the center of the macula halfway between the center and the nasal edge of the field. If field 2 was centered above the center of the macula, as suggested above, field 3M may be reached by rotating the camera without making any vertical adjustment.

Field 4—Superior temporal. The lower edge of the field is tangent to a horizontal line passing through the upper edge of the optic disc, and the nasal edge of the field is tangent to a vertical line passing through the center of the disc. It is convenient to take field 6 immediately after field 4 by rotating the camera nasally.

Field 6—Superior nasal. The lower edge of the field is tangent to a horizontal line passing through the upper edge of the optic disc, and the temporal edge of the field is tangent to a vertical line passing through the center of the disc.

Field 5—Inferior temporal. The upper edge of the field is tangent to a horizontal line passing through the lower edge of the optic disc and the nasal edge of the field is tangent to a vertical line passing through the center of the disc.

Field 7—Inferior nasal. The upper edge of the field is tangent to a horizontal line passing through the lower edge of the optic disc, and the temporal edge of the field is tangent to a vertical line passing through the center of the disc.

A stereoscopic fundus reflex photograph is taken at each seven-field visit to document media opacities. The photographer is asked to use his or her discretion to achieve a limbal diameter of approximately 13 mm on the finished slide. The best stereo effect is obtained by moving the

A

B

C

D

FIGURE 8-22
The modified seven standard fields (**(A)** OD, **(B)** OS) used to document diabetic retinopathy. All fields are taken in stereo. Fields 1M and 3M are positioned to include the macula. Fields 4–7 do not include the optic nerve. The modified three fields (**(C)** OD, **(D)** OS) used for age-related macular degeneration evaluation include a view of the macula in all three fields. Good stereoscopic effect is essential for the accurate assessment of retinal thickening.

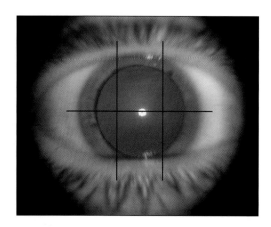

FIGURE 8-23
Stereo fundus reflex photographs are taken by moving the camera laterally approximately 3 mm between exposures. Two exposures are taken with the camera ocular cross-hairs alternately positioned midway between the center and edges of the pupil.

camera laterally approximately 3 mm between exposures. The lateral shift can be obtained by moving the joystick, sliding the camera, or using the Allen stereo separator. A fixation target should be positioned to direct the subject's gaze in the primary (straight ahead) position, so that the optic nerve does not appear directly behind the lens (Figure 8-23).

FLUORESCEIN ANGIOGRAPHY PROCEDURE
The fluorescein angiography procedure contains stereoscopic views of two fields at specified times after injection. These fields include the macula (field 2) of both eyes and the optic disc field (field 1M) of the study eye. To obtain stereo pairs that are correctly oriented in the filmstrip for stereoscopic viewing (i.e., do not have reversed stereoscopic effect), the right member of each pair must be taken first, followed by the left member. Stereoscopic red-free photographs are taken of field 2 in each eye before the injection of the fluorescein dye. The reading center receives the original negatives.

Fluorescein Injection. After the red-free photographs of both eyes have been taken, the camera is positioned for field 2 of the study eye. Fluorescein is injected rapidly (less than 5 seconds if possible) into the anticubital or other convenient vein according to usual clinic procedures.

Timing: Early Phase. The first photograph of the early phase is taken at time "0"—that is, at the moment injection of the fluorescein dye begins. The second photograph is taken at the moment the injection is complete. These photographs constitute a stereo pair and are referred to as the *control* photographs. They serve to document the integrity of the interference filters. The time shown on the second frame documents the rate of injection.

Ideally, the control photographs are followed by a series of 10–16 exposures taken at 1- to 2-second intervals, beginning approximately 15 seconds after the start of fluorescein injection (sooner if fluorescein appears sooner or delaying the initial exposures until fluorescence begins when a slow circulation time is expected). The usual result is five to eight stereo pairs after the control pair, typically culminating approximately 40–45 seconds after the start of injection.

Timing: Mid-Phase. After the early photographs are completed, the photographer takes stereo pairs of field 2 and then of field 1M of the study eye at approximately 60–90 seconds. At this point, the camera is positioned in front of the fellow eye, and a stereo pair is taken of field 2 at approximately 2 minutes. At this point, the camera is repositioned back to the study eye, and a stereo pair of field 2 is taken between 2 and 3 minutes.

Timing: Late-Phase.   A stereo pair of field 2 in the study eye is taken at 5 minutes. Two final stereo pairs are taken of field 2 in both eyes at 10 minutes.

Image Labeling and Handling

The reading center may specify the format for labeling and mounting of color slides, film-based angiograms, or digital files. Typically, the color slides are individually labeled with the study participant identification number, visit number, field location, eye photographed, and other study information. The slide pages are also labeled to accurately identify each slide set. Some reading centers have started to produce all of the slide and slide page labels for each study visit on one label sheet to help photographers expedite the labeling process.

The slides are typically located in heavy gauge, transparent pages with side-loading pockets. These clear pages allow for slide grading without removing slides from the pages, and the side-loading pockets help keep the slides "locked" into the pages because the slides press against each other. Some examples of the typical slide and filmstrip mounting formats are demonstrated in Figure 8-24.

When cutting the fluorescein angiogram negatives into strips, the photographer should take care not to separate the members of a stereo pair (i.e., not to leave one member of the pair at the end of one strip and the second member of the pair at the beginning of the next strip) (Figure 8-25).

Stereo Fundus Photography

Good-quality stereo fundus photographs are often required by reading centers to accurately assess areas of retinal thickening or neovascularization. For example, grading protocols may require the assessment of the presence or absence and extent of diabetic macular edema, or in the case of ARMD, the areas of retinal thickening may be measured as part of the grading process.

When obtaining stereo pairs, care should be taken that at least one member of the pair is of good, technical quality with crisp focus. In many cases, it is possible to obtain good quality in both members of the pair, but if this is not the case, the aim should be to obtain good quality in one member and some stereo separation between the members, accepting somewhat poorer quality in the second member of the pair, if necessary.

Dilation of the pupil to at least 6 mm is important to permit good quality stereo photography. If the pupils cannot be dilated to at least 4 mm, adequate stereoscopic effect may not be possible. The cornea should be undisturbed by prior examination with diagnostic contact lens.

The technique described by Allen used for taking stereo fundus photographs is shown in Figure 8-26.[32] An Allen stereo separator or manual lateral movement of the camera may be used to obtain the required, nonsimultaneous stereo pairs. If the manual method is used, the camera should not be rotated; instead, it should be moved from left to right with the joystick (or by sliding the camera base on its table, if preferred). It is customary to take the left member of the pair first, but this is optional (for angiograms to be viewed in strips, the right member is taken first). The first member of the pair is taken as far to one side of the pupil as possible, while maintaining good illumination and a clear image. If the separator is used, it is then flipped to the other side, and the second photograph is taken if its quality is good. If the quality is not good, refocusing with

A

B

FIGURE 8-24
Stereo color slides are mounted into plastic pages in positions that approximate their anatomic positions. Some studies require seven standard fields be taken of each eye **(A, B)**, whereas others require nine standard fields **(C)**. When only three fields are required, they are mounted as indicated by the shaded slides.

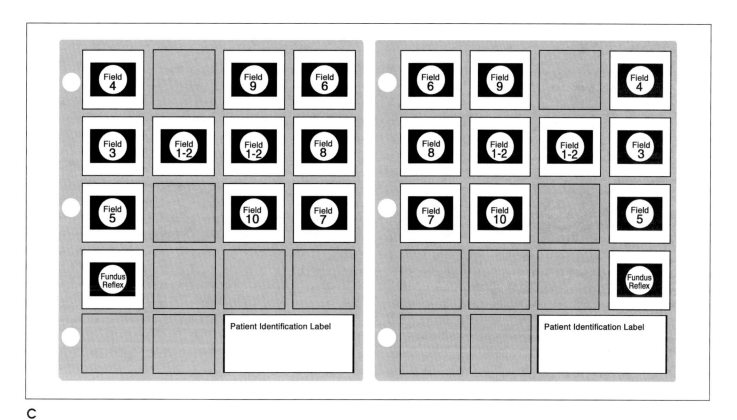

C

FIGURE 8-24 *(continued)*

spherical or astigmatic correction or slight vertical movement of the camera (to avoid lens opacity), or both, may be needed. Such vertical movement does not impair the stereoscopic effect. Somewhat less than optimal focus and clarity is acceptable, if necessary, in the second member of the pair to maintain the stereoscopic effect. The same principles apply when the manual technique is used. If the stereo separator is used, it should be set between 2.25–2.75 mm. Approximately 2 mm is the minimum separation between members of the stereo pair to be aimed for when moving the joystick or sliding the camera.

Digital System Certification

As ophthalmic photography continues to move away from film-based images toward digital images, reading centers face different challenges that may require digital system certification. Once original color slides placed into plastic pages were received, now digital files either electronically or on recordable media are received. Reading centers need to be certain that they can interface with a wide variety of digital system software and hardware components. Complete information about each camera system used to capture digital images may be collected, and digital system evaluation software may be run on the digital system as part of the certification process and periodically throughout the study to monitor system elements critical to accurate assessment of digital images.

Additionally, the reading center may require modifications to the system, for example, the addition of a compact disk writer or that "dial-in" access be present to allow system vendors and reading center technical staff access to the system, before completing certification.

A

B

FIGURE 8-25
The original fluorescein angiogram negatives are cut into strips of six images per strip **(A)**. Care must be taken when cutting the film so that no stereo pairs are cut in half **(B)**. Paying careful attention during photography helps reduce this problem: The right member of each pair must be taken first, followed by the left member.

FIGURE 8-26
Maximum stereo separation is obtained using Allen's technique. One member of the stereo pair is taken from the left edge of the pupil. The camera is then moved laterally to the opposite side of the pupil where the second picture is taken.

References

1. Gass J, Donald M. Stereoscopic Atlas of Macular Diseases: Diagnosis and Treatment (4th ed). St. Louis: Mosby, 1997.
2. Berkow JW, Flower RW, Orth DH, Kelley JS. Fluorescein and Indocyanine Green Angiography: Technique and Interpretation. San Francisco: American Academy of Ophthalmology, 1997.
3. Yanuzzi LA, Flower RW, Slakter JS, eds. Indocyanine Green Angiography. St. Louis: Mosby, 1997.
4. Covey SR. The 7 Habits of Highly Effective People. New York: Simon & Schuster, 1989;98.

5. Isselbacher KJ, Braunwald E, Wilson JD, et al. (eds). Harrison's Principles of Internal Medicine (13th ed). New York: McGraw-Hill, 1994;2.
6. Diabetic Retinopathy Study Research Group. Indications for photocoagulation treatment of diabetic retinopathy, DRS Report No. 14. Int Ophthalmol Clin 1987;27:239.
7. Kertes P, Conway M. Clinical Trials in Ophthalmology: A Summary and Practice Guide. Lippincott Williams & Wilkins, 1998.
8. Early Treatment of Diabetic Retinopathy Study Research Group. Photocoagulation for diabetic macular edema, ETDRS Report No. 1. Arch Ophthalmol 1985;103:1796.
9. Macular Photocoagulation Study Group. Krypton laser photocoagulation for idiopathic neovascular lesions: results of a randomized clinical trial. Arch Ophthalmol 1990;108:832.
10. Macular Photocoagulation Study Group. Persistent and recurrent neovascularization after laser photocoagulation for subfoveal choroidal neovascularization of age-related macular degeneration. Arch Ophthalmol 1994;112:489.
11. Branch Vein Occlusion Study Group. Argon laser scatter photocoagulation for prevention of neovascularization and vitreous hemorrhage in branch vein occlusion: a randomized clinical trial. Arch Ophthalmol 1986;104:34.
12. Branch Vein Occlusion Study Group. Argon laser photocoagulation for macular edema in branch vein occlusion. Am J Ophthalmol 1984;98:271.
13. The Miami Study Group. Cystoid macular edema in aphakic and pseudophakic eyes. Am J Ophthalmol 1979;88:45.
14. Nussbaum JJ, Pruett RC, Delori FC. Historic perspectives—macular yellow pigment: the first 200 years. Retina 1982;1:296.
15. Eagle RC Jr. Mechanisms of maculopathy. Ophthalmology 1984;91:613–625.
16. Hayreh S. The choriocapillaris. Albrecht von Graefes Arch Klin Exp Ophthalmol 1974;192:165.
17. Justice J Jr, Lehmann RP. Cilioretinal arteries: a study based on review of stereo fundus photographs and fluorescein angiographic findings. Arch Ophthalmol 1976;94:1355.
18. Rosenbauer T. Reading Trout Streams. An Orvis Guide. New York: Lyons & Burford, 1988;10.
19. Flower RW, Hochheimer BF. A clinical technique and apparatus for simultaneous angiography of the separate retinal and choroidal circulation. Invest Ophthalmol 1973;12:248–261.
20. Soubrane G, Seres A, Coscas G, Flower RW. Suggested terminology for different phases of indocyanine green angiogram. Retina 2000;3:319–320.
21. Yanuzzi LA, Slakter JS, Sorenson JA, et al. Digital indocyanine green videoangiography and choroidal neovascularization. Retina 1992;12:191–223.
22. Guyer DR, Yanuzzi LA, Slakter JS, et al. Diagnostic indocyanine green videoangiography. In SJ Ryan (ed), Retina (3rd ed). Vol. 2. St. Louis: Mosby, 2001;943–966.
23. Murphy RP, Lin SB, Glaser BM. Feeder vessel treatment for age-related macular degeneration (ARMD) with subfoveal fibrovascular choroidal neovascularization. Invest Ophthalmol Vis Sci 2001;42(4):S231(abst).
24. Uyama M, Matsunaga H, Matsubara T, et al. Indocyanine green angiography and pathophysiology of multifocal posterior pigment epitheliopathy. Retina 1999;19:12–21.
25. Fardeau C, Herbort CP, Kullmann N, et al. Indocyanine green angiography in birdshot chorioretinopathy. Ophthalmology 1999;106:1928–1934.
26. Bouchenaki N, Morisod L, Herbort CP. Vogt-Koyanagi-Harada syndrome: importance of rapid diagnosis and therapeutic intervention. Klinische Monatsblatter fur Augenheilkunde 2000;216:290–294.
27. Schwoerer J, Secretan M, Zografos L, Piguet B. Indocyanine green angiography in fundus flavimaculatus. Ophthalmologica 2000;214:240–245.
28. Townsend-Pico WA, Meyers SM, Lewis H. Indocyanine green angiography in the diagnosis of retinal arterial macroaneurysms associated with submacular and preretinal hemorrhages: a case series. Am J Ophthalmol 2000;129:33–37.
29. Ohno-Matsui K, Morishima N, Ito M, Tokoro T. Indocyanine green angiographic findings of lacquer cracks in pathologic myopia. Jpn J of Ophthalmol 1998;42:293–299.
30. Matsuo T, Itami M, Shiraga F. Choroidopathy in patients with sarcoidosis observed by simultaneous indocyanine green and fluorescein angiography. Retina 2000;20:16–21.
31. Valmaggia C, Speiser P, Bischoff P, Niederberger H. Indocyanine green versus fluorescein angiography in the differential diagnosis of arteritic and nonarteritic anterior ischemic optic neuropathy. Retina 1999;19:131–134.
32. Allen L. Ocular fundus photography. Am J Ophthalmol 1964;57:13–28.

Chapter 9

Fundus Photography: Descriptive Interpretation

Patrick J. Saine and Timothy J. Martin

A. Introduction
B. Normal Fundus
C. Fundus: Normal Variations
D. Posterior Pole
E. Optic Disc
F. Vascular Abnormalities
G. Retinal Hemorrhages
H. Retinal Potpourri
I. Surgical Fundus

Introduction

Examining your initial fundus photographs is a bit like reviewing travel snapshots taken in a foreign land. You remember having taken the trip (the photographs in front of you are proof that you were there), and yet the images seem strangely different. On reviewing them, you discover new shapes, colors, and details that you may have failed to notice at the moment of exposure. And the more you study the images—the more you see!

This chapter uses fundus images of common retinal characteristics to orient you to the new landscape you photograph. Our intent is a short introduction to the visual characteristics of the normal and diseased fundus; this chapter is not meant to be a comprehensive guide to retinal abnormalities. You can learn more about the retina by reviewing your clinical photographs with your referring physician, by studying a comprehensive fundus atlas, and by attending continuing education seminars in ophthalmic photography. A greater understanding of the eye in normal and diseased states enhances your fundus photography results.

Landmarks in the normal fundus and its variations begin the chapter. Abnormal maculae and optic discs are described, as are vascular abnormalities and various types of hemorrhages. We conclude with a potpourri of retinal abnormalities and a look at fundus photographs after retinal surgery.

Normal Fundus

The easiest fundus landmark for orientation is the optic disc (Figure 9-1). This somewhat oval, pink structure is located approximately 15 degrees nasal to the central visual axis (fovea). The optic disc overlies the scleral canal and is made up of a number of elements entering or leaving the eye:

FIGURE 9-1
Normal fundus, right eye. (FundusMap, a multi-image computer composite photo-illustration, by Richard E. Hackel, University of Michigan, Ann Arbor, MI.)

1. Blood vessels: The central retinal artery emerges from the center of the disc and immediately divides to deliver blood to the four quadrants of the retina. The superior and inferior temporal branches (arcades) sweep around the fovea and roughly define the macula. The retinal veins form a similar pattern as they exit the eye at the optic disc. The optic disc can therefore always be found by tracing these vessels to their point of convergence.
2. Axons: The optic disc contains more than a million axons; these "wires" are cell processes that begin in the inner retina and converge to form the optic nerve, making a right-angle turn to exit the eye on their way to the brain. The fine capillaries that support these axons give the disc its pink color. These axons—"end on"—make up the neural rim of the optic disc, which in most individuals surrounds a central, whitish depression of variable size (the optic cup).

The visual axis of the eye intersects the retina at the fovea, the center of the macula. Photoreceptors are highly concentrated here to deliver the sharpest, clearest vision. The fovea is centered between the temporal vascular arcades and can be identified as a circular pigmented area slightly

FIGURE 9-2
Normal variations. **A.** "Blonde" fundus, with transparent, lightly pigmented retinal pigment epithelium (RPE), showing the deep choroidal vessels. **B.** Highly pigmented RPE. **C.** Tigroid fundus shows variations in RPE. **D.** Congenital hypertrophy of the RPE. **E.** Myelinated nerve fiber layer. **F.** Asteroid hylosis.

larger than the disc. The large number of axons extending radially from the center of the fovea cause a mound of increased retinal thickness, often identified by circular light reflexes on the smooth, innermost transparent retinal layer (the internal limiting membrane). To provide the clearest optical performance, axons from the temporal retina are carefully routed around the fovea. This strategy is the basis of the arc-shaped pattern of the nerve fiber layer. The axons can often be seen as fine striations sweeping toward the disc, especially above and below the disc, where the nerve fiber layer is thickest.

In lightly pigmented patients, the deeper choroidal circulation is evident. These vessels have a more random pattern and do not normally communicate with retinal vessels.

Fundus: Normal Variations

The pigmentation (and thus transparency) of the retinal pigment epithelium (RPE) may vary considerably among normal individuals, generally correlating with the degree of pigmentation elsewhere (e.g., skin, hair). Thus, in the blonde fundus, the choroidal vessels are easily seen (Figure 9-2A). In darkly pigmented individuals, all choroidal details are hidden by the relatively opaque RPE (see Figure 9-2B). In some subjects, there may be marked variations of pigmentation within the same fundus (see Figure 9-2C).

Congenital hypertrophy of the RPE (see Figure 9-2D) appears as characteristic grouped areas of darkly pigmented "spots" often described as "bear tracks." This finding does not cause visual symptoms but is important because it must be distinguished from melanoma or other pigmented fundus lesions.

The optic nerve consists of more than a million "wires" (axons) that begin in the retina and travel over the inner retina (as the nerve fiber layer) to exit the eye as the optic nerve. As the axons exit the eye, they acquire an insulating coating (myelin), which increases the speed and efficiency of data transfer. Occasionally, otherwise normal individuals show aberrant myelinization of axons in the nerve fiber layer, producing the feathery, superficial, white areas, extending along the path of the nerve fiber layer (see Figure 9-2E).

In asteroid hyalosis, opaque white concretions (calcium soaps) are scattered throughout the vitreous. Despite their impressive appearance, they generally do not cause visual symptoms, although they can interfere with visualization of the retina (see Figure 9-2F).

Posterior Pole

As opposed to the water-tight retinal vessels, the vessels in the choriocapillaris are inherently "leaky," although Bruch's membrane prevents this fluid from entering the subretinal space by providing the outer blood-retinal barrier. Bruch's membrane is a complex layer between the RPE and the choroid and is composed of elements from the base of the RPE and the choriocapillaris. A number of diseases damage Bruch's membrane and the RPE. In age-related macular degeneration, fluid may collect under the RPE, appearing as "soft drusen" (Figure 9-3A). Fluid also collects under the RPE in central serous retinopathy, a disease of young patients, and breaks through the RPE to collect under the neurosensory retina (see Figure 9-3B). Discontinuities in Bruch's membrane occur in many clinical entities, allowing choroidal vessels to grow into the sub-RPE and subretinal space (subretinal neovascular membrane). Age-related macular degeneration is a common cause of subretinal neovascularization and hemorrhage (see Figure 9-3C).

Myopic individuals of any age may also develop choroidal neovascular membranes. It is thought that in such large, myopic eyes, Bruch's membrane is stretched tenuously thin (as suggested by the failure of the RPE to reach completely to the disc margin, resulting in a "myopic halo" around the disc), and is prone to breakage (see Figure 9-3D).

Many different diseases may cause the retinal vessels to become leaky, allowing blood components to seep into the deep retinal tissues. As the fluid portion resorbs, chalky-white hard exudates or "edema residues" are left behind. In the fovea, the dense radiating axons (Henle's nerve fiber layer) enclose the edema and create radial or wedge-shaped patterns. In other areas, rings of edema residue encircle the leaky spots (see Figure 9-3E). Diabetic retinopathy is a common cause of these hard exudates.

Many ocular disorders may be associated with the growth of membranes at the innermost level (toward the center of the eye) of the retina. Contraction of these membranes results in macular pucker, or wrinkling, distorting vision (see Figure 9-3F).

FIGURE 9-3
The posterior pole. **A.** Age-related macular degeneration with soft drusen. **B.** Central serous chorioretinopathy. **C.** Subretinal neovascularization. **D.** Myopic halo or scleral crescent. **E.** Circinate retinopathy. **F.** Epiretinal membrane.

Optic Disc

In glaucoma, visual field defects result from axonal death. Axonal loss can be identified in the fundus as loss of the nerve fiber layer striations and enlargement of the central cup in the optic disc (Figure 9-4A). In other forms of optic atrophy, the optic cup may change little, but the normally pink neural rim becomes pale (see Figure 9-4B).

Acute disorders of the optic disc often result in swelling of the axons and supporting tissue, causing elevation of the disc and blurring of the disc margins (see Figure 9-4C). The cerebrospinal fluid that bathes the brain and spinal column also surrounds the optic nerve right up to the globe. Intracranial diseases can raise the pressure of this fluid and can cause bilateral disc swelling. Other common causes of disc swelling include anterior ischemic optic neuropathy and optic neuritis.

The optic disc may also be elevated by rock candy–like hyaline material buried in the axons of the optic disc. Visual field loss can occasionally result, but the finding is usually benign. In older individuals, this refractive material can often be seen poking through the surface of the disc (see Figure 9-4D). In young patients, the material may be completely buried, and the disc elevation may be difficult to distinguish from true disc swelling (see Figure 9-4E).

FIGURE 9-4
The optic disc. **A.** Glaucomatous optic nerve. **B.** Optic atrophy. **C.** Optic disc edema. **D.** Drusen of the optic nerve. **E.** Buried drusen. **F.** Coloboma of the optic nerve.

Congenital malformations of the optic disc (such as an optic nerve coloboma) can result in bizarre appearances, with variable visual dysfunction (see Figure 9-4F).

Vascular Abnormalities

Infarction of the retina can occur if intravascular material (an embolus) lodges in the central retinal artery or its branches. Hollenhorst plaques are cholesterol crystals that commonly originate in the large carotid arteries in the neck and can be seen as glistening white, refractile material, often at arterial bifurcations (Figure 9-5A). More proximal blockage of the central retinal artery can be identified acutely as an opaque, pale, macular swelling accentuating the choroidal red of the foveola, known as the *cherry red spot*. After infarction, the normally transparent arterial wall may become opaque, appearing as a ghost vessel (see Figure 9-5B).

Retinal ischemia from vascular disorders, such as diabetes, may incite neovascularization. These new blood vessels grow into the vitreous from the disc (see Figure 9-5C) or elsewhere (see Figure 9-5D), resulting in vitreous hemorrhages and retinal traction detachments. A common early

FIGURE 9-5
Vascular abnormalities. **A.** Hollenhorst plaque.
B. Central retinal artery occlusion.
C. Neovascularization of the optic nerve.
D. Neovascularization "elsewhere." **E.** Venous beading secondary to radiation. **F.** Arterial-venous crossing change. (**E** and **F** reproduced with permission from Timothy Bennett, Penn State Geisinger Health Systems, Hershey, PA.)

sign of ischemic diabetic retinopathy is segmental narrowing of retinal veins, creating venous beading. Figure 9-5E shows venous beading in a patient with radiation retinopathy.

Systemic hypertension causes stiffening and thickening of the retinal arterial walls, resulting in segmental narrowing, as well as the appearance of venous discontinuity at artery-vein crossings (A-V nicking) (see Figure 9-5F).

Retinal Hemorrhages

Hemorrhages may occur at any retinal level. The shape of the hemorrhages is determined by the orientation and shape of the surrounding tissue structures at that level. Blood beneath the sensory retina (subretinal) can separate layers and spread out (Figure 9-6A). Dot and blot hemorrhages are rounded by the deep structures in the retina (see Figure 9-6B). The orientation of the nerve fiber layer creates elongated flame-shaped hemorrhages (see Figure 9-6C). Blood on the surface of the retina (preretinal) obscures retinal details (see Figure 9-6D), with its shape determined by the apposition of the vitreous hyaloid face and the forces of gravity (see Figure 9-6E).

FIGURE 9-6
Retinal hemorrhages. **A.** Subretinal blood. **B.** Dot and
blot hemorrhages. **C.** Nerve fiber layer hemorrhages.
D. Preretinal hemorrhage. **E.** Boat-shaped hemor-
rhage. (**E** reproduced with permission from Richard E.
Hackel, University of Michigan, Ann Arbor, MI.) **F.**
Shaken baby syndrome. (**F** reproduced with permis-
sion from Timothy Bennett, Penn State Geisinger
Health System, Hershey, PA.)

Figure 9-6F is a fundus photograph depicting the characteristic
trauma-induced hemorrhages that occur in the shaken baby syndrome.

Retinal Potpourri

Presumed ocular histoplasmosis presents with punched-out chorioretinal scars and peripapillary atrophy (Figure 9-7A). Patients are generally
asymptomatic unless they develop a third common finding: macular
choroidal neovascular membranes.

Ischemic retinal disorders may cause fluffy, superficial, white, cotton-
wool spots. These lesions are the result of swelling and opacification of
the nerve fiber layer and may obscure the retinal details. Cotton-wool
spots are likely areas of focal nerve fiber layer ischemia and are common
in diabetic, hypertensive, and human immunodeficiency virus retinopathy (see Figure 9-7B).

A common cause of blindness in human immunodeficiency–infected
patients is cytomegalovirus retinitis (see Figure 9-7C). Prompt treatment may prevent its progression to multiple retinal holes and retinal
detachment.

FIGURE 9-7
Other retinal appearances. **A.** Presumed ocular histoplasmosis syndrome. **B.** Human immunodeficiency virus retinopathy. **C.** Cytomegalovirus retinitis. **D.** Retinal nevi. **E.** Angioid streaks. **F.** Retinitis pigmentosa.

Choroidal nevi (see Figure 9-7D) are similar to moles on the skin. They are common and generally benign but must be distinguished from choroidal melanoma.

Angioid streaks are radial cracks in Bruch's membrane (see Figure 9-7E). Because they are red and radiate from the disc, they may be mistaken for blood vessels (thus, "angioid"). Choroidal neovascular membranes may develop.

Retinitis pigmentosa represents a spectrum of retinal degenerative disorders, often characterized by a peculiar "bony spicule" pigmentation of the peripheral retina (see Figure 9-7F).

Surgical Fundus

Neovascularization in ischemic vascular disorders (especially diabetes) can frequently be prevented by selective destruction of ischemic retina with laser photocoagulation. Fresh laser spots appear as pale, "soft" white spots (Figure 9-8A), with time developing into well-defined white areas with variable pigmentation (see Figure 9-8B).

FIGURE 9-8
The surgical fundus. **A.** Laser treatment. **B.** Laser treatment with time. **C.** Macular hole with operculum. **D.** Retinal detachment. **E.** Retinal appearance of a scleral buckle. **F.** Silicone oil vitreous replacement.

Macular holes may develop if abnormal vitreous attachment and traction creates a "divot" in the foveola. A cuff of retinal detachment is frequently seen (see Figure 9-8C).

Any break in the sensory retina may allow vitreous fluid to seep underneath, causing a retinal detachment (see Figure 9-8D). Surgery is required to close the break, often by using an external element to indent the globe beneath the break (see Figure 9-8E). In complicated cases, viscous silicone oil may be required to mechanically "steam roller" the retina back into position (see Figure 9-8F).

Ophthalmic photography integrates specialized photographic procedures with the clinical needs of the ophthalmologist. Successful ophthalmic photographers understand how and why their photographs are used.

Appendix A

Useful Abbreviations for the Ophthalmic Photographer

Patrick J. Saine and Marshall E. Tyler

AAO	American Academy of Ophthalmology
AC	anterior chamber
ACL	anterior chamber lens
AIDS	acquired immunodeficiency syndrome
AION	anterior ischemic optic neuropathy
ALK	automated lamellar keratoplasty
ALP	argon laser photocoagulation
AMPPE	acute multifocal placoid pigment epitheliopathy
ANSI	American National Standards Institute
ANV	angle new vessels
APD	afferent pupillary defect
ARMD	age-related macular degeneration
ARN	acute retinal necrosis
ASAP	as soon as possible
ASCC	anterior subcapsular cataract
ASORN	American Society of Ophthalmic Registered Nurses
ATPO	Association of Technical Personnel in Ophthalmology
AVM	anterior venous malformation
BAO	branch artery occlusion
BDR	background diabetic retinopathy
b.i.d.	twice a day
Bit	Binary digit
BLL	both lower lids
BMP	Bitmap
BOPA	British Ophthalmic Photographic Association
BP	blood pressure
BRAO	branch retinal artery occlusion
BRVO	branch retinal vein occlusion
BUL	both upper lids
BVO	branch vein occlusion
C/D	cup to disc ratio
CAO	central artery occlusion
Cat.	cataract
CC	color correction (filter)
CC	with correction
$\overline{CC}$	cubic centimeters
CD-ROM	compact disk–read only memory
CD-RW	compact disk–rewriteable
CF	count fingers
CME	cystoid macular edema

CMV	cytomegalovirus
CNVM	choroidal neovascular membrane
COA	certified ophthalmic assistant
COAG	chronic open-angle glaucoma
COMS	Collaborative Ocular Melanoma Study
COMT	certified ophthalmic master technician
COT	certified ophthalmic technician
CPR	cardiopulmonary resuscitation
CR	chorioretinal
CRA	central retinal artery
CRA	certified retinal angiographer
CRAO	central retinal artery occlusion
CRVO	central retinal vein occlusion
cSLO	confocal scanning laser ophthalmoscope
CSME	clinically significant macular edema
CSR	central serous retinopathy (choroidopathy)
CSCR	central serous chorioretinopathy
CVO	central vein occlusion
CVOS	central vein occlusion study
CWS	cotton-wool spots
DCCT	Diabetes Control and Complications Trial
DICOM	Digital Imaging and Communications in Medicine
DM	diabetes mellitus
DOB	date of birth
DR	diabetic retinopathy
DRS	Diabetic Retinopathy Study
Dx	diagnosis
ECCE	extracapsular cataract extraction
EI	exposure index
EM	electron microscopy
EOM	extraocular movement
ER	emergency room
ERM	epiretinal membrane
ETDRS	Early Treatment of Diabetic Retinopathy Study
EUA	examination under anesthesia
f/u	follow-up
FA	fluorescein angiography
FAZ	foveal avascular zone
FOPS	fellow of the Ophthalmic Photographers' Society
FP	fundus photographs
FPD	fibrous proliferation at disc
FPE	fibrous proliferation elsewhere
FTP	file transfer protocol
gtt	drop
GIF	graphics interchange format
H&D	Hurter & Driffield (characteristic curve, film)
HCL	hard contact lens
HE	hard exudates
HIV	human immunodeficiency virus
HM	hand motion
HTML	hypertext mark-up language
HTTP	hypertext transfer protocol
Hx	history
ICCE	intracapsular cataract extraction
ICG	indocyanine green
ICG-A	indocyanine green angiography

IDDM	insulin-dependent diabetes mellitus
IEEE	Institute of Electrical and Electronics Engineers
IN	inferior nasal
INV	iris new vessels
IOFB	intraocular foreign body
IOL	intraocular lens
ION	ischemic optic neuropathy
IOP	intraocular pressure
IR	infrared
IRMA	intraretinal microaneurysm
ISO	International Standards Organization (film speed)
IT	inferior temporal
IV	intravenous
IVFA	intravenous fluorescein angiography
JCAHPO	Joint Commission on Allied Health Personnel in Ophthalmology
JOPS	Japanese Ophthalmic Photographers' Society
JPCNV	juxtapapillary choroidal neovascularization
JPEG	Joint Photographic Experts Group
K	Kelvin (color temperature)
LASIK	laser-assisted in situ keratomileusis
KLPC	krypton laser photocoagulation
LLL	left lower lid
LP	light perception (visual acuity)
LUL	left upper lid
MA	microaneurysm
MB	megabyte
Meg	megabyte
ME	macular edema
ml	milliliters
MM	malignant melanoma
MPS	Macular Photocoagulation Study
N/I	no improvement
N/V	nausea and vomiting
NAG	narrow-angle glaucoma
ND	neutral density
NEMA	National Electrical Manufacturers Association
NFL	nerve fiber layer
NIDDM	non–insulin-dependent diabetes mellitus
NL	normal
NLP	no light perception (visual acuity)
nm	nanometer
NPDR	nonproliferative diabetic retinopathy
NV	near vision
NV	neovascularization
NVD	neovascularization at disc
NVE	neovascularization elsewhere
OD	ocular dexter (right eye)
ONH	optic nerve head
OPS	Ophthalmic Photographers' Society
OS	ocular sinister (left eye)
OS	operating system
OU	ocular uterque (both eyes)
P/O	postoperative
PA	physician assistant
PC	posterior chamber

PCL	posterior chamber lens
PDR	proliferative diabetic retinopathy
PED	pigment epithelial detachment
PH	pinhole (visual acuity)
PK	penetrating keratoplasty
p.o.	by mouth
POAG	primary open-angle glaucoma
POHS	presumed ocular histoplasmosis syndrome
PPDR	preproliferative diabetic retinopathy
Pre-op	preoperative
PRK	photoreactive keratectomy
PRM	preretinal membrane
PRMF	preretinal macular fibrosis
p.r.n.	as needed
PRP	panretinal photocoagulation
PS	PostScript
PSC	posterior subcapsular cataract
PSD	Photoshop document
PTK	phototherapeutic keratectomy
PVD	posterior vitreous detachment
PXE	pseudo-xanthoma elasticum
QD	every day
QH	every hour
q.i.d.	four times a day
R/O	rule out
RAM	random access memory
RD	retinal detachment
RK	radial keratotomy
RLF	retrolental fibroplasia
RLL	right lower lid
ROM	read only memory
ROP	retinopathy of prematurity
RP	retinitis pigmentosa
RPE	retinal pigment epithelium
RPED	retinal pigment epithelium detachment
RUL	right upper lid
Rx	prescription
S/P	status post
SB	scleral buckle
$\overline{\text{SC}}$	without correction
SCL	soft contact lens
SCSI	Small Computer Systems Interface
SE	soft exudates
SLO	scanning laser ophthalmoscope
SLR	single lens reflex
SN	superior nasal
SRNV	subretinal neovascularization
SRNVM	subretinal neovascular membrane
ST	superior temporal
STAT	immediately
Sx	symptoms
TAPP	applanation pressure by tonometry
t.i.d.	three times a day
TIFF	tagged image file format
TTL	through the lens
Tx	treatment

USB	universal serial bus
UV	ultraviolet
VA	visual acuity
VB	venous beading
WA	wide angle
WHO	World Health Organization
WNL	within normal limits
Ws	watt seconds
WYSIWYG	"what you see is what you get"
XHTML	extensible hypertext mark-up language

Appendix B

Professional Societies of Interest to the Ophthalmic Photographer

Patrick J. Saine and Marshall E. Tyler

Association Espanola de Technicos Especialistas en Fotografia Cientifica (AETEFC)
Senor Manuel Soler Martinez, President
5 Congreso International de la Imagen Cientifica
Plaza Luc de Tena, No. 13
28045—Madrid
Spain
Tel: +34 1 539 7768

Australian Institute of Medical and Biological Illustration
Michael Shapter
Box 5590 Mail Centre
Townsville QLD 4810 Australia
http://www.aimbi.org.au/

BioCommunications Association, Inc. Central Office
(Formerly Biological Photographic Association)
115 Stoneridge Drive
Chapel Hill, NC 27514-9737
Tel/Fax: 919-967-8246
Email: BCAoffice@aol.com
www.bca.org

British Ophthalmic Photographic Association (BOPA)
c/o Richard Hildred
Medical Imaging
The Priory Hospital
Priory Road
Birmingham B5 7UG
United Kingdom
www.bopa.org.uk

Deutsche Gesellschaft fur Photographie (DGPh)
Horst Wesche
Unfallchirurgische Klinik
Fotodocumentation
Medizinische Hochschule Hannover
Konstanty-Gutschow-Strasse 8
D-3000 Hannover 61
Germany
Tel: 0511-532-3842

Foreninge fur Medicinsk och Tecknisk Fotografi (FMTF)
Ole Roos
Department of Biomedical Communications
Sahlgren Hospital
413 45 Goteborg
Sweden
Tel: 031 60 2326

Japanese Ophthalmic Photographers' Society (JOPS)
C/O Chika Kanagami
Department of Ophthalmology
School of Medicine
Kyorin University
6-20-2 Shinkawa Mitaka City
Tokyo 181
Tel: +81-422-47-5511

Nederlandse Vereniging voor Medische Audiovisuele Communicatie
(NV-MAC)
Secretariaat
Schaepmanlaan 17, 5344 BA Oss
Tel: 04120-23357
http://www.medfac.leidenuniv.nl/medische_fotografie/rmf.htm

Ophthalmic Phototographers' Society (OPS)
OPS Membership Office
Barbara J. McCalley
213 Lorene Street
Nixa, MO 65714
417-725-0181; 800-403-1677
www.opsweb.org

Royal Photographic Society (RPS)
Andrew Rolland
Department of Medical Photography
St. George's Hospital
Blackshaw Road
London SW17 0QT
United Kingdom
Tel: 081 672 1255 ext. 51462/56101

Selskabet for Medicinsk of Biologisk (SMBI)
Preben Holst
The John F. Kennedy Institute
Department of Medical Genetics
G1 Landevej 7
Dk-2600 Glostrup
Denmark
Tel: 4245 2228 ext. 224

Societe Francaise d'Iconographie Medicale et Scientifique (SFIMS)
Jean Pierre Delmas
Service Audio-Visual
Faculte de Medecine Lyon Sud
69921 Oullins Cedex
France
Tel: 78 51 0826

Appendix C

Companies of Interest to the Ophthalmic Photographer

Patrick J. Saine and Marshall E. Tyler

Adobe Systems Incorporated
345 Park Avenue
San Jose, California 95110-2704
http://www.adobe.com

Agfa, Division of Miles
100 Challenger Road
Ridgefield Park, NJ 07660
http://www.agfa.com

Akorn, Inc.
100 Akorn Drive
Abita Springs, LA 70420
http://www.akorn.com

Alcon Laboratories, Inc.
6201 South Freeway
Ft. Worth, TX 76134
http://www.alconlabs.com

American Paper Optics
2005 Nonconnah Blvd., Suite 27
Memphis, TN 38132
http://www.3dglassesonline.com

Angiographics/Angiolith Premium Films
80 Oak Street, PO Box 430
Newton, MA 02164
Email: Angiolith@aol.com
http://www.angiolith.com

Bardes Products, Inc.
5245 Clinton Ave.
Milwaukee, WI 53223-4717
800-223-1357
http://www.bardes.com

Belrose Refracting Equipment
3734 Oakton St.
Skokie, IL 60076
847-675-2300

Byers Industries, Inc.
6955 Southwest Sandburg St.
Portland, OR 97223

Canon USA, Inc.
1 Canon Plaza
Lake Success, NY 11042-1119
516-328-5000
http://www.canon.com

Carl Zeiss Canada, Ltd.
45 Valleybrook Dr.
Don Mills, ON M3B2S6
http://www.zeiss.com

CFS Imaging
PO Box 648
Fair Lawn, NJ 07410-5248
800-499-2291
Email: Info@CFSImaging.com
http://CFSImaging.com

Ciba Vision Ophthalmics
11460 Johns Creek Pkwy.
Duluth, GA 30136
http://www.cibavision.com

Clement Clarke International Limited
Edinburgh Way, Harlow
Essex, CM20 2TT,
United Kingdom
http://www.clement-clarke.com

DA-LITE Screen Co., Inc.
PO Box 137
Warsaw, IN 46581-0137
http://www.dalite.com

National Electrical Manufacturers Association
2101 L Street, N.W. Suite 300
Washington, DC 20037 USA
http://medical.nema.org

Eastman Kodak Co., Inc.
343 State Street
Rochester, NY 14650
http://www.kodak.com

Escalon Medical Imaging
2440 South 179th Street
New Berlin, WI 53146
800-433-8197
http://www.escalonmed.com/

Eye Supply USA
10770 N. 46th St. Suite C-700
Tampa, FL 33617
800-521-5257
http://www.eyesupplyusa.com

FUJI Photo Film, USA, Inc.
555 Faxter Road
Elmsford, NY 10523
http://www.fujifilm.com

Heidelberg Engineering
5661 Palmer Way, Suite G
Carlsbad, CA 92008
http://www.heidelbergengineering.com

Humphrey Instruments, Inc.
5160 Hacienda Drive
Dublin, CA 94568
877-486-7473
http://www.zeiss.com/us
http://www.humphrey.com

Ilford Photo Corp.
70 W. Century Road
Paramus, NJ 07653-1490
201-265-6000
http://www.ilford.com

Insight Instruments, Inc.
175 E. Crystal Lake Ave.
Lake Mary, FL 32746
http://www.insightinstruments.com

Interzeag, Inc.
100 Otis St.
Northboro, MA 01532-2438
http://www.interzeag.com

Justice Ophthalmics
825 Ridge Lake Blvd.
Suite 300
Memphis, TN 38120
800-842-1574
http://www.justiceop.com
http://www.ocunet.com

Kowa Optimed, Inc.
20001 South Vermont Ave.
Torrance, CA 90502
310-327-1913
http://www.kowa.com

Larson Viewer
PO Box 0192
Sheboygan, WI 53082

Laser Diagnostic Technologies, Inc.
9550 Waples St., Suite 105
San Diego, CA 92121
http://www.laserdiagnostic.com

Loersch Corporation
1530 E. Race St.
Allentown, PA 18103
610-264-5641

Massie Research Laboratories, Inc.
6761 Sierra Court, Suite E
Dublin, CA 94568
925-560-2465
http://www.retcam.com

MRP Group, Inc.
49 Blanchard Street
Lawrence, MA 01843
http://www.mrpgroup.com

National Instrument Service Corp.
336 S. Fulton Ave.
Mount Vernon, NY 10553
914-667-8260
niscl@netzero.net

New Vision Technology
653 Hutchison Street
Vista, CA 92084
http://www.3d-web.com

Nidek Incorporated
2460 Embracadero Way
PO Box 50488
Palo Alto, CA 94303
800-223-9044
http://www.nidek.com

Nikon Inc. Instrument Group
1300 Walt Whitman Rd.
Melville, NY 11747-3012
http://www.nikonusa.com

Ophthalmic Imaging Systems, Inc.
221 Lathrop Way, Suite I
Sacramento, CA 95815
916-646-2020
http://www.oisi.com

Optos North America
199 Forest Street
Marlborough, MA 01752
http://www.optos.com

PhotoSystems Inc.
7200 Huron River Dr.
Dexter, MI 48130
800-521-4042

Polaroid Corp.
575 Technology Square
Cambridge, MA 02139-3587
http://www.polaroid.com

Qualix Direct
1065 E. Hillsdale Blvd., Suite 245
Foster City, CA 94404
http://www.qualixdirect.com

Reel 3-D Enterprises, Inc.
PO Box 2368
Culver City, CA 90231
http://www.stereoscopy.com/reel3d

Reliance International
http://www.reliance-medical.com

StereoGraphics, Inc.
PO Box 2309
2171 E. Francisco Blvd.
San Rafael, CA 94901-5536
http://www.stereographics.com

Stereo World
National Stereoscopic Assoc., Inc.
Box 14801
Columbus, Ohio 43214
http://www.stereoview.org

Technical Enterprises
1401 Bonnie Doone
Corona Del Mar, CA 92625-1717
http://members.home.net/stereophoto/

Topcon America Corporation
65 West Century Road
Paramus, NJ 07652
201-261-9450
http://www.topcon.com

TTI Medical
7026 Koll Center Pkwy., Suite 207
Pleasanton, CA 94566-3105

Twin Chimney Publishing
63 Wellington Circle
Lebanon, NH 03766
http://www.twinchimney.com

Vision Imaging Systems, Inc.
1140 Rt. 22 West
Mountainside, NJ 07092
http://www.visimaging.com

VRex, Inc.: The 3D Stereoscopic Imaging Company
85 Executive Blvd.
Elmsford, NY 10523
http://www.vrex.com

Wilson Ophthalmic Corp.
PO Box 496
Mustang, OK 73064
800-222-2020

Zeiss Humphrey Systems (Carl Zeiss)
5160 Hacienda Drive
Dublin, CA 94568
877-486-7473
http://www.zeiss.com/us
http://www.humphrey.com

Index

Note: Page numbers followed by *f* indicate figures; numbers followed by *t* indicate tables.